Dementia

MEDICINE IN OLD AGE

Volumes already published

Hearing and balance in the elderly
R. Hinchcliffe, *Editor*

Bone and joint disease in the elderly
V. Wright, *Editor*

Peripheral vascular disease in the elderly
S. T. McCarthy, *Editor*

**Clinical pharmacology and drug treatment in
the elderly**
K. O'Malley, *Editor*

Clinical biochemistry in the elderly
H. M. Hodkinson, *Editor*

Immunology and infection in the elderly
R. A. Fox, *Editor*

Gastrointestinal tract disorders in the elderly
J. Hellemans and G. Vantrappen, *Editors*

Arterial disease in the elderly
R. W. Stout, *Editor*

Urology in the elderly
J. C. Brocklehurst, *Editor*

Prevention of disease in the elderly
J. A. Muir Gray, *Editor*

Blood disorders in the elderly
M. J. Denham and I. Chanarin, *Editors*

Skin problems in the elderly
L. Fry, *Editor*

Affective disorders in the elderly
E. Murphy, *Editor*

Volumes in preparation

Cardiology in the elderly
R. J. Luchi, *Editor*

Medical ethics and the elderly
R. J. Elford, *Editor*

Dementia

EDITED BY

Brice Pitt
MD FRCPsych
Professor of Psychiatry of Old Age
St Mary's Hospital, London

CHURCHILL LIVINGSTONE
EDINBURGH LONDON MELBOURNE AND NEW YORK 1987

CHURCHILL LIVINGSTONE
Medical Division of Longman Group UK Limited

Distributed in the United States of America by
Churchill Livingstone Inc., 1560 Broadway, New
York, N.Y. 10036, and by associated companies,
branches and representatives throughout the world.

First published 1987

ISBN 0 443 03264 5
ISSN 0264-5602

British Library Cataloguing in Publication Data
Dementia. — (Medicine in old age,
  ISSN 0264–5602)
  1. Dementia
  I. Pitt, Brice   II. Series
  616.89   RC524

Library of Congress Cataloging in Publication Data
Dementia.
  (Medicine in old age)
  Includes bibliographies and index.
  1. Dementia.   2. Alzheimer's disease.
I. Pitt, Brice.   II. Series.
[DNLM: 1. Alzheimer's Disease — in old age.
2. Dementia — in old age.   WM 220 D3762]
RC521.D45   1987   618.97'68982   86–9650

Produced by Longman Singapore Publishers (Pte) Limited
Printed in Singapore

Introduction

To a great extent the medicine of today and tomorrow is the medicine of old age. In every hospital in the Western World old patients predominate. In the past it was too readily assumed that either the medicine of old age was confined to degenerative disease and was uninfluenced by diagnosis and treatment; or that it was identical to the medicine of young and middle age and required no special study. Neither view is correct. It is now becoming clear that the diseases which strike old people, the symptoms and the signs which are induced, and the response to treatment are distinctive. Years of growth, maturation and decline alter the response of the host to disease and to its management in ways which require special study. As this fact has been grasped medical science and research-minded clinicians have embarked on the study of the diseases of late life and have documented their characteristic features. Progress has been slow, partly because of an initial lack of sense of urgency, and difficulty in attracting research workers and funds; partly because of the complexities of defining normal values in old age and of attributing deviations from the normal to any one cause. Methodological and statistical problems have compounded the difficulties. But over the years there has been a very real and impressive growth of knowledge of the medicine of late life.

Some years ago the idea was conceived of collecting this new knowledge, system by system, in a series of volumes to be entitled 'Medicine in Old Age'. These books were addressed to physicians in all Western countries and in all medical disciplines who dealt with elderly patients. The contributors included physiologists, pathologists, epidemiologists and community physicians, as well as general internal physicians, geriatricians, psychiatrists and specialists in the various systems of the body. The response accorded to the first few volumes in the series was most encouraging, and the publishers are continuing and expanding the series.

This enterprise is supervised by an Editorial Board composed of practising clinicians and academics on both sides of the Atlantic. The Board selects the topics and appoints the guest editors for each volume and has been fortunate in its choice as editors of leaders in each field. These have been able in turn to attract contributions of high merit from many countries, thus putting into the hands of the reader a series of highly authoritative volumes. These bring together a wealth of knowledge and the best of modern practice in the care of elderly patients, retaining the critical spirit in the evaluation of the data which is characteristic of medicine in all age groups. The volumes are intended to stand mid-way between the immediacy of the scientific journal and the urbanity of the standard text book, combining freshness with authority. It is hoped that the profession will find them of value.

Birmingham 1984   Bernard Isaacs

Preface

'O! Let me not be mad, not mad, sweet heaven;
Keep me in temper: I would not be mad!'

King Lear's vain cry is equally in vain for at least five per cent of those aged over 65 in the developed countries (data on the far fewer elderly who survive into the senium in the third world are meagre) and one in five of those over 80. Old age is a time when one infirmity after another is added to such vicissitudes as widowhood and dwindling life expectancy, but none matches dementia in its devastation of the capacity for self-care, its erosion of relationships and its demands on the family and the community. Without dementia other disabilities associated with ageing can very often be managed at home, within the resources of personality, finances, accommodation, family and neighbourly care and the health and social service provision available. But dementia, a major disability in its own right, exacerbates all other disabilities. Demented people tend to lack foresight and common sense, are careless and accident-prone, and are always forgetful. Consequently dementia is the dominant single factor (at least, in Britain) in the institutionalisation of the elderly. One in 20 old people in Britain is in a 'home' or hospital, but one in five of the demented. The prime support of the four who stay at home is the family. Recent studies have spelt out how much the family, especially the key supporter, may be strained by such care, and research into what helps them to do so or diminishes their tolerance is growing, and the practical implications are where possible being applied.

Not long ago the medical attitude to the demented elderly was either indignant or resigned. Indignation was felt towards 'rejecting' families and inefficient social services, and there was much in-fighting between GPs, general hospital doctors, geriatricians and psychiatrists and labelling of unwanted patients as bed-blockers, 'social' admissions or misplaced. Psychiatrists tended to express their resignation by the use of lengthy waiting-lists for long-stay beds. Now, while the basic problem has not changed at all and the world grows older, the challenge of dementia as a disease particularly prevalent in the elderly, rather than as an inevitable accompaniment of ageing, is being faced, and approaches to the problem are more positive and energetic. The publication in 1977 of the Medical Research Council's report which approved the scientific community's study of dementia was something of a breakthrough. The extension of the concept of Alzheimer's disease made, as it were, 'an honest woman' of senile dementia, and symbolised this awakening of scientific interest.

The discovery that cholinergic neurones in the CNS are especially afflicted by Alzheimer's disease, with relative preservation of pre-synaptic neurones, offered prospects for its alleviation comparable to the benefits to sufferers from Parkinson's disease from L-Dopa. While this promise is as yet unfulfilled, there has been a surge of research into other neurotransmitter systems and other aspects of cerebral functioning. Advances in imaging techniques enable not just the structure of the brain to be far better visualised than with former, largely superseded invasive methods, but can demonstrate its metabolic activity. The contribution of an organism, such as a prion, to Alzheimer's disease as well as to the spongy encephalopathies has yet to be excluded. Advances in genetics and immunology will certainly increase understanding of dementia and possibly its treatment, as may discoveries consequent on the inevitable spate of searches for the 'philosopher's stone' of a drug that may arrest or cure it. Diverse other paths of enquiry may lead somewhere, or prove to be blind alleys; aluminium, for example, which once seemed a likely factor in Alzheimer's disease, then not, is at the heart of the senile plaque, and its significance there has still to be discovered.

Epidemiological studies are essential to ascertain risk factors and the elusive mild or early dementia on which hopes of effective therapy largely depend. Internationally agreed diagnostic criteria are essential if like is to be compared with like, and the US/UK studies and DSM III are pointers in the right direction. Nosology is now taken very seriously. Do clinical pictures and courses match neuropathological findings, and how much are the different dementias entities? There is good evidence that there are (at least) two disorders to which the term Alzheimer's disease properly applies on neuropathological findings post-mortem, yet clinically and biochemically somewhat different and running different courses. Psychologists are developing and refining psychometric instruments to make them more sensitive, specific, comprehensive, acceptable, reliable and valid; automated and computerised testing is part of this development.

Social and psychological factors are probably of little importance in the genesis of dementia, but determine how and when it presents. Psychological treatments such as reality orientation therapy, reminiscence and behavioural modification may be only mildly effective but can improve the morale of the carers. Much thought is now given to the milieu in which the demented are best cared for, and a wide variety of imaginative, appropriate and humane developments in community supports and activities, sheltered housing and 'homes' is now to be found in all sorts of places. There is evidence that improvements in care are increasing the life expectancy of the demented. However, such care costs, and the cost of dementia as well as that of ensuring a happy old age in ageing societies taxes the economy ever more.

Clearly dementia concerns almost everyone. A wide range of professions are involved, and all are needed. However, it is heartening that among the psychiatrists there are enough willing to concentrate on the mental health problems of the elderly and thus, inevitably, dementia, to form an important and growing sub-specialty of psychiatry. Happily, liaison is the forte of many psychogeriatricians, who may be seen as Jacks of all trades, able to involve a variety of experts if necessary on their patients' behalf.

This book deals with all these topics, as well as the disorders which impinge on and overlap dementia such as delirium, depression and disorders of movement. I am most sincerely grateful to the distinguished contributors who have not only been willing to participate, but have made my task as Editor so easy, by for the most part meeting deadlines with model manuscripts! I am also most grateful to Churchill Livingstone, especially Sylvia Hull, Georgina Bentliff and my colleagues on the Editorial Advisory Board, for their advice, stimulation and encouragement.

London 1987   Brice Pitt

Contributors

G. E. Berrios MA DPhil Sci MD FRCPsych DPM
Consultant and University Lecturer in Psychiatry, Department of
Psychiatry, University of Cambridge; Director of Medical Studies and
Fellow, Robinson College, Cambridge

John A. O. Besson BSc MB ChB DPM MRCPsych
Senior Lecturer and Honorary Consultant Psychiatrist, Department of
Mental Health, Aberdeen University

Dan G. Blazer II MD MPH PhD
Professor of Psychiatry, Division of Social and Community Psychiatry,
Director, Affective Disorders Program, Department of Psychiatry,
and Assistant Professor, Department of Family and Community
Medicine, Duke University Medical Center

Alex B. Christie MB ChB FRCP(Glasg) FRCPsych DPM
Consultant Psychiatrist, Crichton Royal, Dumfries

John R. M. Copeland MA MD FRCP FRCPsych DPM
Professor and Head, Department of Psychiatry, University of Liverpool

David Dodwell MB ChB MRCPsych MSc
Lecturer in Psychiatry, Department of Psychiatry, University of
Manchester

Colin Godber BA BM BCh MPhil FRCP FRCPsych
Consultant Psychogeriatrician, Moorgreen Hospital, Southampton

Vladimir Hachinski MD FRCP(Can)
Professor of Neurology, Department of Clinical Neurological Sciences,
University of Western Ontario; Director, Stroke and Aging Group, Robarts
Research Institute, London, Canada

A. S. Henderson MD FRACP FRCPsych FRANZCP MRCP
Director, National Health and Medical Research Council Social
Psychiatry Research Unit, The Australian National University, Canberra,
Australia

Philip J. Henschke MB BS FRACP FRCP(Can) FACRM
Consultant in Geriatric Medicine, Repatriation General Hospital, Daw
Park, South Australia; Senior Clinical Lecturer, Department of Medicine,
Flinders University, Bedford Park, South Australia

Martin J. Kendall MD MRCP
Senior Lecturer in Clinical Pharmacology, Department of Therapeutics
and Clinical Pharmacology, University of Birmingham

Don C. Kendrick BA Dip Psychol PhD FBPsS
Reader in Clinical Psychology, The University, Hull

R. H. S. Mindham MD FRCP(Ed) FRCPsych
Nuffield Professor of Psychiatry, University of Leeds

Alison Norman BA Dip Soc Admin Dip MHSW
Deputy Director, Centre for Policy on Ageing, Nuffield Lodge Studio,
London

Brice Pitt MD FRCPsych
Professor of Psychiatry of Old Age, St Mary's Hospital, London

Felix Post MD FRCP FRCPsych
Emeritus Physician, The Bethlem Royal Hospital and The Maudsley
Hospital, London

Martin Rossor MA MRCP
Consultant Neurologist, National Hospital and St Mary's Hospital, London

C. L. Scholtz PhD FRCPA
Consultant Neuropathologist, The London Hospital

R. J. Smith BSc MPhil MSC
Research Clinical Psychologist, Leeds Western AHA; Honorary Research
Fellow, Department of Psychiatry, University of Leeds

Samuel B. Thielman MD
Assistant Professor and Head, Section of Geriatric Psychiatry,
Department of Psychiatry and Health Behavior, Medical College of
Georgia, Augusta, USA

Richard U'Ren MD CM
Director, Outpatient Psychiatry and Psychogeriatrics Clinics and
Associate Professor, Department of Psychiatry, Oregon Health Sciences
University, Portland, Oregon, USA

J. P. H. Wade MA MD MRCP
Senior Registrar, The National Hospital for Nervous Diseases and St
Bartholomew's Hospital, London

R. T. Woods MA MSc ABPsS
Lecturer in Clinical Psychology, Institute of Psychiatry, London

Contents

1. Introduction   1
   Richard U'Ren
2. The nosology of the dementias: an overview   19
   G. E. Berrios
3. The diagnosis of dementia in old age   52
   J. R. M. Copeland
4. Psychological assessment   69
   D. C. Kendrick
5. Electrophysiological and brain imaging investigations   90
   John Besson
6. Alzheimer's disease: aetiology   109
   P. J. Henschke
7. Alzheimer's disease: neuropathology   118
   Carl Scholtz
8. Alzheimer's disease: neurobiochemistry   140
   Martin Rossor
9. Alzheimer's disease: epidemiology   154
   A. S. Henderson
10. Alzheimer's disease: the clinical picture   174
    David Dodwell
11. Alzheimer's disease: the prognosis   197
    A. B. Christie
12. Multi-infarct dementia   209
    J. P. H. Wade and V. C. Hachinski
13. Dementia in disorders of movement   229
    R. J. Smith and R. H. S. Mindham
14. Delirium and dementia   241
    Brice Pitt
15. Depression and dementia   251
    Samuel B. Thielman and Dan G. Blazer
16. Drugs for dementia   265
    Martin Kendall

17. Psychological management of dementia   281
    Robert Woods
18. Psychogeriatric and social services for the demented   296
    Colin Godber
19. Caring for the carers   317
    Alison Norman
20. Epilogue: research prospects   330
    Felix Post
Index   337

Introduction

HISTORY OF THE CONCEPT OF DEMENTIA

Great advances in medicine have come about when a clinical syndrome has been defined in a reliable way and the associated pathological changes described. The concept of dementia has evolved from the struggle to define the signs and symptoms now called the dementia syndrome and the quest to discover its various causes. As with other syndromes, such as delirium, much of the history of dementia is a reflection of attempts to separate it from other disorders and to give it an identity of its own.

The word dementia, derived from the Latin *demens*, did not originally have the specific connotation that it does today. It meant 'being out of one's mind' and, as such, was a general term for insanity or madness. It referred to any behaviour or state of mind considered irrational, unusual, abnormal or incomprehensible (Mahendra, 1984).

Throughout most of recorded history intellectual decay and melancholy were assumed to be invariable features of ageing. In fact, the first account of a syndrome of mental illness may have been senile deterioration, described by Prince Ptah-Hotep around 3000 BC. The Ebers papyrus, dating from 1500 BC., has descriptions of senile deterioration and alcoholism. Hippocrates, though credited with recognizing what we now define as psychiatric problems, did not propose a separate diagnostic category for dementia; it may have been included under melancholia, a term that covered all varieties of chronic mental disorder (Menninger et al, 1963).

According to Lipowski (1981), the encylopedist Aulus Celsus deserves credit for first using the words 'delirium' and 'dementia' in his *De re medicina*, published around AD 30. Aretaeus the Cappadocian, at the end of the first century AD, mentions 'the dotage which is the calamity of old age' in discussing the differential diagnosis of what may have been mania. Mania, he observes, 'intermits, and with care ceases altogether', whereas 'dotage commencing with old age never intermits but accompanies the patient until death' (Rosen, 1968). Aretaeus may have been the first to use the equivalent of the term 'senile dementia' — dotage — and to distinquish it from 'secondary' dementia (Menninger et al, 1963).

Juvenal, in his satires, written between BC 100 and 128, described a man afflicted with dementia as one 'who . . . no longer knows the names of his slaves or recognizes the friend with whom he has dined the night before, or those whom he has begotten and brought up. And by cruel will he disinherits his own and makes over all his property to Phiale' (Lipowski, 1981). Oribasius, physician to the emperor Julian, described *meiosis encephalon*, or cerebral atrophy, a disease that he thought was associated with baldness and manifested by loss of intellectual capacity and weakness of movement (Rosen, 1968).

The Oxford English Dictionary informs us that the word 'dementia' as a noun was first used in 1806 to render Pinel's 'demence' into English, though the earlier word 'demency' was used in 1522 by the poet John Skelton. The OED's authority is open to question, however. In 1592, writing about insanity as a defence, Richard Cosin, Vicar-General of Canterbury and a member of Parliament, used the word dementia and defined it as 'a passion of the mind, bereaving it of the light of under-standing: or . . . when a man's perceivance and understanding of all things is taken away, and may be englished distracted of wit, or being beside himselfe.' Ninety years later William Salmon described a case of a man 'decayed in his Intellectuals' who showed marked forgetfulness, persever-ation and emotional lability, all suggesting multi-infarct dementia (Hunter & MacAlpine, 1963).

In the Dark and Middle Ages, through the Renaissance, and well into the 18th century, dementia is mentioned in most systems of psychiatric classification, though the precise meaning of the word is often unclear. For example, Avicenna spoke of oblivio: loss of memory due to lesions of the posterior ventricle; in addition to oblivio, Fernel mentioned 'amentia': loss or absence of intellingence; Platter wrote of memoria imminuta — gross loss of memory (Menninger et al, 1963). Thomas Willis held that delirium and dementia were the same; his descriptions sound more like what we would call delirium than dementia. He did, however, identify a chronic mental disorder that he called 'stupidity', a condition characterized by defects of memory, understanding and judgment (Lipowski, 1981).

Medicine entered a new era with Sydenham, who originated the idea of disease as a syndrome, a constellation of related symptoms with a charac-teristic prognosis (Kendall, 1975). Until then, illness was assumed to have arisen from a single pathogen, often a disturbed balance of humours. Sydenham rejected previous speculations and insisted on a strict empiricism in the study of disease. His suggestion, that diseases be reduced to definite species with the same care that botanists describe plants, was taken up with passion by Francois Boissier de Sauvages, who proceeded to tabulate 2400 diseases, most of them individual symptoms (Kendall, 1975). In his *Noso-logie methodique*, published posthumously in 1771, the eighth form of disease was dementia, under which were listed the majority of mental illnesses, including not only dementia but also mania, melancholia, nostalgia and demonomania. In 1777 William Cullen published an elaborate classification system using the Linneian format of classes, orders, genera and species. Under Vesaniae (or forms of insanity) are listed three species of amentia: congenita, senilis and acquisita (Menninger et al, 1963).

At the end of the 18th century, Philippe Pinel, better known for his humane treatment of mental patients in the wake of the French Revolution, reacted against the elaborate classification systems of the time and reduced the nosology of insanity to five categories: mania with delirium, mania without delirium, melancholia, dementia and idiotism. Pinel believed that all five types were interchangeable: one person might show any of the five forms during his or her lifetime. His description of dementia does not correspond exactly to our present-day concept of it. He mentions 'complete forgetfulness of every previous state' and impaired judgment; but other symptoms — 'repeated acts of extravagance' and 'rapid succession or uninterrupted alternation of insulated ideas' — could just as well refer to mania, schizophrenia or even delirium. His term 'idiotism' — an obliteration of the intellectual faculty — also includes signs of dementia (Pinel, 1962). Pinel at that point had not differentiated mental subnormality from dementia. It remained for Esquirol, his student, to do that in 1838 (Mahendra, 1984).

Esquirol also limited mental disorders to a parsimonious five categories. One was dementia, which could take one of three forms: acute, chronic, senile. The senile form was associated with advancing age, but the chronic form, Esquirol asserted, could be caused by masturbation, excessive study or drunkenness. However, his description of senile dementia, while still overinclusive, corresponds in many respects to our own. He maintained that it starts with enfeeblement of memory, particularly recent memory, and that it progresses slowly. He also described the apathy, the progressive difficulty with attention, the 'slow and impractical' movements seen in the condition (Esquirol, 1976). By 1838, then, the clinical description of senile dementia was essentially completed (Torack, 1983).

The 19th century was dense with systems of classification and large heroic figures. The German titans — Neumann, Kahlbaum and Griesinger — believed that there was one mental disease — insanity — and that the various clinical syndromes were but stages of a unitary morbid process (Menninger et al, 1963). Dementia was considered to be the terminal stage of the process. In 1837 the British psychiatrist Prichard divided dementia into primary and secondary forms and proposed that the illness could be divided into four stages, but the aetiology was still ascribed to moral rather than to physical causes (Lipowski, 1981).

Proponents of the position that mental illnesses were actually brain diseases, buoyed by Bayle's discovery of a specific condition — general paresis of the insane — with an organic basis and by Broca's discovery that certain localized brain lesions resulted in distinctive forms of aphasia, helped to drive moral and religious ideas of causation out of psychiatric thinking. Another step forward was taken by Theodor Ziehens, who divided psychoses on the basis of the presence or absence of an intellectual defect. His classification of 'acquired defect psychosis', in which he included senile dementia, the dementia of syphilis, dementias secondary to other brain diseases and to functional psychoses, as well as epileptic and alcoholic dementia — the very diseases that would comprise a present-day list of the aetiologies of the dementia syndrome — has a decidedly modern ring (Menninger et al, 1963).

It was Emil Kraepelin's classification system that swept the field at the end of the 19th century and became the basis for our modern nosological thinking. In the famous 6th edition of his textbook (published in 1899, translated 1902) Kraepelin separated dementia praecox from the other dementias (paralytica and organic), a decision that greatly narrowed the scope of the concept of dementia. Senile dementia was included under yet another category of 'involution psychosis' along with melancholia and 'presenile delusional insanity' — probably what we would call paranoia today — but his description of senile dementia was similar to Esquirol's (Defendorf, 1902).

The discovery of both the cause and the neuropathological basis of syndromes has always lagged behind their clinical delineation. The case of dementia is no exception. Syphilis, still the most important infection of the nervous system which is encountered in clinical practice, is an instructive case in point. Haslam, an apothecary at the Bethlem Hospital in London, is usually given credit for the first description of general paralysis. In 1798 he reported a case of a man, dying at the age of 42, who suffered from grandiose delusions, strokes, inarticulate speech, cognitive impairment and physical deterioration. It was, however, the French physician Bayle, working in an insane asylum in the suburbs of Paris, who in 1822 in the aftermath of the Napoleonic Wars described fully the characteristic signs and symptoms of general paresis, drew attention to the stages of the disease and commented on the characteristic brain changes. For the first time a group of patients whose disease could be recognized clinically and anatomically was separated from other madmen. Bayle was convinced that the symptoms of general paresis did not occur as part of any other mental illness, an opinion that was not immediately accepted. As late as 1862, for instance, Griesinger was still insisting that general paralysis was the main complication of insanity (Ackerknecht, 1968). Bayle was never able to discover the aetiology of the disease he did so much to define. He thought that syphilis *might* be a cause of general paresis, but only one among many. The frequent occurrence of the disease in soldiers and officers of the Napoleonic Wars led him to speculate about psychosocial causes, among which he included privation, the terrors of war, excessive drinking, and even disappointment following the defeat of Napoleon.

The opinion that general paralysis was caused by syphilis was first proposed by Esmarch and Jessen in 1857 but it took a long time before this view was accepted and proved. For example, as late as 1877 Krafft-Ebing mentioned heredity, dissipation, smoking, head trauma, weak nerves and exhaustive attempts to make a living as possible causes of general paresis. Henry Maudsley absolutely rejected the syphilogenic theory of paresis, as did the great Virchow in 1898. It was only after Nissl and Alzheimer described the uniform microscopic changes in the brains of paretic patients in 1904, and the demonstration of spirochetes in the brains of the afflicted by Noguchi and Moore in 1913, that a specific cause for a general paresis, then a very common mental disorder, was finally accepted (Bruetsch, 1975).

Leonardo da Vinci had recognized that arteriosclerosis occurred in blood vessels, but it was another Bayle, François, who was the first, in 1677, to relate it to strokes (McHenry, 1969). In 1694 Baglivi attended (and later dissected) the famous Malpighi when Malpighi was struck down by a stroke that affected the right side of his body. After 40 days, however, 'he got clear of the Apoplexy, and Palsie' but it was observed that he continued to suffer much 'in his Memory and Reason and melted into tears upon the slightest occasion' (Major, 1945). By the time the 6th edition of Kraepelin's textbook was published, it was established with some authority that arteriosclerosis could be distinguished from senile dementia and was associated with a form of insanity characterized by headache, vertigo, irritability, loss of memory, aphasia, circumscribed paralyses and periods of remission (Defendorf, 1902). The groundwork had been laid earlier by Alzheimer who, in 1894, had reported the characteristic microscopic changes associated with arterio-sclerosis of the brain and along with Kraepelin had correlated them with the clinical findings (Mahendra, 1984; Defendorf, 1902).

Nevertheless, throughout much of the present century, controversy about the role of cerebral arteriosclerosis in dementia remained. Kraepelin himself was at first wary of attributing senility to arteriosclerotic changes, as Grie-singer had done in 1845. It remained for European investigators to provide the critical evidence (and only recently) that dementia was related not to the degree of arteriosclerosis in cerebral vessels or even to cerebral ischaemia but to the amount of brain parenchyma destroyed and that the role of arteriosclerosis in the causation of dementia had been overestimated (Worm-Peterson & Pakkenberg, 1967; Tomlinson et al, 1970).

Although the clinical description of senile dementia was completed by the first third of the 19th century, the necessary anatomical and histopatholog-ical correlations came, as in the case of both syphilis and arteriosclerosis, much later. The first mention of ventricular dilatation was in 1795 by the British pathologist Baillie. Cortical atrophy was described in 1864 by Wilks, who thought that it was caused by chronic alcoholism, syphilis and senile dementia (Torack, 1983). And Wille, in 1873–4, made one of the first attempts to distinguish senile dementia from general paresis (Mahendra, 1984).

Blocq and Marinesco in 1892 first described what we now know as senile plaques, although they were then called 'neuroglia nodules', in the brain of an epileptic man. Redlich re-described these same lesions in 1898 as 'miliary sclerosis'. It was Simchowitz who first proposed the term 'senile plaque' in 1911 (Ferraro, 1975). But it was Alzheimer in 1904 who reported their presence in cases of senile dementia. Since he believed that the major problem in cerebral atrophy was arteriosclerosis, however, and because he assumed that the plaques were glial tissue, he did not get excited. It was only in 1906, with the aid of the new Bielschowsky stain, that he identified something new: neurofibrillary tangles — and reported his findings to a meeting of the Southwest German Society of Alienists a year later. Alzheimer was sure he had discovered a new disease entity, a form of dementia occurring in the presenium. Kraepelin was again sceptical about the distinction between senile and presenile dementia on the basis of age alone and commented, 'The anatomic findings suggest . . . an especially severe form of senile dementia.' But he finally accepted Alzheimer's argument and endorsed the existence of presenile dementia, a term actually proposed by Binswanger in 1898, in the 8th edition of his textbook (1910), thereby guaranteeing, through his immense stature, its longevity (Torack, 1978). It only remained for Simchowicz in 1910 to describe the granulovacuolar changes in the large pyramidal cells of the hippocampus to complete the triad of neuropathological changes we now associate with Alzheimer's disease (Ferraro, 1975).

By the turn of the century, as Mahendra (1984) has pointed out, the use of the word dementia had become much more specific than it had been earlier: dementia usually occurred in older age but sometimes earlier; its principal causes — syphilis, arteriosclerosis, Alzheimer's disease — could be identified and distinguished from each other; it was due to brain disease. Although the foundations of the dementia syndrome as we know it today were firmly in place, then, 80 years ago, the entire field of organic psychiatry fell into relative neglect throughout much of that time. This was caused, in large part, by the influence of Freud and his followers, who caused American psychiatry to swerve in the direction of psychological explanations for mental illness and toward psychotherapy. But it was also caused by the father of descriptive psychiatry himself, Kraepelin, whose brilliant descriptions and solid classifications seemed to leave little room for therapeutic efforts or optimism.

In the last 25 years, and especially in the past ten, organic psychiatry has been on the move again, and the concept of dementia is once again in flux. A few recent developments will be mentioned briefly.

New causes of the dementia syndrome have been recognized, including depression, which in the form of pseudodementia may mimic dementia (Kiloh, 1961), progressive supranuclear palsy (Steele et al, 1964) and normal pressure hydrocephalus (Adams et al, 1965). Binswanger's disease has been rediscovered (Pullicino et al, 1983) and angular gyrus syndrome, which can be confused with Alzheimer's disease, has been described (Benson, 1979; Benson et al, 1982). Criteria for the syndrome of dementia have recently been made clearer and more precise. The DSM-III in the

American system of classification represents an advance in conceptualization in that the global term 'chronic organic brain syndrome', which lumped together more specific brain syndromes and which connoted irreversibility, has been eliminated; and dementia, a syndrome that refers to a constellation of signs and symptoms without reference to aetiology, is clearly distinguished from senile and presenile dementia as well as from multi-infarct dementia, both of which are known brain diseases (DSM-III, 1980; Lipowski, 1984). Also, criteria for the diagnosis of Alzheimer's disease (senile and presenile dementia) have been tightened (McKhann et al, 1984). There have been differences about how dementia, especially Alzheimer's disease, should be staged, debate about whether or not the dementias can be reliably and logically classified into cortical and subcortical types — the evidence seems to be against it (Mayeux et al, 1983) — and even controversy about what to call Alzheimer's disease. The American Psychiatric Association favours 'primary degenerative dementia', the ICD-9 advocates the term 'senile dementia' for patients over the age of 65, many neurologists prefer 'senile dementia, Alzheimer's type', and the term 'hippocampal dementia' has recently been proposed as an alternative to Alzheimer's disease (Ball et al, 1985). There is controversy about whether or not there is more than one form of Alzheimer's disease since, in its presenile form, the clinical course may be more malignant, parietal lobe involvement more noticeable, and the number of neurofibrillary tangles in the brain at autopsy more pronounced (Boundareff, 1983; Mann et al, 1984). There is argument about what proportion of cases of Alzheimer's disease are familial and what proportion are sporadic (Breitner & folstein, 1984).

Differences of opinion, re-definition, refinements and new knowledge are all, of course, signs of a robust, engaging and rapidly growing area of investigation far removed from the atmosphere of indifference that prevailed, at least in American psychiatry, in this field earlier in the century.

DEMENTIA AND OLD AGE

In 1899 Kraepelin wrote: 'Senility brings with it, for everyone, a certain degree of mental and physical deterioration, so that the borderline between physiological senility and the state of mental alienation cannot always be a sharp one' (Defendorf, 1902). Where this borderline is, or whether it even exists, has been a matter much debated.

The literature on the psychology of ageing is immense (see Birren & Shaie, 1977; Siegler, 1980). All of it is complicated, much of it controversial (Shaie, 1974; Horn & Donaldson, 1976). There is now general agreement, however, that a number of cognitive functions decline slowly with age in most, though not all, individuals. These impairments are neither uniform nor extensive, however (LaRue, 1982). The ability to solve problems, learn, remember and abstract show the most changes with age (see Woods, 1982;

Katzman & Terry, 1984). There is little decline in vocabulary, information, comprehension and other verbal skills, at least until the age of 70 or 75, after which even impairment of verbal abilities may occur, albeit gradually (Eisdorfer & Wilkie, 1973; Blum et al, 1973). Factors other than intrinsic brain changes impair cognitive function, also: for instance, impairments of vision and hearing, the use of pharmacologic agents, and pressure of time all affect memory and learning in older individuals adversely.

Of the three types of memory function, immediate memory is not significantly impaired in elderly persons nor is remote memory. It is on tests of recent memory that the elderly perform less well than younger individuals do. Elderly individuals typically have a harder time than younger control subjects in recalling words on a list, remembering elements of a paragraph, recalling pairs of words or remembering visual designs (LaRue, 1982). The neurobiological bases for these changes are poorly understood, though an increase in central processing time has been implicated (see Katzman & Terry, 1983). Brain cell mass and absolute numbers of neurons decrease with age, but correlations between these changes in cognitive impairment are very low. It may turn out that lower levels of functioning neurotransmitter substances such as acetylcholine and gamma-aminobutyric acid correlate more highly with cognitive function than do structural changes (Perry & Perry, 1982).

Memory loss is usually the most prominent troublesome symptom of senile dementia — for relatives if not for the patient. The degree of memory impairment of course depends on the stage of the disease. Immediate memory, for example, may be normal in patients with mild to moderate senile dementia, and remote memory may be surprisingly well maintained, at least in response to over-learned information, such as dates, world events and significant personal experiences (LaRue, 1982). As the disease progresses into its later stage, however, these remote memories disappear also.

As with the normal elderly, it is recent memory that suffers the most in patients with senile dementia. Patients in all but the earliest stages of the disease will usually have trouble recalling more than a word or two (from a list of four or five) and difficulty repeating significant elements of a paragraph read aloud to them. Miller (1971) has shown that patients with mild presenile dementia have a much harder time than normal controls in recalling common words from a list that are presented at the beginning, as compared with the later part, of the trial, indicating impairment of recent memory. LaRue (1982) has suggested that, while both normals and demented patients have difficulty with recent memory, the two groups can be distinguished by the more extreme amount of dysfunction on simple tests of new learning and recall of unfamiliar material that demented patients show.

How easy it would be for clinicians if individuals in their care could easily be separated into normal and demented categories on the basis of two or three simple memory tests! Mild forgetfulness is an extremely common complaint among older people (Sluss et al, 1980). Most older people do not expect their memory to be as acute as it was when they were young however, and persistent subjective complaints about memory are more often associated with depression than dementia (Kahn, 1975). Except in the earliest stages of the disease and perhaps only when asked about specific aspects of memory functioning, patients with senile dementia often do not complain of memory problems (Wells, 1978). Most moderately and severely impaired patients with senile dementia, when asked how their memory is, will deny impairment (but there are exceptions). Fortunately, perhaps, loss of memory and loss of insight into one's condition often parallel each other.

In 1962 Kral introduced the phrase 'benign senescent forgetfulness'. This term was applied to individuals whose memory problems were characterized by a forgetfulness for some of the details of an experience but a good memory for the experience itself. They were usually able to recall the details at a later time, were cognizant of their forgetfulness and made efforts to compensate for their momentarily deficient memory through circumlocution or apologies (Kral, 1962). Their deficit, Kral said, progressed 'relatively slowly': only one of 20 subjects in this group developed the more severe form of memory disorder as time went on (Kral, 1978).

In contrast, a second group of individuals had 'malignant senescent forgetfulness'. They showed, initially, more impairment on memory tests and had a higher mortality rate at the end of four years than did the benign group. These individuals frequently forgot not only details but also the important events and experiences themselves and were unaware of their deficiencies. Kral speculated that a defect in the process of association — encoding — which underlies the recall of names and information was responsible. This speculation has now been supported by recent work which shows that many older people do, in fact, practise fewer visual and auditory associations than younger individuals when given words to memorize (Craik, 1977). Kral further conjectured that the two groups, benign versus malignant, might be quantitatively rather than qualitatively different: the benign form of memory impairment might result, he suggested, if atrophic changes affected the hippocampal-fornix-mammillary system only mildly, whereas the malignant form might be seen if changes affected those same structures more severely.

In a later report on a larger sample, Kral (1978) confirmed his original report. In this report, also, patients with malignant senescent forgetfulness had a higher mortality rate and a shorter survival time than individuals with the benign syndrome.

Kral's work has been criticized on the ground that his distinctions between the two conditions lack specific criteria for discrimination (LaRue, 1982) but his original observations seem to be holding up, at least so far. From the limited studies available so far, it appears that the milder a patient's cognitive impairment is at the time of initial evaluation, the less likely it is that he/she will deteriorate cognitively during a follow up period when compared to patients with more severe degrees of impairment. One study showed that none of 17 patients with very mild cognitive impairment on the Global Deterioration Scale (Reisberg et al, 1982) showed any impairment over a 27-month period, whereas patients with more severe degrees of cognitive impairment deteriorated much faster over the follow-up period (Reisberg, 1982). Using the Clinical Dementia Rating scale (Hughes et al, 1982), the original investigators reported that, of 14 individuals classified as questionably impaired at the initial evaluation, only four were rated as suffering form 'mild' dementia six to nine months later. Berg et al (1984), using the same scale, found that 21 of 43 subjects with mild (as contrasted with questionable or moderate) dementia progressed to the moderate or severee stages within a year. One patient was lost to follow up and the other 21 patients remained only mildly impaired and showed no evidence of further deterioration.

More discriminating scales for rating not only memory impairment and disorientation but also judgment, interests and the ability to carry on activities of daily life have been published since Kral's work. On the Clinical Dementia Rating scale (Hughes et al, 1982), for example, Kral's benign senescent forgetfulness would probably be classified as questionable dementia and the malignant form would be characterized as mild to moderate dementia. On the Global Deterioration Scale (Reisberg et al, 1982), the benign form of memory disorder would be called the 'the forgetfulness phase' of cognitive impairment.

In summary, the following conclusions can be drawn about the relationship of ageing, benign senescent forgetfulness and dementia:

— The majority of older individuals show mild cognitive changes, particularly in recent memory, when compared to younger individuals, but these changes are neither uniform or extensive.
— Most normal older people living in the community have complaints about their memory. Among patients, persistent memory complaints are more likely to be symptomatic of depression than dementia.
— The majority of individuals suffering from benign senescent forgetfulness who would be classified as suffering from only very mild or questionable cognitive impairment on other rating scales do not show significant deterioration, at least over a one- to three-year period.
— Senile dementia, in its very earliest phases, is indistinguishable, clinically and neuropsychologiacally, from the normal cognitive changes of ageing. Obviously there is an area of overlap between normal memory changes with age and early Alzheimer's disease, a no-man's-land where it is unclear at what point normal variation ends and abnormalities begin. Terry (1978) and Roth (1981) have also suggested that there is no clear line of demarcation between normal ageing and the earliest stages of senile dementia. Neither histopathologically (i.e., plaques and

tangles) nor neurochemically are there any qualitative differences between normal elderly subjects and patients with senile dementia. Rather, the differences are quantitative: senile dementia is a threshold phenomenon — it results when, for unknown reasons, a particular level of brain lesions is reached.

There is no doubt that further work will be concentrated on efforts to help clinicians and researchers alike discern the earlier stages of senile dementia more clearly than they are able to do now. A relatively simple psychological test battery has recently been published that claims to discriminate between normal elderly subjects and individuals suffering from mild cognitive impairment with a high degree of accuracy (Storandt et al, 1984). Further refinements in computerized tomographic methodology, with particular attention to ventricular and parenchymal changes (Albert et al, 1984a; Albert et al, 1984b) and the use of the positron emission tomography (Ferris & Leon, 1983) may also shed light on this problematic issue.

From the standpoint of the clinician who is faced with determining if someone is dementing or not, a thorough history with special attention to signs of memory, intellectual and personality deterioration and the extent to which these changes impair the person's ability to carry on in daily life is still the most important part of the inquiry. This should be followed by a physical examination with particular attention to the neurological aspects. A formal mental status examination — with close attention to the subtle signs of early dementia such as mild dysphasia, unexpected and unusual problems with spelling, difficulty with tasks that require some effort, or momentary lapses in modulation of social behaviour — should be carried out and supplemented by either the Mini-Mental State Examination (MMSE) (Folstein et al, 1975) or one of the simpler memory-orientation tests (Pfeiffer, 1975). For most patients, as a matter of routine, blood work that includes a complete blood count, a chemistry panel and thyroid function tests should be requested. Abnormalities on history, physical or mental status testing should of course inspire a search for one the many causes of the dementia syndrome. In doubtful cases, referral for neuropsychological testing and/or a return appointment with re-evaluation every 6 to 12 months with a repeated mental status examination is recommended.

THE IMPORTANCE OF ALZHEIMER'S DISEASE

The accelerating interest in dementia, and particularly in Alzheimer's disease, is based on several developments in recent years. The most significant may be the way that Alzheimer's disease, senile dementia and their relationship to ageing have been reconceptualized. For most of this century, Alzheimer's disease, with its onset before age 65, and senile dementia, with its appearance after 65, were considered to be distinct and separate entities.

Alzheimer's disease together with Pick's disease was described as 'quite rare' in a standard American textbook in 1966 (Redlich & Freedman, 1966). Not more than 100 cases of both diseases together had been described in the literature up till that time. Senile dementia was considered to be an extreme variant of the normal changes that accompany advancing age and, since intellectual deterioration was considered to be an almost inevitable consequence of ageing, there was little to attract medical attention and interest. Furthermore, arteriosclerosis of the cerebral vessels — hardening of the arteries' — was throught to be the commonest cause of senile brain disease. In 1967, Busse could write that, of first admissions to hospital in patients over 65, 45% were ill primarily because of cerebral arteriosclerosis (Busse, 1967).

Arteriosclerosis was decisively knocked out of the running as the prime cause of dementia by several reports between 1960 and 1970 which demonstrated that arteriosclerosis was greatly overestimated as a cause of dementia and that the majority of patients dying with dementia in fact showed the characteristic plaques and tangles of Alzheimer's disease in their brains, although some degree of overlap (15–20%) existed between the two conditions (Corsellis, 1962; Tomlinson et al, 1970).

Slater and Roth in 1963 noted, 'The clinical features of Alzheimer's disease are admittedly different from those of senile dementia but pathologically no sharp distinction exists.' However, several sentences later a qualifier creeps in: 'There is more overlap between the clinical features of senile and presenile dementia than the literature would lead one to believe' (Slater & Roth,1969). Although the idea that Alzheimer's disease and senile dementia were the same disease with different ages of onset was not new, especially to neuropathologists, this view was not generally accepted until recently. Katzman, in his often-cited editorial of 1976, argued that because of the similarity of the clinical picture and the identical nature of the histopathology, distinctions between Alzheimer's disease and senile dementia were arbitrary and no longer useful. And Terry, in a conference a year later that set the tone for much of the subsequent interest and work in dementia, said, 'One must conclude that . . . SDAT and presenile Alzheimer's disease are at least very similar if not identical' (Terry, 1978).

Once Alzheimer's disease was firmly linked with senile dementia (the disturbingly high prevalence of which was also becoming apparent) it was clear that Alzheimer's disease was no longer uncommon. It was, in fact, perhaps the fourth or fifth most common cause of death among the elderly in the United States (Katzman & Karasu, 1975): a rare disease had been transformed into an alarmingly common one.

There was a third reconceptualization also, perhaps the most important of all, that allowed this area to advance. It had been known — and documented (Birren et al, 1963) — for a long time that senility or senile brain disease was not an inevitable accompaniment of ageing. Yet the notion that senility was a normal part of ageing remained widespread. Butler's (1975) attack on the myth of senility — the clearest expression of a changing point of view — was a timely and badly needed effort to dispel this long-held misconception. Butler insisted that senility was a wastebasket term for all problems of the aged and should be discarded. He argued forcefully that 'senility', when it occurs, was a result of brain disease or depression and was potentially treatable. The extension of this view was that 'senility' was abnormal, not normal, and that its usual causes were diseases, not just ageing. And by then it was known, earlier in Britain than in the United States, that the commonest cause of senility was Alzheimer's disease.

Recent discoveries in neurochemistry and neurobiology have also heightened interest in the dementias. The discovery of dopamine deficiency due to neuronal loss in the substantia nigra in Parkinson's disease (see Parkes & Marsden, 1973) raised hopes that similar neurochemical deficiencies and neuro-anatomical sites might be identified in other degenerative deseases also. In the mid-1970s three different laboratories reported low levels of the marker enzyme for acetylcholine, choline acetyltransferase, in the brains of patients dying with Alzheimer's disease, a finding that has been confirmed several times since (Bowen et al, 1976; Davies & Maloney, 1976; Perry et al, 1977). Subsequent investigators also reported abnormalities in acetyl-cholinesterase, dopamine-beta-hydroxylase (the marker enzyme for nor-ephinephrine), serotonin, dopamine and the neuropeptide somatostatin (see Rosser, 1982). The deficiency of acetycholine has been the most promising clue to an understanding of Alzheimer's disease and the target of most therapeutic efforts thus far.

Gajdusek's work (Gajdusek & Gibbs, 1972) on the transmissibility of kuru and Creutzfeldt-Jakob disease raised the possibility that other chronic degenerative diseases, including Alzheimer's, might be due to transmissible agents. Prusiner's discovery and isolation of prions from the brains of sheep with scrapie (Prusiner, 1982) and the brains of humans with Creutzfeldt-Jakob disease (Bockman et al, 1985) has added weight at this tantalizing suggestion (Prusiner, 1984). The possibility that Alzheimer's disease may have a genetic basis, originally proposed by investigators in Scandinavia (Larrson et al, 1963), has been given impetus by the work of Heston (1981), who found an increased probability of occurrence of Alzheimer's disease among siblings and parents of Alzheimer's disease patients compared to normal families. And his confirmation of another observation — that relatives of patients with Alzheimer's disease have a higher incidence of Down's syndrome than the normal population — suggests that chromosome 21 may play some part in the genesis of Alzheimer's disease.

Besides the neurochemical, infections and genetic models of causation, models attempting to explain the causation of Alzheimer's disease have focused on abnormal proteins, aluminium toxicity, and various problems with blood flow and glucose utilization (see Wurtman, 1985). The multiplicity of theories about senile dementia, Alzheimer's type, is, in fact, a reflection of the vigour of current research efforts and represents a great contrast to the situation not too long ago, when the aetiology of Alzheimer's disease in a standard American psychiatric textbook was nowhere discussed (Noyes & Kolb, 1958).

Parallel to advances in biology and chemistry have been spectacular advances in technology, thus making the investigation of dementia and Alzheimer's disease not only easier and more rewarding but also rendering other procedures, such as pneumo-encephalography, obsolete. Computerized axial tomography — 'the most significant advance in the use of X-rays for diagnosis since their discovery' (Lishman, 1978) — has become a standard evaluation procedure for dementia in the last ten years. The use of nuclear magnetic resonance techniques and positron emission tomography will extend the range of basic technology even further and — in the case of the positron emission tomography scan — more dynamically than any of the older procedures.

Particularly in the United States, which has considered itself young both in history and population, the reality that the population is ageing has begun to impress itself on politicians, sociologists and physicians alike. The percentage of older people in the American population, estimated at 4% in 1900 and 11% in the 1980s, is projected to be 17% in the year 2030. Declining mortality and fertility rates means inevitably that the population will continue to age. Furthermore, old age, once a relatively unusual state, has become a general expectation for most people. In fact, the population of elderly over 75 years of age and especially over 85 years in increasing proportionately faster than the group over 65 years as a whole. In the 1980s people over 85 comprise 9% of all older individuals, whereas, the Census Bureau anticipates, in the year 2040 the figure will rise to 14.5%. Of course it is among the elderly that the highest rates of physical disability, functional incapacity and dementia occur (Watts & McCally, 1984).

The extraordinary costs of caring for the elderly are also beginning to be felt. About 60% of nursing-home residents in the United States have significant cognitive impairment, for example. Most of this is caused by Alzheimer's disease, and the cost runs into billions of dollars each year. It is estimated that 25–40% of individuals will spend at least some time in a nursing home before their deaths (Vicente et al, 1979; Palmore, 1976) and there is evidence, too, that patients with Alzheimer's disease are living longer than they used to be (Blessed & Wilson, 1982). These statistics mean more than just an awakening to an already existing state of affairs. They reflect the palpable existence of a population that did not exist before, 'an unprecedented new population of persons who are suffering from multiple chronic illnesses, functional disabilities and dependence' (McCally et al, 1984).

The role of the news media in calling attention to dementia and to Alzheimer's disease should not be underestimated. A number of articles in national newspapers and newsmagazines, well-written and accurate, have made the public, as well as physicians, more aware of many aspects of dementia and Alzheimer's disease: its prevalence, the possible reversible causes, signs and symptoms, prognosis, what families should expect in the way of evaluation and care, and what research efforts are being undertaken. A recent article in the *New York Times* 23 November 1983), for example, called attention to the 'mind-destroying disease that currently afflicts two million Americans and devastates the lives of perhaps ten million of their relatives' (Brody, 1983).

The role of the federal government in providing money, incentives, and otherwise serving as a catalyst for clinical and research work in ageing and in dementia must be recognized also. The creation of the National Institute on Aging in 1974, one of whose major aims has been the understanding of Alzheimer's disease, was a major step in promoting interst in research in the area. A joint workshop in Alzheimer's disease that was sponsored by the National Institute on Aging and two other federal agencies in 1977 was a landmark in that, at the conference and the publication of the proceedings that followed, the idea that senile dementia and Alzheimer's disease were one disease was consolidated (Katzman et al, 1978). The conference also drew attention to the concept that Alzheimer's disease and senile dementia should be treated as diseases and not just as variants of normal ageing. The National Institute on Aging has recently designated and funded several medical schools as Alzheimer's Disease Research Centers in order to promote even more intensive research into all aspects of the disease (Butler & Emr, 1983). And federal spending for ageing and research, in all agencies combined, has grown from US$4 million in 1976 to US$37 million today (Clark et al, 1984).

The interest in dementia, in both the United States and Great Britain, is also part of the larger development of geriatrics in those two countries. But that story has been told elsewhere and will not be repeated here (Beck & Vivell, 1984; Adams, 1975).

REFERENCES

Ackerknecht E 1968 A short history of psychiatry. Hafner, New York, p 70
Adams G 1975 Eld health; origins and destiny of British geriatrics. Age and Ageing 4: 65–68
Adams R D, Fisher C M, Hakim S, Ojemann R G, Sweet W H 1965 Symptomatic occult hydrocephalus with 'normal' cerebrospinal fluid pressure: a treatable syndrome. New England Journal of Medicine 273: 117–126
Albert M, Naeser M A, Levine H L, Garvey H A 1984a Ventricular size in patients with pre-senile dementia of the Alzheimer's type. Archives of Neurology 41: 1258–1263
Albert M, Naeser M A, Levine H L, Garvey H A 1984b Mean CT density numbers in patients with senile dementia of the Alzheimer's type. Archives of Neurology 41: 1264–1269
Ball M J et al 1985 A new definition of Alzheimer's disease: a hippocampal dementia. Lancet 1: 14–16
Beck J C, Vivell S 1984 Development of geriatrics in the United States. In: Cassel C, Walsh J R (eds) Geriatric medicine, vol 2. Springer, New York, ch 5, p 59–81
Benson D F 1979 Aphasia, alexia and agraphia. Churchill Livingstone, London, p 169–170

Benson D F, Cummings J L, Tsai S Y 1982 Angular gyrus syndrome simulating
Alzheimer's disease. Archives of Neurology 39: 616–620
Berg L et al 1984 Predictive features in mild senile dementia of the Alzheimer type.
Neurology 34: 563–569
Birren J E, Butler R N, Greenhouse S W, Sokoloff L, Yarrow M R 1963 Human Aging.
National Institute of Mental Health, Bethesda
Birren J E, Shaie K W 1977 Handbook of the psychology of aging. Van Nostrand
Reinhold, New York
Blessed G, Wilson I D 1982 The contemporary natural history of mental disorder in old
age. British Journal of Psychiatry 141: 56–67
Blum J E, Clark E T, Jarvik L F 1973 The New York State Psychiatric Institute study of
aging twins. In: Jarvik L F, Eisdorfer C, Blum J E (eds) Intellectual functioning in
adults. Springer, New York, p 13
Bockman J M, Kingsbury D T, McKinley M P, Bendheim P E, Prusiner S B 1985
Creutzfeldt-Jakob disease prion proteins in human brains. New England Journal of
Medicine 312: 73–78
Bondareff W 1983 Age and Alzheimer's disease. Lancet 1: 1447
Bowen D M, Smith C B, White P, Davison A N 1976 Neurotransmitter-related enzymes
and indices of hypoxia in senile dementia and other abiotrophies. Brain 99: 459–496
Breitner J C S , Folstein M F 1984 Familial nature of Alzheimer's disease. New England
Journal of Medicine 311: 192
Brody J E 1983 A disease afflicting the mind. New York Times, 23 November
Bruetsch W L 1975 Neurosyphilitic conditions: general paralysis, general paresis, dementia
paralytica. In: Reiser M F (ed) American handbook of psychiatry, vol 4: Organic
disorders and psychosomatic medicine. Basic Books, New York, ch 5, p 134–151
Busse E W 1967 Brain syndromes associated with disturbances in metabolism, growth, and
nutrition. In: Freedman A M, Kaplan H I (eds) Comprehensive textbook of psychiatry,
Williams & Wilkins, Baltimore, ch 19.2 p 726–740
Butler R N 1975 Why survive? Being old in America. Harper & Row, New York
Butler R N, Emr M 1983 An American perspective. In: Reisberg B (ed) Alzheimer's
disease. Free Press, New York, ch 58, p 461–464
Clark M et al 1984 A slow death of the mind. Newsweek, 3 December
Corsellis J A N 1962 Mental illness and the ageing brain. Oxford University Press, Oxford
Craik F I M 1977 Age differences in human memory. In: Birren J E, Shaie K W (eds)
Handbook of the psychology of aging. Van Nostrand Reinhold, New York, p 384–420
Davies P, Maloney A J 1976 Selective loss of central cholinergic neurones in Alzheimer's
disease. Lancet 2: 1403
Defendorf A R 1902 Clinical psychiatry: a textbook for students and physicians. Abstracted
and adapted from the 6th German edition of Kraepelin's Lehrbuch der Psychiatrie.
Macmillan, London
Diagnostic and statistical manual of mental disorders III 1980 American Psychiatric
Association, Washington D C
Eisdorfer C, Wilkie F 1973 Intellectual changes with advancing age. In: Jarvik L F,
Eisdorfer C, Blum J E (eds) Intellectual functioning in adults. Springer, New York, p 21
Esquirol J E D 1976 Des malades mentales, vol 2. Arno, New York, p 261
Ferraro A 1975 The neuropathology associated with psychoses of aging. In: Reiser M F
(ed) American handbook of psychiatry, vol 4: Organic disorders and psychosomatic
medicine. Basic Books, New York, ch 4, p 90–133
Ferris S H, de Leon M 1983 The PET scan in the study of Alzheimer's disease.
In: Reisberg B (ed) Alzheimer's disease. Free Press, New York, ch 36, P 291
Folstein M F, Folstein S E, McHugh P R 1975 'Mini-mental state': a practical method of
grading the cognitive state of patients for the clinician. Journal of Psychiatric Research
12: 189–198
Gajdusek D C, Gibbs C J 1972 Transmissible virus dementias and kuru: the two
spongiform virus encephalopathies of man. Bulletin de l'Institut Pasteur 70: 117–144
Heston L L, Mastri A R, Anderson V E, White J 1981 Dementia of the Alzheimer type.
Archives of General Psychiatry 38: 1085–1090
Horn J L, Donaldson G 1976 On the myth of intellectual decline in adulthood. American
Psychologist 31: 701–719

Hughes C P, Berg L, Danziger W L, Coben L A, Martin R L 1982 A new clinical scale for the staging of dementia. British Journal of Psychiatry 140: 566–572

Hunter R, Macalpine I 1963 Three hundred years of psychiatry 1535–1860. Oxford University Press, London

Kahn R L, Zarit S H, Hilbert N M, Niederehe G 1975 Memory complaint and impairment in the aged. Archives of General Psychiatry 32: 1569–1573

Katzman R 1976 The prevalence and malignancy of Alzheimer's disease. Archives of Neurology 33: 217–218

Katzman R, Karasu T V 1975 Differential diagnosis of dementia. In: Fields W (ed) Neurological and sensory disorders in the elderly. Stratton Intercontinental Medical Book Corporation, New York, p 103–134

Katzman R, Terry R D, Bick K L 1978 Alzheimer's disease: senile dementia and related disorders. Raven Press, New York

Katzman R, Terry R 1983 Neurology of aging. Davis, Philadelphia, p 16–26

Kendell R E 1975 The role of diagnosis in psychiatry. Blackwell, Oxford

Kiloh L G 1961 Pseudo-dementia. Acta Psychiatrica Scandinavica 37: 336–351

Kral V A 1962 Senescent forgetfulness: benign and malignant. Canadian Medical Association Journal 86: 257–260

Kral V A 1978 Benign senescent forgetfulness. In: Katzman R, Terry R D, Bick K L (eds) Alzheimer's disease: senile dementia and related disorders. Raven Press, New York, p 47–51

Larsson T, Sjogren T, Jacobson G 1963 Senile dementia. Acta Psychiatrica Scandinavica 39 (suppl 167): 3–259

LaRue A 1982 Memory loss in aging. In: Jarvik LF, Small G W (eds) The Psychiatric Clinics of North America 5: 89–103

Lishman W A 1978 Organic psychiatry. Blackwell, Oxford

Lipowski Z J 1981 Organic mental disorders: their history and classification with special reference to DSM-III. In: Miller N E, Cohen G D (eds) Clinical aspects of Alzheimer's disease and senile dementia. Raven Press, New York, p 37–45

Lipowski Z J 1984 Organic mental disorders — an American perspective. British Journal of Psychiatry 144: 542–546

McCally M, Greeenlick M, Beck J C 1984 Research in geriatrics: needs and priorities. In: Cassel C, Walsh J R (eds) Geriatric medicine, vol 2. Springer, New York, p 451–463

McHenry L C 1969 Garrison's history of neurology. Thomas, Springfield, P 86

McKhann N G, Drachman D, Folstein M, Katzman R, Price D, Stadlan E M 1984 Clinical diagnosis of Alzheimer's disease. Neurology 34: 939–943

Mahendra B 1984 Dementia. Lancaster, MTP Press, ch 1, p 1–18

Major R H 1945 Classic descriptions of disease. Thomas, Springfield, p 476–477

Mann D M A, Yates P O, Marcyniuk B 1984 Age and Alzheimer's disease. Lancet 1: 281–282

Mayeux R, Stern Y, Rosen J, Benson D F 1983 Is'subcortical dementia'a recognizable clinical entity? Annals of Neurology 14: 278–283

Menninger K, Mayman M, Pruyser P 1963 The vital balance. Viking Press, New York, p 419–489

Miller E 1971 On the nature of the memory disorder in presenile dementia. Neuropsychologia 9: 75–81

Noyes A P, Kolb L C 1958 Modern clinical psychiatry, 5th edn. Saunders, Philadelphia

Palmore E 1976 Total chance of institutionalization among the aged. Gerontologist 16: 504–507

Parkes J D, Marsden C D 1973 The treatment of Parkinson's disease. British Journal of Hospital Medicine 10: 284–294

Perry R, Perry E 1982 The ageing brain and its pathology. In: Levy R, Post F (eds) The psychiatry of late life. Blackwell, Oxford, ch 1, p 9–67

Perry E K, Perry R H, Blessed G, Tomlinson B E 1977 Necropsy evidence of central cholinergic deficits in senile dementia. Lancet 1: 189

Pfeiffer E 1975 Short portable mental status questionnaire for the assessment of organic brain deficit in elderly patients. Journal of the American Geriatric Society 23: 433–441

Pinel P 1962 A treatise on insanity. Hafner, New York

Prusiner S B 1982 Novel proteinaceous infectious particles cause scrapie. Science 216: 136–144

Prusiner S B 1984 Some speculations about prions, amyloid and Alzheimer's disease. New England Journal of Medicine 310: 661–663

Pullicino P, Eskin T, Ketonen L 1983 Prevalence of Binswanger's disease. Lancet 1: 939

Redlich F C, Freedman D X 1967 The theory and practice of psychiatry. Basic Books, New York, P 712

Reisberg B 1982 Office management and treatment of primary degenerative dementia. Psychiatric Annals 12: 631–637

Reisberg B, Ferris S H, DeLeon M J, Crook T 1982 The global deterioration scale for assessment of primary degenerative dementia. American Journal of Psychiatry 139: 1136–1139

Rosen G 1968 Madness in society. University of Chicago Press, Chicago, P 229–262

Rossor M N 1982 Dementia. Lancet 2: 1200–1204

Roth M 1980 Aging of the brain and dementia: an overview. In: Amaducci L, Davison A N, Antuono P A P (eds) Aging of the brain and dementia. Raven Press, New York, p 1–21

Shaie K W 1974 Transition in gerontology — from lab to life: intellectual functioning. American Psychologist 29: 802–807

Siegler I C 1980 The psychology of adult development and aging. In: Busse E W, Blazer D G (eds) Handbook of geriatric psychiatry. Van Nostrand Rheinhold, New York, ch 8, p 169–221

Slater E, Roth M 1969 Clinical psychiatry, 3rd edn. Williams & Wilkins, Baltimore, P 612

Sluss T K, Rabins P, Gruenberg E M, Reedman G 1980 Memory complaints in community residing men. Gerontologist 20 (Pt II): 201

Steele J C, Richardson J C, Olszewski J 1964 Progressive supranuclear palsy. Archives of Neurology 10: 333–359

Storandt M, Botwinick J, Danziger W L, Berg L, Hughes C P 1984 Psychometric differentiation of mild senile dementia of the Alzheimer type. Archives of Neurology 41: 497–499

Terry R D 1978 Aging, senile dementia and Alzheimer's disease. In: Katzman R, Terry R D, Bick K L (eds) Alzheimer's disease: senile dementia and related disorders. Raven Press, New York, p 11–14

Tomlinson B E, Blessed G, Roth 1970 Observations on the brains of demented old people. Journal of the Neurological Sciences 11: 205–242

Torack R M 1978 The pathologic physiology of dementia. Springer, Berlin, p 1–16

Torack R M, 1983 The early history of senile dementia. In: Reisberg B (ed) Alzheimer's disease. The Free Press, New York, ch 2, p 23–28

Vicente L, Wiley J A, Carrington R A 1979 The risk of institutionalization before death. Gerontologist 19: 361–366

Watts D, McCally M 1984 Demographic perspectives. In: Cassel C, Walsh J R (eds) Geriatric medicine, vol 2. Springer, New York, ch 1, p 3–15

Wells C E 1978 Chronic brain disease: an overview. American Journal of Psychiatry 135: 1–12

Woods R 1982 The psychology of ageing: assessment of defects and their management. In: Levy R, Post F (eds) The psychiatry of late life. Blackwell, Oxford, ch 2, p 68–113

Worm-Peterson J, Pakkenberg H 1967 Atherosclerosis of cerebral arteries, pathological and clinical correlations. Acta Neurologica Scandinavica 43 (suppl 31): 112–113

Wurtman R J 1985 Alzheimer's disease. Scientific American 252: 62–74

The nosology of the dementias: an overview

INTRODUCTION

While the number of publications on the dementias has of late increased geometrically, the clinician seems no better able to understand and manage this group of conditions.

The therapeutic predictions of the 1970s' (e.g. the acetylcholine story) have come to grief. Epidemiological study has not yet confirmed whether there is in fact an approaching 'epidemic' of dementia (Plum, 1979) or whether the problem is smaller than statistical extrapolations might suggest (Weissman et al, 1985).

Lured by the psychometry of cognition (Branconnier & Devitt, 1983) diagnosticians have concentrated on the disturbances of memory and language to the detriment of the non-cognitive symptomatology of dementia (Berrios, 1986).

The 'cognitivist' view, adequate at the actuarial level, has probably reached its limits of resolution in relation to differential diagnosis. Dementia remains both an underdiagnosed (Garcia et al, 1984) and an overdiagnosed psychiatric category (Marsden & Harrison, 1972; Nott & Fleminger, 1975; Ron et al, 1979).

HISTORICAL NOTE ON THE NOSOLOGY OF THE DEMENTIAS

The term and concept of dementia have existed since before the 19th century. The term was used to refer both to a syndrome of psychological dilapidation (clinical meaning) and to the related state of civil and legal incapacity (forensic meaning) (Berrios, 1986a). This quality of usage underlies much of the semantic and clinical confusion found in later writings.

The category senile dementia (amentia senilis) has been in use in the West since an earlier period, but until the end of the 18th century it had a predominant social meaning (dotage). The condition may in fact have been statistically uncommon due to the enviromental constraints imposed upon survival during these earlier periods.

During the late 18th century no distinction was made between functional and organic disorders in psychiatry, and the term dementia had the widest possible referent. It was not attached to a specific set of diagnostic criteria and often the same clinical tests (e.g. number counting and knowledge of coinage) were used to ascertain the presence of both acquired dementia and mental handicap (Scheerenberger, 1983). During this period the category senile dementia is found in most nosologies (e.g. Cullen, 1827). Age and memory impairment were utilized as the nosological criteria.

During the early 19th century and in the wake of the medical reorganization of clinical psychiatry (Berrios, 1984) dementia became separated from the states of cognitive incompetence caused by congenital causes (i.e. idiocy). Three forms of dementia were distinctly described: senile, organic and vesanic and the differentiation between the first two was made in terms of age and aetiology.

The discovery of the general paralysis of the insane, which affected the individual at any age, provided a workable model of dementia (Berrios, 1985). For the first time a given symptomatology could be related to acquired brain pathology. The development of an organic view of dementia encouraged the redefinition of the 'vesanic' dementias as states of psychosocial defect related to chronic insanity.

Up to the second half of the 19th century, however, the differential diagnosis between the three forms of dementia was not considered as essential. This resulted from the fact that dementia was conceived of as a final common pathway, and aetiological and post-mortem criteria were still unclear. The lists of potential causal factors were overcomprehensive, and the usefulness of the pathological changes was reduced by non-specific post-mortem changes. Preoccupation with this technical problem only developed during the 1880s (Berrios, 1985).

Delirium and the confusional states were redefined as states of altered consciousness during the second half of the 19th century (Berrios, 1981, 1982); dementia was conceptualized as a state of memory decay according to the new models of Richet & Ribot (Berrios, The memory disorders: unpublished findings); advances in the neuropathology of senile dementias began to be made.

At the turn of the century these factors brought about marked changes in the concept of dementia. Advances in the psychometry of memory showed that the vesanic dementias were not 'real' dementias, and the adoption of the 'neuropathological' basis for the intellectual decay of senescence paved the way for the acceptance of the 'irreversibility' criterion.

Up to this period taxonomic and clinical factors and an unprejudiced attention to the psychopathology of the dementias had encouraged the classification of these conditions as 'exogenous psychoses'. Neuropathological and clinical observation led to the description of Alzheimer's and Pick's disease and of presbyophrenia (Berrios, 1986).

By the late 19th century advances had also taken place in relation to the mechanisms of brain circulation. The concepts of hypoxia and cerebral infarction gave rise (during the 1890s) to the concept of atherosclerotic dementia. The clinical territory of this noble category soon grew at the expense of the other types of dementia.

Clinical and social factors led to the creation of groupings based on age or symptomatology, such as the presenile states, melancholic pseudo-dementia (Berrios, 1985) and presbyophrenia (Berrios, 1985a). The psychologization of the psychoses encouraged the reinterpretation of the vesanic dementias as defect states without organic impairment.

PSYCHOPATHOLOGY

The characterization of dementia as a global cognitive failure cannot differentiate it reliably (in the cross-sectional diagnosis) from other states of compromised cognition. Diagnostic discrimination could be improved by utilizing longitudinal indicators (e.g. symptom-staging, evolution of the memory impairment, onset pattern of the cerebrocortical syndromes) and by including new criteria in the definition of the condition (e.g. language disorder and psychotic symptoms).

Since the cognitive aspects of dementia are dealt with elsewhere in this book, this section will only touch upon symptoms unrelated to memory impairment.

Psychotic symptoms

Psychotic symptoms occur with certain frequency in dementia (Berrios & Brook, 1984, 1985; Ballinger, 1982; Wertheimer, 1974; Allison, 1962; Jonsson et al, 1972). The view taken by the present writer is that these are not just interloping phenomena but reflect an as yet unclarified neurophysiological dysfunction intrinsic to the dementia state.

In the past a number of hypotheses have been put forward to explain the psychotic symptoms away (Berrios, The psychotic symptoms of dementia: unpublished findings). They have been considered as resulting from intercurrent delirium, disordered REM activity breaking into consciousness, cortical disinhibition, enhancement of personality traits by the dementing process, coexisting endogenous psychoses (i.e. late-onset schizophrenia or bipolar disorder), drug toxicity and even psychodynamic factors.

It is likely that these explanations may be occasionally relevant, but they cannot explain the more persistent psychotic phenomena (e.g. presbyophrenia) (Berrios, 1986).

Language disorder in dementia

Language impairment is considered as one of the central symptoms of dementia (Kirschner et al, 1984). The main features of such impairment are listed as poverty of expression, loss of ability to name objects and loss of fluency. Less frequently stereotypies and interloping phenomena such as perseveration, echolalia, syntactic disintegration and emission of strange noises and shouting can also be observed.

Disagreement exists, however, as to whether this symptom cluster constitutes a form of aphasia. A number of pathogenic mechanisms have been described: cortical atrophy (giving rise to pathological changes in the expression and comprehension of speech), arousal collapse, memory dysfunction, thought disorder and perceptual decline. It is possible that all contribute to the peculiar disintegration of spoken, written and read language found in the demented patient.

Research in this area is marred by the changes in language parameters caused by ageing. Speech discrimination and comprehension of spoken language are affected in ways that can go unnoticed in colloquial communication. Speech becomes more fluent, but prosody (i.e. the melodic aspect of language) acquires a wooden quality. Active lexicon (i.e. the ability to recall and incorporate words in speech) eteriorates, whereas passive lexicon (i.e. the ability to recognize terms) increases with age.

In the patient with dementia (of the so-called cortical-type) marked changes in language function can be found (Stengel, 1964). It has been suggested that its deterioration follows a pattern of dedifferentiation according to which linguistic losses are in direct relationship to linguistic complexity (i.e. higher functions suffer first) (Emery & Emery, 1983).

It is also possible to identify specific dysfunctions: for example inability to name uncommon objects worsens (Barker & Lawson, 1968) and this can be rendered more salient by controlling for reaction time (Lawson & Barker, 1968). When patients with Alzheimer's disease are compared with normal controls and with stroke patients on the Western Aphasia Battery (Kertesz, 1979), it is found that the first group is different on all parameters. Transcortical sensory and Wernicke's types of aphasia are also common in the Alzheimer group but, interestingly, Broca's aphasia is very infrequent. Fluency is not impaired, while the opposite is true of comprehension and naming (Appell et al, 1982).

The extent of the language impairment does not correlate with age but with length of hospitalization. Language disorder in the context of dementia tends to predict earlier death (Kaszniak et al, 1981; Berrios & Brook, 1985). Aphasia scores have also been found to predict severity of the dementia a year later (Berg et al, 1984).

BENIGN SENESCENT FORGETFULNESS

A common problem in the diagnosis of dementia concerns its differentiation from the memory impairment seen in the 'normal' elderly. It would seem that lesser degrees of mnestic decay do occur with ageing, but it is unclear how they relate to the memory defect of dementia.

Kral (1959) introduced the terms benign and malignant forgetting. The benign form described recall failures of relatively unimportant facts or parts of an experience (i.e. names, dates, places); information forgotten on one occasion was susceptible to later retrieval and tended to belong to the remote past; insight into own occasional lapses was the rule and subjects were apologetic and overcompensatory.

Malignant forgetting, on the other hand, was characterized by poor retention time, inability to recall events from the recent past, with both incidental and central aspects of memories being wiped out; patients also showed paramnesic or confabulatory recall and orientation failures involving, progressively, time, place and person (Kral, 1978).

Kral's distinction appeals to common sense. His data, however, seem insufficient to support the view that benign and malignant forgetting are qualitatively different (Miller, 1977). Operational difficulties also limit its clinical use. The clinical description of the criteria is vague, and the account of the memory difficulties too subjective. Hence a great deal of overlap between the two forms of forgetting is found in clinical practice, and it is not uncommon for cases diagnosed as suffering from benign forgetting to develop dementia (LaRue & Jarvik, 1980; Mayeux et al, 1985).

REVERSIBLE DEMENTIAS

Vitamin B_{12} deficiency, hypothyroidism, space-occupying lesion, chronic subdural haematoma, normal pressure hydrocephalus and some endogenous psychoses can cause brain dysfunction of sufficient severity to precipitate reversible cognitive impairment (in some cases the impairment may be reversible only during the earlier stages). Their multiplicity, however, has prevented the formulation of a unified pathogenic mechanism. In general, however, it is claimed that these dementing processes are of the 'subcortical' type (see below).

Vitamin B_{12} deficiency

Deficiency of cobalamin can cause haematological and neurological disease. Cobalamin is needed to add a methyl group to homocysteine to yield methionine (Lindenbaum, 1980). Its deficiency may lead to demyelinization (reversible during the early stages) and neuropathic degeneration of peripheral nerves, of posterior and lateral spinal tracts, and of brain.

Both delirium and dementia can be seen in relation to B_{12} deficiency (Evans et al, 1983). These states can be accompanied by abnormal e.e.g. (slowing) (Walton et al, 1954) and are commonest in patients with a history of gastric surgery, particularly when the source of intrinsic factor (a glycoprotein secreted by the gastric parietal cell) has been tampered with or anastomosis or drainage operations have led to changes in intestinal flora (Melzer & Vernea, 1959; Becker & Caspary, 1980; Alexander-Williams et al, 1977; Roos & Willanger, 1977; Roos, 1978).

Nutritional deficiencies in the elderly (Schorah & Morgan, 1985) and in the psychiatrically infirm (Eisborg et al, 1979) may also contribute to a reduced concentration of vitamin B_{12}. Ageing per se, however, does not reduce the absorption of this (McEvoy et al, 1982) or indeed of other vitamins (Scileppi et al, 1984).

Patients with avitaminosis B_{12} do not always show megaloblastic changes (Strachen & Henderson, 1965; Zucker et al, 1981; Carney & Sheffield, 1978; Garey et al, 1984). It is therefore advisable to ascertain the plasma level of the vitamin in patients presenting with dementia of rapid onset (without cortical syndrome), history of gastric surgery and abnormal e.e.g.

Therapeutic response depends upon early detection. Folate deficiency may also be present (Carney, 1967; Enk et al, 1980; Botez & Reynolds, 1979). It is wise in these cases to include both vitamins in the therapy. Patients must remain in maintenance therapy for life.

Hypothyroidism

Slowness, lethargy, memory impairment and paranoid symptoms have been described as part of the myxoedematous syndrome since the 19th century (Ord, 1888). About 5% of cases will show a syndrome indistinguishable from dementia and often accompanied by paranoid ideation, irritability and psychomotor retardation. Cognitive assessment usually shows a degree of dysfunction (Reitan, 1953). Patients who have reached this level of mental impairment, however, show also the concomitant physical signs (Swanson et al, 1981).

Difficulties arise in the case of thyroid disease of late onset, as the physical changes of ageing may mask some of the physical signs of hypothyroidism (Reed & Bland, 1977). Occasionally, it is only the appearance of hypothermia, mutism or stupor that will alert the clinician.

Although considered as a reversible state, the dementia of hypothyroidism often responds incompletely to treatment. Thyroxine will arrest (or improve) the evolution of the dementia (Crown, 1949; Olivarus & Roder, 1970) but formal testing and observation of behaviour may show that the patient has been left with a degree of cognitive impairment.

Space-occupying lesion

Localization, nature and rate of growth of the brain tumour determine the clinical predominance of either specific or non-specific symptoms (Howell, 1979; Mulder & Swenson, 1974). The former usually relate to the site and lateralization of the mass; the latter to the rate of growth, the total mass effect and the premorbid personality of the affected individual (Thomas, 1983).

Tumours (primary or metastatic) are the commonest form of space-occupying lesion followed by haematomas and, more rarely, vessel malformations, cysts and parasites.

Type and location of the tumour vary according to age. Posterior fossa is a favourite location for primary neoplasias in the child; in the elderly, tumours are more often supratentorial and metastatic (Annegers et al, 1981). The incidence of brain tumours steadily increases with age and peaks at 75, when the figure reaches 90 cases per hundred thousand population (Schoenberg et al, 1978). Post-mortem figures are higher owing to the fact that slow-growing meningiomas may be asymptomatic during life.

Malignant astrocytoma, the commonest tumour in adult life, becomes infrequent after 65. Malignant glia tumours and meningiomas are common in the elderly; the commonest are the metastatic growths. Craniopharyngioma, when it occurs in the elderly, is often accompanied by signs of cognitive impairment (Russell & Pennybacker,1961).

Tumours in the elderly can present acutely, subacutely and, not uncommonly, in an insidious manner (Cairncross & Posner,1984). Acute and subacute presentations, either with epilepsy, focal motor or sensory signs or cerebrovascular accidents (caused by tumour bleeding) are easily recognizable, and patients thus affected can be rarely (if ever) considered as having dementia. Uncommon cortical syndromes, however, presenting with aphasic (mainly Wernicke's) syndromes may catch the clinician unawares.

From the point of view of this chapter, however, the third group (slow-growing space-occupying lesions) is the most relevant, as their clinical presentation is that of gradual cognitive deterioration without localizing signs. In this case it is not uncommon for the patient to be considered as suffering from dementia. Tumours of the frontal lobe (Avery, 1971; Angelergues et al, 1955) and particularly of the corpus callosum (Selecki, 1965) have a marked tendency to cause retardation and cognitive impairment.

Neurological examination may show in a number of cases mild lateralized motor or sensory signs. Affective disorder, irritability, personality change, inability to cope are equally common and often may precede the actual memory impairment and inattention. The appearance of 'late onset' epilepsy in the elderly patient already showing a degree of cognitive impairment must always be followed by a determined search for a space-occupying lesion. It is true of course that Alzheimer's disease may occasionally be accompanied by seizural activity, but this occurs late in the evolution of the condition.

Once the diagnosis has been made and treatment started, it is important to remember that whole-brain radiation therapy, often used to treat multiple metastasis, may also cause dementia; this occurs in about 25% of treated patients within 18 to 24 months after cessation of the therapy (Cairncross et al, 1980).

In general, neurosurgeons tend to be conservative with regard to slow-growing tumours in the elderly. If the psychiatric symptomatology is accompanied by severe epilepsy or motor impairment (curtailing psychosocial competence), resection of the tumour may, however, be attempted.

Another complication of neoplastic growth which may cause dementia is the so-called limbic encephalitis (Corsellis et al, 1968). This is a syndrome with fatal outcome which holds an obscure relationship to systemic malignancy (with or without brain metastasis). Its main symptoms are memory impairment and occasional psychotic phenomena. An opportunistic herpes simplex infection has been suggested as the mediating mechanism (Glaser & Pincus, 1969). The particular predilection of the virus for the limbic system has been explained by a specific susceptibility of the latter to viral attack (Damasio & Van Hoesen, 1985).

Chronic subdural haematoma (CSH)

Although a form of space-occupying lesion, CHS is dealt with under a separate heading because it exhibits characteristic symptomatology (Patrick & Gates, 1984; Brocklehurst, 1982).

The main point to remember is that the clinical presentation of CSH in the elderly is different from that of the acute subdural haematoma (Cameron, 1978). History of head trauma is often absent; indeed, tearing of subdural veins (and bleeding) can occur in the elderly following trivial blows to the head or sudden movements which may induce a degree of angular acceleration. Clots can develop bilaterally and this may prevent the shift of calcified middle-line structures in the plain skull X-ray. Periods of mutism, akinesis and episodic confusion are not uncommon. The CAT scan of the head may be temporarily unhelful as the clot becomes isodense with respect to surrounding brain tissue (Jacobson & Farmer,1979).

Surgical evacuation of the clot, provided that it is performed early, is effective. Late interventions may leave the patient with a degree of cognitive impairment.

Normal pressure hydrocephalus (NPH)

This fascinating and obscure syndrome is, in its pure form, relatively uncommon. Although officially named in 1965 (Adams et al, 1965; Temey, 1976) it has been known at least since 1943 (David et al, 1943).

An important mechanism in the pathogenesis of this form of communicating hydrocephalus (Pickard, 1982) is a reduced rate of CSF absorption at the superior sagittal sinus.

Far less clear is the mechanism culpable for the dilation of ventricles in the presence of apparently normal CSF pressure. The conventional 'hydraulic pressure hypothesis' made use of Pascal's Law (the same that applies to the insufflation of balloons) (Adams et al, 1965). This hypothesis, however, cannot explain a number of the features of NPH (Frank & Tew, 1982); it also necessitates that sometime during the development of the syndrome there must be a period of high CSF pressure (Sjaastad & Nornes, 1976).

It is possible therefore that other factors such as hypertension and atherosclerotic vascular disease may be involved (Koto et al. 1977). Thus reductions in cerebral blood flow may give rise to micro-infarction and to a loss of the tensile strength of the brain (Frank & Tew, 1982). There is no firm evidence that a genetic factor is at play (Portenoy et al, 1984).

Clinically, NPH should be suspected in subjects over 45 presenting with rapidly evolving dementia, early urinary incontinence, akinesis, retardation and apraxia of gait (the characteristic 'magnetic gait' of Denny Brown) (Caltagirone et al, 1982). These subject may be found to have a history of meningitis, hypertension, subarachnoid haemorrhage (Yasargil et al, 1973) or Paget's disease (Botez et al, 1977), and on clinical examination show no signs of aphasia, apraxia or agnosia. An idiopathic and a secondary type of NPH have been distinguished (Wolinsky et al, 1973).

Imaging of the brain will show enlarged lateral ventricles (Jacobs & Kinkel, 1976) and a flattening of LeMay's angle. The lumbar CSF pressure is usually normal; it has been reported that removal of CSF caused a temporary improvement of the cognitive impairment. This practice adds little to the diagnosis, may be dangerous and is to be discouraged.

CSF shunting, whether to the venous system, cardiac cavities or lumbar peritoneum, often affords marked improvement. During the late 1960s overenthusiastic shunting led to a marked failure rate; this was due to the fact that patients with Alzheimer's disease (and secondary enlargement of the ventricles) underwent unnecessary shunting (Samuelson et al 1972). It is therefore of the essence that no radiological signs of cortical atrophy (i.e. no 'air' in the convexities) are present before neurosurgery is contemplated (Woods et al, 1974; Stein & Langfitt, 1974; Salmon, 1972; Messert & Wannamaker, 1974).

In patients who fail to respond to shunting, an increase in the number of neurofibrillary tangles has been described (Ball, 1976).

Pseudodementias

Pseudodementia refers to states of reversible cognitive impairment caused by functional psychiatric disease (Bulbena & Berrios, 1986). This category has created some controversy (Reifler, 1982; Mahendra, 1983). The main issue is whether it is only a bad copy of dementia (i.e. the patient is too depressed or preoccupied to respond) or a 'real' impairment.

With regards to the latter it has been reported that depression (or mania) may in fact cause genuine cognitive impairment (Kirstein & Smith, 1981). The adjective 'real' in this context would mean that the 'impairment' is not simply a reflection of the patient's unwillingness to cooperate (Miller, 1975; McAllister, 1983).

There seem to be at least three types of pseudodementia (Bulbena & Berrios, 1986). Phenocopies due to delirium (Allen, 1982) and to hysterical mechanisms (Kiloh, 1961) are probably crude imitations of dementia. But the cognitive impairment observed in relation to depressive (or manic) illness may be real and can be accompanied by reversible soft neurological signs (Bulbena & Berrios, 1986; Kramer, 1982; Caine, 1981; Wells, 1979).

Clinical indicators of the pseudodementia state include agitation, inconsistencies in the cognitive performance, history of affective disorder, response to the sodium amylobarbitone test, positive dexamethasone suppression test, reduced latency of REM (i.e. the first period of rapid eye movement appears too early); absence of dysphasia, apraxia and agnosia, depressed appearance, CAT scan of the head showing no abvious pathological changes (Wells, 1979; Caine, 1981; Grunhaus et al, 1983).

Disordered cholinergic transmission offers a link between depression and memory impairment. Agonist muscarinic activity may lead to affective disorder (indistinguishable from depression, e.g. after treatment with physostigmine) (Risch et al, 1981; Janowsky et al, 1983). Blockading of muscarinic receptors (e.g. with atropine) may cause cognitive impairment in humans and in experimental animals (Deutsch, 1983). Increased cholinergic agonist activity on a hypersensitive muscarinic receptor may cause learning dysfunction (Deutsch, 1983). It could be suggested therefore that cholinergic overstimulation (in some depressed individuals) may cause cognitive impairment by blockading muscarinic receptors. Indeed, similarities between the cognitive impairment of Alzheimer's disease and that of drug-induced cholinergic deficiency have been reported (Fuld, 1984).

Patients in whom depressive pseudodementia is suspected must be energetically treated. In most cases electroconvulsive therapy should be tried as the results are excellent and there is not evidence that it shortens survival or perpetuates the cognitive impairment.

SENILE DEMENTIA OF THE ALZHEIMER TYPE

Alzheimer's disease is the most common of all dementing illnesses, and its clinical picture has become a prototype (Schneck et al, 1982; Gusstafson & Nilsson, 1982). This is not necessarily advantageous to the definition of the dementia syndrome, as views on the psychopathology of Alzheimer's disease have changed since it was first described and may still be changing (Liston, 1979).

Furthermore, subtypes of Alzheimer's disease have been described, and at this stage it is difficult to decide which of these constitutes the central syndrome (McDonald, 1969; Mayeux et al. 1985; Bondareff, 1983). This definitional confusion may explain why, even when strict entry criteria are used, only 70–90% of diagnoses are corroborated during necropsy (Sulka et al, 1983; Eisendorfer & Cohen, 1980; Todorov et al, 1975).

A major factor in these definitional changes has been the abandonment of the 'exogenous psychosis' concept upon which the notion of dementia was originally based (Berrios, 1986). To that view the presence of delusional ideas, hallucinations, manic and melancholic affect, confabulation and motility disorders was as important as the intellectual deterioration itself (Marie, 1906). One of Alzheimer's earliest cases, for example, exhibited hallucinations as one of her main symptoms (McMenemey, 1970).

Concepts

The current definition of the disease is rather narrow and stipulates both neuropathological (Sourander & Sjogren, 1970; Corsellis, 1982) and clinical criteria (Sim et al, 1966). The latter include changes in memory, thinking, judgment, personality, language, praxia and gnosia, but not psychotic symptoms. The old age boundary (65 years) which once separated the presenile form of the illness has been replaced by a clinical and a neuropathological continuum. New disease categories have been described to name sections of the continuum: e.g. senile dementia of the Alzheimer type (SDAT) and 'Alzheimerized' dementia (a continental category) (Constantinidis et al, 1978).

Difficulties in finding a unified view of Alzheimer's disease stem from an ambiguity in the choice of defining criterion. Thus if it is defined in terms of the presence of senile plaques, neurofibrillary tangles and vacuolar degeneration, clinical states other than Alzheimer's meet the criteria (Ulrich, 1985); if, on the other hand, it is defined in terms of the clinical picture, a percentage of cases fails to be confirmed pathologically (e.g angular gyrus syndrome; Benson & Cummings, 1982). Absolution to this problem will probably be found in the identification of ultrastructural differences in neurofibrils (Wischik & Crowther, 1986).

Therapeutic optimism based on the finding that Alzheimer's disease is related to a dysfunction of cholinergic transmission has proved groundless, and not even biological markers based on this deficiency have been developed. For example, there is no difference between Alzheimer patients and controls in terms of the mean values of red blood cell choline and plasma choline (Greenwald et al, 1985) and of CSF acetylcholinesterase (Lal et el, 1984).

Neurotransmitters found to be deficient in Alzheimer's disease include dopamine, noradrenaline, serotonin (Winblad et al, 1982); and GABA in specific areas) (Rossor et al, 1982); deficient neuropeptides include somatostatin (Rossor et al, 1984), angiotensin-converting enzyme (Arregui et al, 1982), and substance P (in some brain areas) (Crystal & Davies, 1982). The functional relevance of these findings in unclear.

The cause of the basic lesion or lesions of Alzheimer's disease remains obscure, although the subcortical structure to which the cholinergic dysfunction relates has been found to be the nucleus basalis of Meynert (Rogers et al, 1985). Six aetiological models have been distinguished (Wurtman, 1985): genetic, abnormal protein, infectious agent, toxin, blood flow and cholinergic. Efforts have also been made to link Alzheimer's disease to the group of disorders caused by virus-like agents, but inoculation of brain tissue from patients suffering from this condition to primates has so far been unsuccessful (Goudsmit et al, 1980). It has also been speculated that a reactivated herpes virus, with predilection for the limbic system, may be involved (Ball, 1982) and that similarities between scrapie and Alzheimer's disease may warrant its use as an animal model (Bruce, 1984).

A genetic factor may be important in relation to a subtype of Alzheimer's disease, and pedigrees have been reported (Feldman et al, 1963). An association with Down's syndrome and haematological malignancies has also been described (Heston & Mastri, 1977; Crapper et al, 1975). Cases reportedly precipitated by trauma (Rudelli et al, 1982) constitute unexplained curiosities, although a significant association between a history of head trauma and Alzheimer's disease has been noticed (Heyman et al, 1984). The same authors also found an increased incidence of thyroid disease amongst the propositi.

Clinical aspects

The clinical features of the earliest stages of dementia are unclear (Henderson & Huppert, 1984; Liston, 1977, 1979), and diagnosis does not seem to depend exclusively upon objective symptomatology. Factors such as age of onset, sex, premorbid personality, level of intelligence and professional status may influence the 'perception of the disease' both by the patient and by those near him/her.

Since the 1950s', it has become customary to identify three stages in the evolution of Alzheimer's disease (Sjogren et al, 1952). The first stage is characterized by incipient memory impairment (with insight), mild to moderate naming difficulty, reduced spontaneity and fixed forward stare; the second by progressive dementia, memory disturbance, generalized disorientation, aspontaneity, amnestic and sensory aphasia, perseveration, agraphia, alexia, increased muscle tone, gait disturbance, apraxia, dysarthria and occasionally Klüver-Bucy syndrome (Lilly et al, 1983). In the third and terminal stage authors included mutism, stupor, rigidity, vegetative state and emaciation ending up in status decerebratus (perhaps less often seen nowadays); life terminated by the development of pressure sores and infections.

Recent research has shown that during the first stage subtle psychophysiological and neurological changes may take place: subjects may show slow, simple and choice reactions times (Pirazolo et al, 1981); long saccadic latencies (Hershey et al, 1983); short stages 3 and 4 during sleep (Loewenstein et al, 1982); slow philothermal responses (rate of leukocyte migration in response to an increase in temperature) (Jarvik, 1982); decreased sensitivity of cranial nerves (Waldton, 1974); visuoperceptual impairment (Eslinger & Benton, 1983) and positive nuchocephalic reflex (particularly in subjects younger that 60) (Jenkyn et al, 1975).

There is however, no reason to believe that this staged, evolutionary view of Alzheimer's disease fits all clinical facts although it tallies with the current view that there is a gradual and ineluctable deterioration of the brain. It is quite likely, however, that a different model of the disease could obtain if different functional modules (e.g. mood, perception, volition, language) were assessed independently. Thus a steplike picture may well replace the apparently smooth decline currently considered as the rule.

Apart from the longitudinal typologies, symptomatic subgrouping have also been suggested. For example, Mayeux et al (1985) describe four groups: benign (little progression); myoclonic (younger onset, severe decline and mutism); extrapyramidal (severe decline and psychotic symptoms) and typical (gradual progression without a distinguishing symptom). Bondareff (1983) in turn has identified two forms of the disease: AD1 with insidious onset, gradual evolution, little involvement of locus coeruleus, limited motor symptomatology and moderate ventricular enlargement and affecting an older age group; and AD2 with rapid evolution, severe motor symptoms, marked enlargement of cerebral ventricles, atrophy of locus coeruleus, accentuated cholinergic deficit and affecting younger subjects.

PICK'S DISEASE

Minimal diagnostic criteria for this condition are progressive dementia and lobar atrophy of fronto-temporal areas. More stringent criteria include the presence of argyrophilic ball-shaped inclusions in the neuronal cytoplasm.

The disease was first described by Arnold Pick as a form of presenile dementia characterized by early development of 'amnestic aphasia' (forgetting of words) and ideomotor apraxia. Pick's contribution is of some importance to the history of dementia, since it showed (as against the view of Griesinger and Wernicke) that 'focalized symptoms can develop in spite of a generalized senile cortical atrophy' (Pick, 1901).

Pick's early patients exhibited temporal lobe atrophy, but the frontal lobes began to feature prominently after he reported the 'Vlass . . . Joseph' case (Pick, 1904). Pick also emphasized (a feature forgotten since) the involvement of the left hemisphere and presence of visual asymbolia due as he believed) to atrophy of the occipital cortex.

Between Pick's descriptions and the phenomenological modifications brought about by Carl Schneider, most of the published work was dedicated to the neuropathology of the condition. Schneider (1927, 1929) recognized three stages in the evolution of the disease. The first consisted of a progressive failure in judgement and thinking; the second started with the appearance of the focal symptoms (e.g. aphasia and apraxia) and third was the terminal stage characterized by deterioration and death. Schneider also recognized a slow (lasting up to 15 years) and a fast form of the condition.

Caron (1934) in his superb monograph reviewed 65 cases and established the current criteria for the disease. He believed that there were sufficient grounds to consider it as a separate entity, with its highest incidence in the

50–60 years period. He confirmed that the most common form of the condition had an insidious onset, with early development of aphasia (always) and agnosia and apraxia (sometimes). Memory impairment developed later and was followed by a cluster of symptoms that included abulia, lethargy, stereotyped speech (echolalia, palilalia) and mutism. Interestingly he related this latter group of symptoms to impairment of subcortical structures.

He also emphasized the circumscribed nature of the atrophic changes, the infrequent presence of senile plaques and the argyrophilic ball-shaped inclusions. With some prescience he wrote that 'it is impossible to claim that Pick's disease is a different condition from Alzheimer's' (Caron, 1934).

Not much has been learnt since (Van Mansvelt, 1945; Goldstein & Katz 1937). Recent studies are still concerned with the possibility of a continuum of 'degenerative cortical neuronal loss'. Pick's disease at one end would be characterized by spongiform degeneration, focal atrophy, Pick's bodies and cells; Alzheimer's disease at the other with generalized atrophy, neurofibrillary tangles and neuritic plaques (Morris et all, 1984). A number of transitional states could be found along the continuum, such as the non-specific dementia syndrome (Kim et al, 1981) and the hereditary dysphasic dementia (Cole et al, 1979).

Two types of Pick's disease have been recognized. A classical type, so-called, characterized by predominant cortical atrophy and the presence of inclusion bodies in the hippocampus; and a second type showing generalized atrophy of both cortical and subcortical structures, especially the caudate nucleus (Muñoz Garcia & Ludwin, 1984). Differences in the extent of the atrophy and in the immunoreactivity of the cytoplasmic bodies do not seem to depend upon sex or duration of the condition. The second type, however, seems more frequent in younger patients.

Neuronal counts in the nucleus basalis of Meynert are also reduced in Pick's disease (Uhl et al, 1983) but, in contrast with Alzheimer's, there is a greater loss of muscarinic receptors (Yates et al, 1980).

Little is known about the aetiology of this condition. Head trauma has been reported as a precipitating factor (Kosaka et al, 1982), The absence of a neurochemical hypothesis has so far denied the possibility of pharmacological management.

TRAUMATIC, METABOLIC AND INFECTIOUS DEMENTIAS

Beyond a certain intensity threshold and in the presence of host vulnerability, any mechanical, metabolic or infective insult to the brain may cause permanent cognitive impairment.

The very protection afforded to the brain by its rigid casing may on occasions facilitate the damage. Likewise its marked dependence on oxygen and nutrients can make the brain vulnerable to overriding falls in blood supply. Infections may also cause generalized impairment depending upon the agent and structure involved: mechanical damage results from oedema-induced distortion and metabolic interference from competition with the invasive agent.

Damage by exogenous factors varies from brain tissue laceration to shearing of white matter to neurochemical dysfunction. Functional collapse may follow any of these lesions. This section will illustrate each of the mechanisms mentioned above.

Dementia pugilistica

Few human sports are more likely to cause brain damage than boxing. Repeated blows to the skull, delivered from all angles, may give rise to direct and contra-coup lesions and to rotational shearing. These lesions may be gross or microscopic and affect both cortical and subcortical structures.

The observation that old boxers showed difficulty in articulation of speech, unsteadiness of gait, memory impairment and spasticity was made over 50 years ago, and the hypothesis put forward that symptoms were due to rupture of the pericapillary spaces of Virchow and Robin (Martland, 1928). Classical papers by Critchley (1957), Spillane (1962) and Corsellis et al (1973) have since outlined the pyramidal, extrapyramidal, cerebellar and psychiatric aspects of the 'punch drunk' syndrome and of its neuropathology.

The earliest clinical manifestation is usually a change in articulation, voice tonality and prosody followed by extrapyramidal slowing. Whilst the motor symptoms occur early, the cognitive impairment may take far longer to appear and when it does may be progressive for reasons which are unclear (but probably not solely dependent upon ageing). Follow-up is therefore important to demonstrate the damage, and the view can no longer be held that absence of gross brain damage immediately after a bout of boxing is sufficient to call into question the existence of the syndrome (Kaplan & Browder, 1954; McCown, 1959).

Neuropathological changes include cortical atrophy, ventricular dilatation, cavum septum pellucidum, detachment of fornix, depigmentation of substantia nigra, neurofibrillary tangles and loss of forebrain cholinergic neurons (Uhl et al, 1982). An absence of senile plaques has been reported, and this dissociation puts paid to the view that neuropathological and clinical findings in dementia pugilistica are but the result of a coincidental superimposition of Alzheimerian changes.

Dialytic dementia

This syndrome, also known as dialysis encephalopathy and progressive myoclonic dialysis encephalopathy, is a progressive (and fatal) condition that may affect patients undergoing haemodialysis; it has a prevalence of about 600 per 100 000.

Its clinical features include disordered speech, myoclonus, seizures, dyspraxia, memory impairment, abnormal e.e.g., osteodystrophy (often painful) and tendency to bone fractures (O'Hare et al, 1983; Chokroverty et al, 1976; Scheiber & Ziesat, 1976, 1978). Partial syndromes are a common presentation, hence a high degree of suspicion must be exercised to enhance early detection.

The Registration Committee of the European Dialysis and Transplant Association reported in 1980 that dialytic dementia occurred more frequently in patients dialysed with unprocessed water (Wing et al, 1980). It has been suggested that the condition may be due to increased aluminium content in grey matter (Alfrey et al, 1976).

Differential diagnoses of dialytic dementia include the cognitive changes caused by the chronic renal failure itself; the confusional syndrome induced by benzodiazepines (Taclob & Needle, 1976); and the acute hypercalcaemia syndrome (Rivera-Vasquez, 1980). In these three states, however, the e.e.g., does not show the typical changes of dialytic dementia: paroxysmal high voltage (100–150 mV), rhythmic and symmetrical delta activity with a frequency range of 3 Hz and prominent on the frontal area. Spike and slow wave activity are also common accompaniments. In the advanced case the e.e.g., becomes disorganized. CAT scan of the brain is unremarkable (Lederman & Henry, 1978).

The syndrome has no specific neuropathology and is said to respond temporarily to diazepam (Snider et al, 1979); the mechanism underlying this response is unknown.

Neurosyphilitic dementia

Luetic infection of the brain may be asymptomatic (with positive CSF serology as the only sign) or symptomatic. The infection may be predominantly meningovascular or parenchymatous, and psychiatric and neurological symptoms can be seen in both. Although far less common than before the advent of the antibiotics, the cerebral forms of syphilis can still be found, and fears have been expressed that the increase in infected subjects (mainly male homosexuals) detected in the 1970s' may in due course give rise to an spate of neurosyphilitic syndromes (Catterall, 1977).

Dementia has featured prominently amongst the psychiatric complications of neurosyphilis. In earlier periods, when effective treatment was not available, sufferers constituted a sizeable proportion of the total number admitted to mental hospitals. Psychiatric symptomatology could then progress unrestrained, and kaleidoscopic presentations gave rise, in the older literature, to debate as to whether neurosyphilitic dementia was always irreversible and whether there were behavioural phenocopies caused by a combination of retardation, apathy, attentional deficit and disturbances of consciousness. This 'pseudodementia' syndrome was offered as the explanation for cases in which remission took place (Valenciano, 1978).

The meningovascular form of neurosyphilis is characterized by a vascular and perivascular inflammation. It may often present with 'cerebral' symptomatology which includes general irritability, impairment of memory, marked apathy, mental confusion and aphasia. The period of latency (time between initial infection and dementia) is shorter for the meningovascular form (2–20 years). Involvement of cranial nerves is frequent (40%) as are 'apoplectic' (infarct) and hydrocephalic complications.

The parenchymatous form has a longer latency (2–40 years) and is characterized by marked involvement of cortical and subcortical structures. It is more frequent in men, and the most common presentation is that of marked cognitive impairment. Dewhurst (1969) found, in a series of 91 cases collected from six hospitals, that in about 8 % the symptom precipitating the admission had been memory lapses and disorientation. On final assessment about 20% of the total sample exhibited the 'simple dementia' type, and a combination of cognitive impairment and depression was the commonest.

The two forms of neurosyphilis are susceptible to treatment. Once the diagnosis has been confirmed and prednisone administered (5 mg 6-hourly in 24 hours) to forestall the Herxheimer reaction, daily intramuscular procaine penicillin (600 000 units) should be given for 21 days. In general the symptoms of cognitive impairment tend to remit at a slower pace than the other psychiatric manifestations.

SPONGY ENCEPHALOPATHIES IN OLD AGE

The group of disorders grouped under the category 'spongiform dementias' is believed to result from the pathological activity of a virus-like agent.

Creutzfeldt-Jakob disease was first described in the 1920s, but some of the clinical and neuropathological features originally mentioned are no longer part of the current concept of the disease. For example, 'Bertha E.' was a 23-year-old woman with a family history of mental handicap who at 21 seems to have suffered from an episode of anorexia nervosa and at 22 of a severe skin disease. On admission she showed catatonic features, twitching, nystagmus, signs of upper and lower motor neuron involvement, confusion and terminal status epilepticus (6 weeks after admission). On necropsy, brain tissue showed neuronal fall-out, cortical disorganization, glial hypertrophy and 'homogenization' of neuronal cytoplasm (vacuolar degeneration) (Creutzfeldt, 1920). This case suggests a number of diagnoses, not least the possibility of a papulosis atrophicans maligna of Kohlmaier-Degos, also caused by a virus-like agent (Strole et al, 1967).

The clinical picture suggested by the earlier reports was therefore that of a fulminating condition, with a superacute course and early death. Its salient features were marked disintegration of behaviour, involvement of cortical functions (aphasia, apraxia, agnosia), dementia, myoclonic jerks, pyramidal, extrapyramidal and cerebellar symptoms and death by inanition following involvement of autonomic functions.

The standard neuropathology was listed as neuronal destruction, hypertrophy of astrocytes and vacuolar degeneration of neurons and glia (giving a spongiform appearance).

Hadlow (1959) suggested that kuru (an illness affecting the Fore people in New Guinea) and scrapie, a degenerative, non-inflammatory disease of sheep and goats, had some features in common, not least their transmissibility and pathogenic mechanism (a virus-like agent).

Gajdusek and Gibbs (1971) established the connection between kuru and Creutzfeldt-Jakob disease and showed that both could be transmitted to New World monkeys. Inoculation studies in a number of species have since showed the transmissibility of the disease (Chou et al, 1980). Marked variability has however been found in the duration of the incubation periods and in the ability of the species (and strains) in question to 'take' the intracerebral injections. These latter observations suggest that there may also be a vulnerability factor, probably genetic in nature. Brown et al (1979a) reported a significant correlation between population density (in Paris) and mortality rate of Creutzfeldt-Jakob disease and suggested that this is consistent with the hypothesis of a human-to-human transmission.

Of the four main spongiform encephalopathies (scrapie, mink encephalopathy, kuru and Creutzfeldt-Jakob disease), the first two affect animals and the third is becoming rare (probably due to changes in the social mores of the Fore people).

Creutzfeldt-Jakob disease

The clinical definition of this condition has not yet been completed (Gibbs & Gajdusek, 1978; Traub et al, 1970). Its prevalence seems to be of about 1 per million or less and its clinical course varied. A proportion of cases have a superacute course (Brown et al, 1979); 20% last for a long time 10–15 years) and the rest distribute themselves between the two extremes (Brown et al, 1984). Both sporadic and familial cases have been described (Cathala et al, 1980).

The acute form is characterized by marked cognitive involvement, myoclonus, typical EEG, non-familial origin and is easily transmissible to other animals. The chronic form, on the other hand, has an earlier onset, is familial in origin, is non-transmissible, has no characteristic EEG, and shows more signs of lower motor neuron involvement.

Stages in the evolution of the condition (and atypical variants) have been described. The first, protean stage may last weeks or months (according to type) and may be easily confused with a psychotic illness. EEG and imaging of the brain are unremarkable, and this normal appearance may not be in keeping with clinical severity (Galvez & Cartier, 1984).

The second stage is characteristic. In the superacute type the first and second stages may overlap. There is then generalized involvement of cortical functions with aphasia (always), apraxia and agnosias; memory impairment and severe disorientation become well established as do the motor symptoms, myoclonus (often found to be entrained to EEG changes if special techniques are utilize) and epilepsy. EEG shows a progressive loss of normal rhythms which are soon replaced by generalized slow activity (Chiofalo et al, 1980).

By then the patient has become bedridden, incontinent and begins to sink into the third stage, characterized by akinesia, stupor and disconnection from the enviroment; i.e. the 'apallic' or decorticated state. Urinary infection, aspiration pneumonia and pressure sores terminate with the patient's life.

Stage two in the slow course cases may last for 5–10 years. In older patients, it may be confused with Alzheimer's or Pick's disease.

There is no treatment for the condition. Reports that amantadine causes temporary improvement are uncontrolled (Sanders 1979). Antiviral agents are equally unhelpful, probably due to the fact that viroid or prion involved (which has not yet been visualized) does not behave like a normal virus. It causes no immunological or inflammatory response in the host and is extremely resistant to disinfecting techniques. This latter feature may explain the occasional reports of cases in which iatrogenic transmission (inoculation via contaminated electrodes) seems to have taken place. During the 1970s fears were expressed that personnel dealing with patients or with contaminated material could become infected. Good counsels, however, prevailed and a list of precautions has since been published (Corsellis, 1979; Cook & Austin, 1978).

VASCULAR DEMENTIAS

The concept of atherosclerotic dementia developed at the end of the 19th century. It arose from contemporary views on the mechanisms that sustained blood supply to the brain and led to the concept that gradual attrition of oxygen could cause dysfunction and eventual neuronal death. This explanatory model was so powerful that it lasted well into the 1960s when advances in knowledge on cerebral microcirculation and metabolism called into question the view that cerebral hypoxia by itself (Raichle, 1983) could cause dementia (Sokolof, 1966).

Although cerebral blood flow (rCBF) as measured by 133-xenon washout shows marked frontal decrease in patients with dementia (Ingvar & Lassen, 1979) there does not seem to be a difference in rCBF between Alzheimer's disease and the various syndromes exhibiting cerebro-vascular pathology (Obrist, 1979; Barclay et al, 1984).

Clinical aspects

Dementia directly related to atheromatous changes is not common (under 20% of all cases of dementia) (Hutton, 1981). Since postmortem studies may show multiple cerebral softenings in cases of dementia, it has been suggested that a threshold of volumetric loss may exist (100 cc of brain tissue) beyond which the appearance of cognitive impairment becomes likely (Tomlinson et al, 1970).

The dementia related to cerebrovascular disease is steplike (discontinuous) in evolution, and the episodic worsenings correspond to successive cerebrovascular accidents (Wells, 1977). Vascular dementias are said to have a longer survival rate than parenchymatous ones (Shah et al, 1969). Systemic hypertension seems to play a role in this process and is known to be related to increased atrophy of brain matter in the elderly (Hatazama et al, 1984).

Some 40–50% of cerebral infarctions are caused by emboli originating from the heart (Blackwood et al, 1969; Torvik & Jorgensen, 1964); another sizeable proportion originate from extracranial arteries; thrombosis of intracerebral arteries ia a relatively uncommon occurrence.

The presence and type of peripheral motor or sensory symptoms depend upon the infarction site. On occasions no eloquent areas of the brain are involved and dementia may develop without peripheral neurological signs. On other occasions pure aphasic syndromes (particularly disconnection states or Wernicke's syndromes with jargonaphasia) may lead to the diagnosis of delirium or schizophrenia.

The phenomenology of multi-infarct dementia has been enshrined in the so-called 'ischaemic score' (Hachinski et al, 1974) (see Chaptear 12). The reliability and validity of this scale is adequate although it comes to grief in cases showing mixed pathology. In general the differential diagnosis between vascular and degenerative dementias is not easy (Bucht et al, 1984) and can be accurately done in about 50% of cases (Loeb, 1980).

The terms vascular or multi-infarct dementia describe more accurately the pathogenesis of the condition than the term 'atherosclerotic' and are to be preferred. One of the consequences of this change is the realization of the uselessness of drugs which are supposed to improve dementia by increasing cerebral blood supply, causing dilation of brain vessels or maximizing neuronal metabolism (Yesavage et al, 1979; Dowson, 1982; Reisberg et al, 1981; Mindus et al, 1976).

The profile of cognitive impairment is different in multi-infarct dementia, vertebrobasilar insufficiency with dementia and Alzheimer's disease in that the latter group persistently shows more intense cognitive impairment (Perez et al, 1975). Patients with vascular dementia seem also to preserve insight more frequently than those with Alzheimer's disease and, if the left frontal area is compromised, they may also present with affective disorder (Robinson et al, 1984). Strokes affecting the dominant hemisphere are more likely to cause dementia (Ladurner et al, 1982). Vertebrobasilar syndromes cause dementia less often than supratentorial ones (Donnan et al, 1978).

Dementia can be caused by pathological involvement of both large and small vessels (Brust, 1983). Infarction caused by embolism of large vessels gives rise to the classical syndromes and often involves cortical areas (Kohlmeyer, 1979). Pathology of small (penetrating) vessels also gives rise to dementia but with a predominant involvement of subcortical structures.

Binswanger's disease

Binswanger described, at the end of the 19th century, a form of white-matter disorder associated with dementia that since then has also been called 'état lacunaire' or 'subcortical arteriosclerotic encephalopathy' (Olszewski, 1962; Tomonaga et al, 1982). It is believed that this state results from pathology of the penetrating basal arteries. The resulting cognitive impairment is sui generis in that it does not show any involvement of cortical functions.

The patient with Binswanger's disease has usually suffered from persistent hypertension and systemic vascular disease (Burger et al, 1976). Its clinical evolution is punctuated by acute strokes, and the symptomatology includes long plateau periods, lengthy clinical course, motor signs, spasticity, seizures, signs of pseudobulbar palsy, hydrocephalus and dementia (Caplan & Schoen, 1978). A diffuse demyelinization of white matter can be demonstrated by CAT scan (Rosenberg et al, 1979; Janota, 1981; Loizou et al, 1981; Zeumer et al, 1980).

The dementia itself is characterized by inertia, lethargy and apathy and, during the earlier states of the condition, by episodes of ebullient behaviour and disinhibition. Memory impairment, hallmark of the dementias, is not invariably present, although when thalamic involvement occurs it is not uncommon for these patients to exhibit a degree of amnesia.

The picture is therefore one of absence of cortical syndromes (e.g. aphasia, apraxia or agnosia) and of marked psychosocial incompetence. Since the pathological changes underlying the condition may on occasions cause a marked reduction in neurophysiological arousal (probably related to a hypodopaminergic state), amphetamines or levodopa, together with rehabilitation, may be of some benefit.

SUBCORTICAL DEMENTIA

Psychosocial incompetence in the elderly is a common cause of psychiatric referral. This molar category refers to a general inability to sustain adequate commerce with the environment; it usually combines a failure to monitor social behaviour and psychomotor routines.

Common causes of psychosocial incompetence include disorientation, amnesia, aphasia, apraxia, social phobias and physical disability. Occasionally, however, incompetence can be observed in patients whose cortical functions and motor behaviour are remarkably unimpaired.

Subjects suffering from Parkinson's disease, progressive supranuclear palsy, Huntington's chorea, thalamic vascular damage, Binswanger's disease, Wilson's disease, normal pressure hydrocephalus, the late effects of carbon monoxide intoxication and other rarer conditions affecting subcortical structures, may exhibit marked psychosocial incompetence similar or worse, on superficial observation, to that seen in Alzheimer's Disease.

On closer examination, however, these patients do not as a rule have aphasia, apraxia or gnostic defect, and exhibit only a minor degree of memory impairment, insufficient as a rule to explain the marked degree of accompanying psychosocial incompetence.

In the early 1970s the term 'subcortical dementia' began to be used to refer to this special form of cognitive impairment (Albert et al, 1974). Patients thus affected were said to show lethargy, reduced arousal, frontal lobe apathy, inability to plan and organize behavioural routines, and general motor slowness. They also showed forgetfulness (rather than memory impairment) and, most importantly, little or no involvement of cortical functions.

There is some controversy concerning the validity and clinical usefulness of this diagnosis (Mayeux et al, 1983; Benson, 1983; Albert, 1978). As with pseudodementia, the term has been criticized on semantic grounds and considered to result from unrigorous clinical thinking. Both categories, however, draw the clinician's attention to problem areas. Subcortical dementia is not a neurophysiological or neuropathological diagnosis (nor is it meant to be). It is a clinical shorthand for states of marked degree of psychosocial incompetence not due to cortical dysfunction in which a reduction in motility and in drive can be observed.

It is of course likely that a number of dementia states diagnosed as 'subcortical' may, on closer examination, prove to have cortical involvement. It is also likely that subcortical dementia is no more than a cross-sectional diagnosis; indeed there is not much evidence that it has longitudinal validity, and subjects with rather typical subcortical symptoms (e.g. Parkinson's disease) may, in the fullness of time, show classical cortical changes (both clinically and neuropathologically) (Mayeux et al, 1983). The clinical converse also obtains, namely Alzheimer's disease may occasionally make its début with a 'subcortical' syndrome.

Clinical aspects

Albert et al (1974) used the term 'subcortical dementia' to refer to four symptoms observed in patients with progressive supranuclear palsy (PSP): forgetfulness, slowing of thought process, emotional or personality changes (apathy or depression with occasional outbursts of irritability) and impaired ability to manipulate knowledge. They reported five cases and reviewed about 45 from the literature. Albert (1978) has also suggested that subtypes of subcortical dementia can be identified and that they may be related to impairment of specific neurochemical pathways. Recent studies of PSP do not seem to consider subcortical dementia as an important feature of the condition (Kristensen, 1985; Jackson et al, 1983).

Mayeux et al (1983) studied 123 consecutive patients, of whom 46 had Alzheimer's disease, 20 Huntington's chorea and 57 Parkinson's disease. The three groups were unmatchable with regards to age, functional impairment and duration of illness, and the authors categorized them in terms of their degree of psychosocial incompetence. Neuropsychological assessement identified no difference in the pattern of cognitive impairment among the three groups. The authors concluded that the term subcortical dementia does not seem to identify a particular defect and that intellectual dysfunction in the three groups was probably due to a combination of cortical and subcortical degeneration. There is little doubt that cortical and subcortical dementias can be found in combination, but their predominance will vary according to the disease (e.g. Alzheimer's or Parkinson's disease). Neuropathological differences can also be found; thus there seems to be more involvement of the nucleus basalis of Meynert in Alzheimer's disease than there is in PSP (Rogers et al, 1985).

Associated pathological states are the limbic dementias (Brun & Gustafson, 1978; Gascon & Gilles, 1973), thalamic dementias (Kompf et al, 1984; Segarra et al, 1974) and diencephalic dementias (McEntee et al, 1976).

Benson (1983) has suggested that the distinction cortical-subcortical may have some therapeutic relevance, as states of subcortical dementia occasionally respond to dopamine agonists and levodopa.

Neuropsychological issues

Confusion arises from the limited knowledge available concerning the cognitive and arousal-related functions of the frontal lobes and the basal ganglia. Most of the information on the role of the frontal lobes comes from studies in patients with massive anatomical damage. For example the so-called 'frontal lobe' syndrome relates to extreme forms of anatomical amputation (e.g. subjects with bullet wounds, old leucotomies or strokes).

If it is to be accepted that the frontal lobe plays a 'supervisory' role in relation to the functional architecture of the brain, then even minor degrees of dysfunction may cause subtle forms of behavioural noise. It follows from this that identification of frontal lobe dysfunction may well depend upon the sensitivity of the clinical tests.

The pathological states related to subcortical dementia, however, are known not to cause major lesions of the frontal lobe, but they may compromise mesocortical (dopaminergic) tracts. It is possible therefore that the subtle inability to plan and organize behaviour so characteristic of patients with subcortical dementia may result from minor involvement of the frontal lobes.

Views on the cognitive function of the basal ganglia are equally controversial. Neurologists, in general, tend to consider these structures as sustaining only motor behavior; the only cognitive role they may concede relates to the construction and execution of motor plans (Marsden, 1982). As opposed to this, psychiatrists and neuropsychologists, involved clinically in the care of schizophrenic patients and of patients who have sustained damage to the basal ganglia (and exhibit behavioural syndromes) feel more inclined to accept that the basal ganglia have a cognitive function.

Cumming and Benson (1984), commenting upon related issues, conclude that the type of neurochological deficits described following lesions of subcortical structures seems to indicate that they have a role in arousal, attention, mood, motivation, memory, abstraction and visuospatial skills. Hence there seems to be a point in retaining the concept of subcortical dementia as a separate syndrome until harder information becomes available.

REFERENCES

Adam R D, Fisher C M, Hakim S, Ojemann R G, Sweet W H 1965 Symptomatic occult hydrocephalus with 'normal' cerebrospinal fluid. New England Journal of Medicine 273: 117–26
Albert M 1978 Subcortical dementia. In: Katzman R, Terry R D, Bick K L (eds) Alzheimer's disease: senile dementia and related disorders. Raven Press, New York, p 173
Albert M L, Feldman R G, Willis A L 1974 The 'subcortical dementia' of progressive supranuclear palsy. Journal of Neurology, Neurosurgery and Psychiatry 37: 121–30
Alexander-Williams J, Betts T A, Pidd S 1977 Psychiatric disturbances and the effects of gastric operations. Clinical Gastroenterology 6: 694–99
Allen R M 1982 Pseudodementia and ECT. Biological Psychiatry 17: 1435–43
Allison R S 1962 The senile brain: a clinical study. Edward Arnold, London
Alfrey A C, LeGendre G R, Kaehny W D 1976 The dialysis encephalopathy syndrome. Possible aluminum intoxication. New England Journal of Medicine 294: 184–88.
Angelergues R, Hecaen H, de Ajuriaguerra J 1955 Les troubles mentaux au cours des tumeurs du lobe frontal. Annales Médico-Psychologiques 113: 577–642
Annegers J F, Schoenberg B S, Okazaki H 1981 Epidemiological study of primary intracranial neoplasms. Archives of Neurology 38: 217–19
Appell J, Kertesz A, Fisman M 1982 A study of language functioning in Alzheimer's patients. Brain and Language 17: 73–91
Arregui A, Perry E K, Rossor M, Tomlinson B E 1982 Angiotensin converting enzyme in Alzheimer's disease: increased activity in caudate nucleus and cortical areas. Journal of Neurochemistry 38: 1490–92
Avary T L 1971 Seven cases of frontal tumour with psychiatric presentation. British Journal of Psychiatry 119: 19–23
Ball M J 1976 Neurofibrillary tangles in the dementia of 'normal pressure' hydrocephalus. Canadian Journal of Neurological Sciences 3: 227–35
Ball M J 1982 Limbic predilection in Alzheimer's dementia: is reactivated herpes virus involved? Canadian Journal of Neurological Sciences 9: 303–305
Ballinger B R, Reid A H, Heather B B 1982 Cluster analysis of symptoms in elderly demented patients. British Journal of Psychiatry 140: 257–62
Barclay L, Zemcov A, Blass J P, McDowell F 1984 Rates of decrease of cerebral blood flow in progressive dementia. Neurology 34: 1555–60

Barker M G, Lawson J S 1968 Nominal aphasia in dementias. British Journal of Psychiatry
114: 1351–56
Becker H D, Caspary W K 1980 Postgastrectomy and postvagotomy syndromes. Springer,
Berlin
Benson D F 1983 Subcortical dementia: a clinical approach. In: Mayeux R, Rosen W G
(eds) The dementias. Raven Press, New York, p 185
Benson D F, Cummings J L 1982 Angular gyrus syndrome simulating Alzheimer's disease.
Archives of Neurology 39: 616–20
Berg L, Danzinger W L, Storandt M, Coben L A, Gado M, Hughes C P, Knesevich J W,
Botwinick J 1984, Predictive features in mild senile dementia of the Alzheimer type.
Neurology 34: 563–9.
Berrios G E 1981 Delirium and confusion in the 19th century: a conceptual history. British
Journal of Psychiatry 139: 439–49
Berrios G E 1982 Disorientation states and psychiatry. Comprehensive Psychiatry
23: 479–90
Berrios G E 1984 Descriptive psychopathology: conceptual and historical aspects.
Psychological Medicine 14: 303–13.
Berrios G E 1985 'Depressive pseudodementia' or 'melancholic dementia': a 19th century
view. Journal of Neurology, Neurosurgery and Psychiatry 48: 393–400
Berrios G E 1986 Presbyophrenia: the rise and fall of a concept. Psychological medicine
16: 267–276
Berrios G E 1985b Presbyophrenia: clinical aspects. British Journal of Psychiatry
147: 76–79
Berrios G E 1986 Dementia: a conceptual history. Archives of Neurology (in press)
Berrios G E, Brooks P 1984 Visual hallucinations and sensory delusions in the elderly.
British Journal of Psychiatry 144: 662–64
Berrios G E, Brook P 1985 Delusions and the psychopathology of the elderly with cognitive
failure. Acta Psychiatrica Scandinavica 72: 296–301
Blackwood W, Hallpike J F, Kocen R S, Mair W G P 1969 Atheromatous disease of the
carotid arterial system and embolism from the heart in cerebral infarction: a morbid
anatomical study. Brain 92: 897–910
Bondareff W 1983 Age and Alzheimer's disease. Lancet 1: 1447
Botez I I, Bertrand G, Leveille J, Marchand L 1977 Parkinsonism, dementia complex,
hydrocephalus and Paget's disease. Canadian Journal of Neurological Sciences 4: 139–42
Botez M L, Reynolds E H 1979 Folic acid in neurology, psychiatry and internal medicine.
Raven Press, New York
Branconnier R J, DeVitt D R 1983 Early detection of incipient Alzheimer's disease: some
methodological considerations on computerized diagnosis. In: Reisberg B (ed) Alzheimer's
disease. Free Press, London, ch 29, p 214
Brocklehurst G 1982 Subdural haematoma. British Journal of Hospital Medicine 27: 170–4
Brown P, Cathala F, Sadowsky D, Gajdusek D C 1979 Creutzfeldt-Jakob disease in
France: II. Clinical characteristics of 124 consecutive verified cases during the decade
1968–1977. Annals of Neurology 6: 430–37
Brown P, Cathala F, Gajdusek C 1979 Creutzfeldt-Jakob disease in France: III.
Epidemiological study of 170 patients dying during the decade 1968–1977. Annals of
Neurology 6: 438–46
Brown P, Rodgers-Johnson P, Cathala F, Gibb C J, Gajdusek C 1984 Creutzfeldt-Jakob
disease of long duration: clinicopathological characteristics, transmissibility and
differential diagnosis. Annals of Neurology 16: 295–304
Bruce M E 1984 Scrapie and Alzheimer's disease. Psychological medicine 14: 497–500
Brun A, Gustafson L 1978 Limbic lobe involvement in presenile dementia. Archiv für
Psychiatrie und Nervenkrankheiten 266: 79–93
Brust J C M 1983 Dementia and cerebrovascular disease. In: Mayeux R, Rosen W G (eds)
The dementias. Raven Press, New York, p 131
Bucht G, Adolfsson R, Winblad B 1984 Dementia of the Alzheimer type and multiinfarct
dementia. Journal of the American Geriatrics Society 32: 491–98
Bulbena A, Berrios G E 1986 Pseudodementia: facts and figures. British Journal of
Psychiatry 148: 87–94
Burger P C, Burch J G, Kinze U 1976 Subcortical arteriosclerotic encephalopathy
(Binswanger's disease). Stroke 7: 626–31

Caine E D 1981 Pseudodementia. Current concepts and future directions. Archives of General Psychiatry 38: 1359–64

Cairncross J G, Kim J H, Posner J B 1980 Radiation therapy for brain metastases. Annals of Neurology 7: 529–41

Cairncross J G, Posner J B 1974 Brain tumors in the elderly. In: Albert M L (ed) Clinical neurology of aging. Oxford University Press, New York, ch 24, p 445

Caltagirone C, Gainotti G, Masullo C, Villa G 1982 Neurophysiological study of normal pressure hydrocephalus. Acta Psychiatrica Scandinavica 65: 93–100

Cameron M M 1978 Chronic subdural haematoma: a review of 114 cases. Journal of Neurology, Neurosurgery and Psychiatry 41: 834–9

Caplan L R, Schoene W C 1978 Clinical features of subcortical arteriosclerotic encephalopathy (Binswanger's disease). Neurology 28: 1206–15

Carney M W P 1967 Serum folate values in 423 psychiatric patients. British Medical Journal 2: 512–16

Carney M W P Sheffield B F 1978 Serum folic acid and B_{12} in 272 psychiatric in-patients. Psychological Medicine 8: 139–44

Caron M 1984 Étude clinique de la maladie de Pick. Vigot, Paris, p 237

Cathala F, Chatelain J, Brown P, Dumas M, Gajdusek D C 1980 Familial Creutzfeldt-Jakob disease. Journal of Neurological Science 47: 343–51

Catterall R D 1977 Neurosyphilis. British Journal of Hospital Medicine 17: 585–604

Chiofalo N, Fuentes A, Galvez S 1980 Serial EEG findings in 27 cases of Creutzfeldt-Jakob disease. Archives of Neurology 37:143

Chokroverty S, Bruetman M E, Berger V, Reyes M G 1976 Progressive dialytic encephalopathy. Journal of Neurology, Neurosurgery and Psychiatry 39: 411–19

Chou S M, Payne W N, Gibbs C J, Gajdusek C 1980 Transmission and scanning electron microscopy of spongiform change in Creutzfelt-Jakob disease. Brain 103: 885–904

Cole M, Wright D, Banker D 1979 Familial aphasia, In: Duvoisin R C (ed) Transactions of the American Neurological Association, Vol 104. Springer, New York, p 811

Cook R H, Austin J H 1978 Precautions in familial transmissible dementia. Archives of Neurology 35: 697–698

Constantinidis J, Richard J, de Ajuriaguerra J 1978 Dementias with senile plaques and neurofibrillary tangles. In: Isaacs A D, Post F (eds) Studies in geriatric psychiatry. Wiley, New York, ch 6, p 119

Corsellis J A N 1979 On the transmission of dementia. A personal view of the slow virus problem. British Journal of Psychiatry 134: 553–59

Corsellis J A N 1982 Plaques, tangles and Alzheimer's disease. Psychological Medicine 12: 449–59

Corsellis J A N 1982, Goldberg G J, Norton A R 1968 'Limbic encephalitis' and its association with carcinoma. Brain 81: 481–96

Corsellis J A N, Bruton C J, Freeman Brown D 1973 The aftermath of boxing, Psychological Medicine 3: 270–303

Crapper D R, Dalton A J, Skopitz M, Scott J W, Hachinski V C 1975 Alzheimer degeneration in Down's syndrome. Archives of Neurology 32: 618–23

Creutzfeldt H G 1920 Über eine eigenartige herdformige Erkrankung des Zentralnervensystems. Zeitschrift für die gesamte Neurologie und Psychiatrie 57: 1–18

Critchley M 1957 Medical aspects of boxing, particularly from a neurological standpoint. British Medical Journal 1: 357–62

Crown S 1949 Notes on an experimental study of intellectual deterioration. British Medical Journal 2: 684–5

Crystal H A, Davies P 1982 Cortical substance P-like immunoreactivity in cases of Alzheimer's disease and senile dementia of the Alzheimer type. Journal of Neurochemistry 38: 1781–84

Cullen W 1827 The works of William Cullen, Vol I, Blackwood, Edinburgh

Cummings J L, Benson F D 1984 Subcortical dementia. Review of an emerging concept. Archives of Neurology 41: 874–79

Damasio A R, Van Hoesen G W 1985 The limbic system and the localization of herpes simplex encephalitis. Journal of Neurology, Neurosurgery and Psychiatry 48: 297–301

David, Hecaen, Fouquet 1943 Démence, distension ventriculaire, disparition progressive des troubles mentaux après ouverture de la lame suroptique. Annales Médico-Psychologiques 101: 435–38

Deutsch J A 1983 The cholinergic synapse and the site of memory, In: The physiological basis of memory. Academic Press, New York, ch 9, p 367

Dewhurst K 1969 The neuroshyphilitic psychoses today. British Journal of Psychiatry 115: 31–8

Donnan G A, Walsh K W, Bladin P F 1978 Memory disorder in vertebrobasilar disease. Proceeding of the Australian Association of Neurology 15: 215–20

Dowson J H 1982 Pharmacological treatment of chronic cognitive deficit: a review. Comprehensive Psychiatry 23: 85–98

Eisborg L, Hansen T, Rafaelsen O J 1979 Vitamin B_{12} concentration in psychiatric patients. Acta Psychiatrica Scandinavica 59: 145–52

Eisendorfer C, Cohen D 1980 Diagnostic criteria for primary neuronal degeneration of the Alzheimer type. Journal of Family Practice 2: 553–57

Emery O B, Emery P E 1983 Language in senile dementia of the Alzheimer type. The Psychiatric Journal of the University of Ottawa 8: 169–178

Enk C, Hougaard K, Hippe E 1980 Reversible dementia and neuropathy associated with folate deficiency 16 years after partial gastrectomy. Scandinavian Journal of Haematology 25: 63–66

Eslinger P J, Benton A L 1983 Visuoperceptual performances in aging and dementia: clinical and theoretical implications. Journal of Clinical Neuropsychology 5: 213–20

Evans D L, Edelsohn G A, Golden R N 1983 Organic psychosis without anemia or spinal cord symptoms in patients with vitamin B_{12} deficiency. American Journal of Psychiatry 140: 218–21

Feldman R G, Chandler K A, Levy L 1963 Familial Alzheimer's disease. Neurology 13: 811–24

Frank E, Tew J M 1982 Normal pressure hydrocephalus: Clinical symptoms, diagnosis, pathophysiology and treatment. Heart and Lung 11: 321–26

Fuld P A 1984 Test profile of cholinergic dysfunction and Alzheimer-type dementia. Journal of Clinical Neuropsychology 6: 380–92

Gajdusek C, Gibbs C J 1971 Transmission of two subacute spongiform encephalopathies of man (kuru and Creutzfeldt-Jakob disease) to New World monkeys. Nature 230: 588–91

Galvez S, Cartier L 1984 Computed tomography findings in 15 cases of Creutzfeldt-Jakob disease with histological verification. Journal of Neurology, Neurosurgery and Psychiatry 47: 1244–46

Garcia C A, Tweedy J R, Blass J P 1984 Underdiagnosis of cognitive impairment in a rehabilitation setting. Journal of the American Geriatrics Society 32: 339–42

Garey P J, Goodwin J S, Hunt W C 1984 Folate and vitamin B_{12} status in a healthy elderly population. Journal of the American Geriatrics Society 32: 719–26

Gascon G G, Gilles F 1973 Limbic dementia. Journal of Neurology, Neurosurgery and Psychiatry 36: 421–30

Gibbs C J, Gajdusek C 1978 Subacute spongiform virus encephalopathies: the transmissible virus dementias. In: Katzman R, Terry R D, Bick K L (eds) Alzheimer's disease: senile dementia and related disorders (Aging, Vol 7), Raven Press. New York, p 559

Glaser G H, Pincus J H 1969 Limbic encephalitis. Journal of Nervous and Mental Disease 149: 59–67

Goldstein K, Katz S E 1937 The psychopathology of Pick's disease. Archives of Neurology and Psychiatry 38:473

Goudsmit J, Morrow C H, Asher D M, Yanagihara R T Masters C L, Gibbs C J, Gajdusek D C 1980 Evidence for and against the transmissibility of Alzheimer's disease. Neurology 30: 945–50

Greenwald B S, Edasery J, Mohs R C, Shah N, Trigos G G, Davis K L 1985 Red blood choline I: choline in Alzheimer's disease. Biological Psychiatry 20: 367–74

Grunhaus L, Dilsaver S, Greden J F, Carroll, B J 1983 Depressive pseudodementia: a suggested diagnostic profile. Biological Psychiatry 18: 215–25

Gustafson L, Nilsson L 1982 Differential diagnosis of presenile dementia on clinical grounds. Acta Psychiatrica Scandinavica 65: 194–209

Hachinski V C, Lassen N A, Marshall J 1974 Multi-infarct dementia. A cause of mental deterioration in the elderly. Lancet ii, 207–9

Hadlow W J 1959 Scrapie and kuru. Lancet ii, 289–90

Hatazama J, Yamaguchi T, Masatoshi I, Yanaoura H, Matsuzawa T 1984 Association of hypertension with increased atrophy of brain matter in the elderly. Journal of the American Geriatrics Society 32: 370–74

Henderson A S, Huppert F 1984 The problem of mild dementia. Psychological Medicine 14: 5–11

Hershey L A, Whicker L, Abel L A, Dell'Osso L F, Traccis S, Grossniklaus D 1983 Saccadic latency measurements in dementia. Archives of Neurology 40: 592–3

Heston L L, Mastri A R 1977 The genetics of Alzheimer's disease. Archives of General Psychiatry 34: 976–81

Heyman A, wilkinson W E, Sttaford J A, Helms M J, Sigmon A H, Weinberg T 1984 Alzheimer's disease: a study of epidemiological aspects. Annals of Neurology 15: 335–41

Howell D A 1979 Clinical and pathological consequences of lumps and swellings inside the cranium. British Journal of Hospital Medicine 21: 60–66

Hutton J T 1981 Results of clinical assessment for the dementia syndrome: implications for epidemiological studies. In: Mortimer J A, Schuman L M (eds) The epidemiology of dementia. Oxford University Press, New York, ch 3, p 62

Ingvar D H, Lassen N A 1979 Activity distribution in the cerebral cortex in organic dementia as revealed by measurements of regional cerebral blood flow. In: Hoffmeister F, Muller C (eds) Brain function in old age, Bayer Symposium VII, Springer, Berlin, p 268

Jackson J A, Jankovic J, Ford J 1983 Progressive supranuclear palsy: clinical features and response to treatment in 16 patients. Annals of Neurology 13: 273–78

Jacobs L, Kinkel W 1976 Computerized axial transverse tomography in normal pressure hydrocephalus. Neurology 26: 501–507

Jacobson P L, Farmer T W 1979 The 'hypernormal' CT scan in dementia: bilateral isodense subdural hematomas. Neurology 29: 1522–24

Janota I 1981 Dementia, deep white matter damage and hypertension: 'Binswanger's disease'. Psychological Medicine 11: 39–48

Jonowksy D S, Risch S C, Gillin J C 1983 Adrenergic–cholinergic balance and the treatment of affective disorder. Progress in Neuropsychopharmacology and Biological Psychiatry 7: 297–305

Jarvik L F 1982 Research on dementia. The philothermal response. Psychiatric Clinics of North America 5: 87–88

Jenkyn L R, Walsh D B, Walsh B T, Culver C M, Reeves A G 1975 The nuchocephalic reflex. Journal of Neurology, Neurosurgery and Psychiatry 38: 561–66

Jonsson C O, Waldton S, Malhammar G 1972 The psychiatric symptomatology in senile dementia assessed by means of an interview. Acta Psychiatrica Scandinavica 55: 103–121

Kaplan H A, Browder J 1954 Observations on the clinical and brain wave patterns of professional boxers. Journal of the American Medical Association 156: 1138–44

Kasznik A W, Fox J, Gandell D L 1981 Predictors of mortality in presenile and senile dementia. Annals of Neurology 3: 246–52

Kertesz A 1979 Aphasia and associated disorders. Taxonomy, localization and recovery. Grune & Stratton, New York

Kiloh L G 1961 Pseudodementia. Acta Psychiatrica Scandinavica 37: 336–51

Kim R C, Collins G H, Parisi J E 1981 Familial dementia of adult onset with pathological findings of a nonspecific nature. Brain 104: 61–78

Kirshner H S, Webb W G, Kelly M P, Wells C E 1984 Language disturbance. An initial symptom of cortical degeneration and dementia. Archives of Neurology 41: 49–96

Kirstein L S, Smith H 1981 Cognitive slowing in primary depression. Journal of Psychiatric Treatment and Evaluation 3: 147–50

Kohlmeyer K 1979 Disorders of brain functions due to stroke. Correlates in regional cerebral blood flow and in computerized tomography. In: Hoffmeister F, Muller C (eds) Brain Function in old age, Bayer Symposium VII. Springer, Berlin, p. 242

Kompf D, Oppermann J, Konig F, Talmon-Gross S, Babaian E 1984 Vertikale Blickparese und thalamische Demenz Nervenarzt 55: 625–36

Kosaka K, Matsushita M, Ilzuka R, Mehraein P 1982 Pick's disease and head trauma. Folia Psychiatrica et Neurologica Japonica 36: 125–35

Koto A, Rosenberg G, Zingesser L H, Horoupian D, Katzman R 1977 Syndrome of normal pressure hydrocephalus: possible relation to hypertensive and arteriosclerotic vasculopathy. Journal of Neurology, Neurosurgery and Psychiatry 40: 73–79

Kral V A 1959 Types of memory dysfunction in senescence. Psychiatric Research Reports 11: 30–34

Kral V A 1978 Benign senescent forgetfulness. In: Katzman R, Terry R D, Bick K L
    (eds) Alzheimer's disease: senile dementia and related disorders. Raven Press, New York
Kramer B A 1982 Depressive pseudodementia. Comprehensive Psychiatry 23: 538–44
Kramer M, German P S, Anthony J C, Von Korff M, Skinner E A 1985 Patterns of mental
    disorder among the elderly residents of eastern Baltimore. Journal of the American
    Geriatrics Association 33: 236–45
Kristensen M O 1985 Progressive supranuclear palsy. Acta Neurologica Scandinavica
    71: 177–189
Ladurner G, Iliff L D, Lechner H 1982 Clinical factors associated with dementia in
    ischaemic stroke. Journal of Neurology, Neurosurgery and Psychiatry 45: 97–101
La Rue A, Jarvik L 1980 Reflexions on biological changes in the psychological performance
    of the aged. Age 3: 29–35
Lal S, Wood P L, Kiely M E, Etienne P, Gauthier S, Stratford J, Ford R M, Dastoor D,
    Nair N P V 1984 CSF acetylcholinesterase in dementia and in sequential samples of
    lumber CSF. Neurobiology of Aging 5: 269–74
Lawson J S, Barker M G 1968 The assessment of nominal aphasia in dementia: the use of
    reaction-time measures. British Journal of Medical Psychology 41: 411–414
Lilly R, Cummings J L, Benson D J, Frankel M 1983 The human Klüver-Bucy syndrome.
    Neurology 33: 1141–5
Lindebaum J 1980 Malabsorption of vitamin B_{12} and folate. Current Concepts in Nutrition
    9: 105–23
Liston E H 1977 Occult presenile dementia. Journal of Nervous and Mental Disease
    164: 263–67
Liston E H 1979 The clinical phenomenology of presenile dementia. Journal of Nervous
    and Mental Disease 167: 329–36
Loeb C 1980 Clinical diagnosis of multiinfarct dementia. In: Amaducci L (ed) Aging of the
    brain (Aging Vol 13). Raven Press, New York, p 251
Loewenstein R J, Weingartner H, Gillin Ch, Kaye W, Eberts M, Mendelson W B 1982
    Disturbances of sleep and cognitive functioning in patients with dementia. Neurobiology
    of Aging 3: 371–77
Loizou L A, Kendall B E, Marshall J 1981 Subcortical arterosclerotic encephalopthy: a
    clinical and radiological investigation. Journal of Neurology, Neurosurgery and Psychiatry
    44: 294–304
Mahendra B 1983 'Pseudodementia',a misleading and illogical concept. British Journal of
    Psychiatry 143:202
Marsden C D 1982 The mysterious motor function of the basal ganglia. Neurology
    32: 514–39
Marsden C D, Harrison M J G 1972 Outcome of investigation of patients with presenile
    dementia. British Medical Journal 2: 249–52
Martland H S 1928 Punch — drunk syndrome. Journal of the American Medical
    Association 91: 1103–1107
Marie A 1906 La démence. Doin, Paris
Mayeux R, Stern Y, Rosen J, Benson D F 1983 Is subcortical dementia a recognizable
    clinical entity? Annals of Neurology 14: 278–283
Mayeux R, Stern Y, Spanton S 1985 Heterogeneity in dementia of the Alzheimer type:
    evidence of subgroups. Neurology 35: 453–61
McAllister T W 1983 Overview: pseudodementia. American Journal of Psychiatry
    140: 528–33
McCown I A 1959 Protecting the boxer. Journal of the American Medical Asociation
    169: 1409–1413
McDonald C 1969 Clinical heterogeneity in senile dementia. British Journal of Psychiatry
    115: 267–71
McEntee W J, Biber M P, Perl D P, Benson D F 1976 Diencephalic amnesia. Journal of
    Neurology, Neurosurgery and Psychiatry 39: 436–41
McEvory A W, Fenwick J D, Boddy K, James O F W 1982 Vitamin B_{12} absorption
    from the gut does not decline with age in normal elderly humans. Age and Ageing
    11: 180–3
McMenemey W H 1970 Alois Alzheimer and his disease. In: Wolstenholme G E W,
    O'Connor M (eds) Alzheimer's disease and related conditions (Ciba Foundation
    Symposium). Churchill Livingstone, Edinburgh, p 5

Melzer V, Vernea J 1959 Aspects psychopathologiques des gastrectomises carencés. Annales Médico-Psychologiques 117: 80–88

Messert B, Wannamaker B B 1974 Reappraisal of the adult occult hydrocephalus syndrome. Neurology 24: 224–31

Miller E 1977 Abnormal aging, Wiley, New York

Miller W R 1975 Psychological deficits in depression. Psychological Bulletin 82: 238–60

Mindus P, Cronholm B, Levander S E, Schalling D 1976 Piracetam-induced improvement of mental performance. A controlled study on normally aging individuals. Acta Psychiatrica Scandinavica 54: 150–60

Morris J C, Cole M, Banker B Q, Wright D 1984 Hereditary dysphasic dementia and the Pick–Alzheimer spectrum. Annals of Neurology 16: 455–66

Mulder D W, Swenson W M 1974 Psychologic and psychiatric aspects of brain tumours. In: Vinken P, Bruyn G W (eds) tumours of the brain and skull. Handbook of clinical neurology, Vol 16. North Holland, Amsterdam, ch 19, p 727

Muñoz Garcia D, Ludwin S K 1984 Classic and generalized variants of Pick's disease: a clinicopathological, ultrastructural and immunocytochemical comparative study. Annals of Neurology 16: 467–80

Nott P N, Fleminger J J 1975 Presenile dementia: the difficulties of early diagnosis. Acta Psychiatrica Scandinavica 51: 210–17

Obrist W D 1979 Cerebral circulatory changes in normal ageing and dementia. In: Hoffmeister F, Muller C (eds) Brain function in old age, Bayer Symposium VII. Springer, Berlin, p 278

O'Hare J A, Callaghan N M, Murnaghan D J 1983 Dialysis encephalopthy: clinical, electroencephalographic and interventional aspects. Medicine 62: 129–41

Olivarus B de F, Roder E 1970 Reversible psychosis and dementia of myxoedema. Acta Psychiatrica Scandinavica 46: 1–13

Olszewski J 1962 Subcortical arteriosclerotic encephalopathy. World Neurology 3: 359–75

Ord W M, Cavafy J, Durham A E, Godlee R J, Goodhart J F, Halliburton W D et al 1888 Report of a committee of the Society nominated to investigate the subject of myxoedema. Transaction of the Clinical Society of London 22: 4298–300

Patrick D, Gates P C 1984 Chronic subdural haematoma in the elderly. Age and Ageing 13: 367–69

Perez F I, Rivera V M, Meyer J S, Gay J R A, Taylor R L, Mathew N T 1975 Analysis of intellectual and cognitive performance in patients with multiinfarct dementia, vertebrobasilar insufficiency with dementia and Alzheimer's disease. Journal of Neurology, Neurosurgery and Psychiatry 38: 533–40

Pick A 1901 (Quoted in Caron, 1934) p 403

Pick A 1904 Zur Symptomatologie der linksseitigen Schlafenlappenatrophie. Monatschrift für Psychiatrie und Neurologie 16: 378–88

Pickard J D 1982 Adult communicating hydrocephalus. British Journal of Hospital Medicine 27: 35–44

Pirazzolo F J, Christensen K J, Ogle K M, Hansch E C, Thompson W G 1981 simple and choice reaction times in dementia: clinical implications. Neurobiology of Aging 2: 113–17

Plum F 1979 Dementia: an approaching epidemic. Nature 279: 372–73

Portenoy R K, Berger A, Gross E 1984 Familial occurrence of idiophatic normal pressure hydrocephalus. Archives of Neurology 41: 335–37

Raichle M E 1983 The pathophysiology of brain ischemia, Annals of Neurology 13: 2–10

Reed K, Bland R C 1977 Masked 'myxedema madness'. Acta Psychiatrica Scandinavica 56: 421–26

Reifler B V 1982 Arguments for abandoning the term pseudodementia. Journal of the American Geriatrics Society 30: 665–68

Reisberg B, Ferries S H, Gershon S 1981 An overview of pharmacological treatment of cognitive decline in the aged. American Journal of Psychiatry 138: 593–600

Reitan R M 1953 Intellectual function in myxoedema. Archives of Neurology and Psychiatry 69: 436–42

Risch S C, Cohen R M, Janowsky D S, Kalin N H, Sitaram N, Gillin J C, Murphy D L 1981 Physostigmine induction of depressive symptomatology in normal human subjects. Psychiatry Research 4: 89–94

Rivera-Vasquez A B, Noriega-Sanchez A, Ramirez-Gonzalez R, Marinez-Maldonado M

1980 Acute hypercalcaemia in haemodialysis patients: distinctions from dialysis dementia. Nephron 25: 243–46

Robinson R G, Kubos K L, Starr L B, Rao K, Price T R 1984 Mood disorder in stroke patients: importance of location of lesion. Brain 107: 81–93

Rogers J D, Brogan D, Morra S S 1985 The nucleus basalis of Meynert in neurological disease: a quantitative morphological study. Annals of Neurology 17: 163–70

Ron M A, Toone B K, Garralda M E, Lishmann W A 1979 Diagnostic accuracy in presenile dementia. British Journal of Pychiatry 134: 161–68

Rosenberg G A, Kornfeld M, Stovring J, Bicknell J M 1979 Subcortical arteriosclerotic encephalopathy (Binswanger): computerized tomography. Neurology 29: 1102–06

Roos D 1978 Neurological complications in patients with impaired vitamin B_{12} absorption following partial gastrectomy. Acta Neurologica Scandinavica (Suppl 69)59: 1–77

Roos D, Willanger R 1977 Various degrees of dementia in a selected group of gastrectomized patients with low serum B_{12}. Acta Neurologica Scandinavica 55: 363–76

Rossor M N, Emson P C, Mountjoy C Q, Roth M, Iversen L L 1982 Neurotransmitters of the cerebral cortex in senile dementia of Alzheimer type. Experimental Brain Research, Suppl 5 153–7

Rossor M N, Iversen L L, Reynolds G P, Mountjoy C Q, Roth M 1984 Neurochemical characteristics of early and late onset types of Alzheimer's disease. British Medical Journal 288: 961–64

Rudelli R, Strom J O, Welch P T, Ambler M W 1982 Posttraumatic premature Alzheimer's disease. Archives of Neurology 39: 570–75

Russell R W R, Pennybacker J B 1961 Craniopharyngioma in the elderly. Journal of Neurology, Neurosurgery and Psychiatry 24: 1–13

Salmon J H 1972 Adult hydrocephalus: evaluation of shunt therapy in 80 patients. Journal of Neurosurgery 37: 423–28

Samuelson S, Long D M, Cho S N 1972 Subdural haematoma as a complication of shunting procedures for normal pressure hydrocephalus Journal of Neurosurgery 37: 548–51

Sanders W L 1979 Creutzfeldt-Jakob disease treated with amantadine. Journal of Neurology, Neurosurgery and Psychiatry 42:960

Scheerenberger R C 1983 A history of mental retardation. Brookes, Baltimore

Scheiber S C, Ziesat H 1976 Clinical and psychological test findings in cerebral dyspraxia associated with haemodialysis. Journal of Nervous and Mental Disease 162-5

Scheiber S C, Ziesat H 1978 Dementia dialytica: a new psychotic organic syndrome. Comprehensive Psychiatry 17: 781–5

Schneck M K, Reisberg B, Ferris S H 1982 An overview of current concepts of Alzheimer's disease. American Journal of Psychiatry 139: 165–73

Schneider C 1927 Über Picksche Krankheit. Monatschrift für Psychiatrie und Neurologie 65:230

Schneider C 1929 Weitere Beitrage zur Lehre von der Pickschen Krankheit. Zeitschrift für die Gesamte Neurologie und Psychiatrie 120: 340–84

Schoenberg B S, Christine B W, Whisnant J P 1978 The resolution of discrepancies in the reported incidence of primary brain tumours. Neurology 28: 817–23

Schorah C J, Morgan D B 1985 Nutritional deficiencies in the elderly. May, 353–60

Scileppi K P, Blass J P, Baker H G 1984 Circulating vitamins in Alzheimer's dementia as compared with other dementias. Journal of the American Geriatrics Society 32: 709–11

Segarra J M, Von Stockert T R, Curtis M 1974 Thalamic dementias. In: Subirana A, Espader J M (eds) Neurology (Excerpta Medica) Amsterdam. (Proceedings of the X International Congress of Neurology, Barcelona, Spain) p 393

Selecki B R 1964 Cerebral mid-line tumours involving the corpus callosum among mental hospital patients. Medical Journal of Australia 2: 954–60

Semple S A, Smith C M, Swasch M 1982 The Alzheimer's disease syndrome. In: Corkin (ed) Alzheimer's disease: a report of progress. Raven Press, New York, p 93

Shah K V, Banks G T, Mersky H 1969 Survival in atherosclerotic and senile dementia. British Journal of Psychiatry 115: 1283–6

Sim M, Turner E, Smith W T 1966 Cerebral biopsy in the investigation of presenile dementia. 1. Clinical aspects. British Journal of Psychiatry 112: 119–25

Sjaastad O, Nornes H 1976 Increased intracranial pressure in so-called 'normal pressure hydrocephalus'. European Neurology 14: 161–77

Sjogren T, Sjogren H, Lindgren A G H 1952 Morbus Alzheimer and morbus Pick. A genetic, clinical and patho-anatomical study. Acta Psychiatrica et Neurologica Scandinavica, Suppl 82: 1–115

Snider W D, DeMaria A A, Mann J D 1979 Diazepam and dialysis encephalopathy. Neurology 29: 414–5

Sokolof L 1966 Cerebral circulatory and metabolic changes associated with ageing. Proceeding of Association for Research into Nervous and Mental Disease 41: 237–54

Sourander P, Sjogren H 1970 The concept of Alzheimer's disease and its clinical implications. In: Woltenholme G E W, O'Connor M (eds) Alzheimer's disease and related conditions, (A CIBA Foundation Symposium). Churchill Livingstone, Edinburgh, p 11

Spillane J D 1962 Five boxers. British Medical Journal 2: 1205–1210

Stein S C, Laggfitt T W 1974 Normal pressure hydrocephalus: predicting the results of CSF shunting. Journal of Neurosurgery 41: 463–70

Stengel E 1964 Psychopathology of dementia. Proceedings of the Royal Society of Medicine 57: 911–14

Strachan R W, Henderson J G 1965 Psychiatric syndromes due to avitaminosis B_{12} with normal blood and marrow. Quarterly Journal of Medicine 34: 303–17

Strole W E, Clark W H, Isselbacher K L 1967 Progressive arterial occlusive disease (Kohlmeier–Degos). New England Journal of Medicine 276: 195–201

Sulka R, Matti H, Paetan A, Wilkstrom J, Palo J 1983 Accuracy of clinical diagnosis in primary degenerative dementia: correlations with neurological findings. Journal of Neurology, Neurosurgery and psychiarty 46: 9–13

Swanson J W, Kelly J J, McConahey W M 1981 Neurological aspects of thyroid dysfunction. Mayo Clinic Proceedings 56: 504–12

Taclob L, Needle M 1976 Drug induced encephalopathy in patients on maintenance haemodialysis. Lancet ii, 704–5

Temey G 1976 Psychometrie et hydrocephalie normotensive. Bulletin de Psychologie 30: 468–76

Thomas D G T 1983 Brain tumours. British Journal of Hospital Medicine 25: 148–58

Todorov A V, Go R C P, Constantinidis J, Elston R C 1975 Specificity of the clinical diagnosis of dementia. Journal of Neurological Sciences 26: 81–98

Tomlinson B E, Blessed G, Roth M, 1970 Observations on the brains of demented old people. Journal of Neurological Science 11: 205–242

Tomonaga M, Yamanouichi H, Tohgi H, Kameyama M 1982 Clinicopathological study of progressive subcortical vascular encephalopthy (Binswanger type) in the elderly. Journal of the American Geriatrics Society 30: 524–9

Torvik A, Jorgensen L 1964 Thrombotic and embolic occlusions of the carotid arteries in an autopsy material. Part 1: Prevalence, location and associated disease. Journal of Neurological Science 1: 24–39

Traub R, Gajdusek C, Gibbs C J 1977 Transmissible virus dementia: the relation of transmissible spongiform encephalopathy to Creutzfeldt-Jakob disease. In: Kinsbourne M, Smith L (eds) Aging and dementia. Spectrum, New York, ch 5, p 91

Uhl G R, McKinney M, Hedreen J C 1982 Dementia pugilistica: loss of basal forebrain cholinergic neurons and cortical cholinergic markers (abstract). Annals of Neurology 12:99

Uhl G R, Hilt D C, Hedreen J C 1983 Pick's disease (lobar sclerosis): depletion of neurons in the nucleus basalis of Meynert. Neurology 33: 1470–73

Ulrich J 1985 Alzheimer changes in nondemented patients younger than sixty five, Annals of Neurology 17: 273–77

Valenciano L 1978 Paralisis general progresiva. Imprenta Provincial, Murcia, Spain

Van Mansvelt J 1954 Pick's disease, Leoff, Enschede

Waldton S 1974 Clinical observations of impaired cranial nerve function in senile dementia. Acta Psychiatrica Scandinavica 50: 539–547

Walton J N, Kiloh L G, Osselton J W 1954 The electroencephalogram in pernicious anaemia and subacute combined degeneration of the spinal cord. Electroencephalography and Clinical Neurophysiology 6: 45–64

Weissmann M M, Myers J K, Tischler G L, Holzer III C E, Leaf P J, Orvaschel H, Brody J A 1985 Psychiatric disorders (DSM III) and cognitive impairment among the elderly in a US urban community. Acta Psychiatrica Scandinavica 71: 366–79

Wells C E 1978 Role of stroke in dementia. Stroke 9: 1–3

Wells C E 1979 Pseudodementia. American Journal of Psychiatry 136: 895–900

Wertheimer J 1979 La démence sénile et son évolution. Revue Médicale Suisse Romande 94: 545–54

Winblad B, Adolfsson R, Carlsson A, Gottries C G 1982 Biogenic amines in brains of patients with Alzheimer's disease. In: Corkin S (ed) Alzheimer's disease: a report of progress (Aging, Vol 19), Raven Press, New York, p 25

Wing A J, Brunner F P, Brynger H, Chantler C, Donckerwolcke R A, Gurland H J, Jacobs C, Krammer P, Selwood N H 1980 Dialysis dementia in Europe. Lancet i, 190–92

Wischik C M, Crowther R A 1986 Subunit structure of the Alzheimer tangle. British Medical Bulletin 42: 51–56

Wolinsky J S, Barnes B D, Margolis M T 1973 Diagnostic tests in normal pressure hydrocephalus. Neurology 23: 706–13

Woods J H, Bartlet D, Joes A E, Udvarhelye G B 1974 Normal pressure hydrocephalus: diagnosis and patient selection for shunt surgery, Neurology 24:517

Wurtman R J 1985 Alzheimer's disease. Scientific American 252: 48–56

Yasargil M G, Yonekawa Y, Zumstein B, Stahl H L 1973 Hydrocephalus following spontaneous subarachnoid hemorrhage. Journal of Neurosurgery 39: 474–79

Yates C M, Simpson J, Maloney A F J, Gordon A 1980 Neurochemical observations in a case of Pick's disease. Journal of Neurological Science 48: 257–63

Yesavage J A, Tincklenberg J R, Hollister L E, Berger P A 1979 Vasodilator in senile dementias. Archives of General Psychiatry 36: 220–23

Zeumer H, Schonsky B, Sturm K W 1980 Predominant white matter involvement in subcortical arteriosclerotic encephalopathy. Journal of Computerized Axial Tomography 4: 14–19

Zucker D K, Livingston R L, Nakra R, Clayton P J 1981 B_{12} deficiency and psychiatric disorders: case report and literature review. Biological Psychiatry 16: 197–205

The diagnosis of dementia in old age

INTRODUCTION

In 1978 the author wrote, 'It is incontrovertible that for the elderly accurate diagnosis can be life-saving. The distinction between depressive illness and senile dementia may govern the decision between curative and palliative treatment'. Seven years later there would seem little reason to change that statement. Although the assessment of the mental state for research has undergone refinement with the introduction of computerized diagnostic systems, and knowledge of the chemical disorders of dementia has increased, longitudinal studies of the type required to validate clinical judgment have not been reported. Methods for the assessment of dementia are still based, to a large extent, on clinical impression and established usage. Their validity has not been proven. In our own studies we have accumulated data on some 2000 community subjects and several hundred more aged over 65 residing in different types of institutional care. Some results from our longitudinal studies are now becoming available. Aspects of this chapter will be based upon experience with these studies.

PROBLEMS IN THE DIAGNOSIS OF DEMENTIA

It should be realized at the beginning that many of the problems of diagnosing dementia have been exaggerated. This may have resulted from an inadequate examination of patients, especially those seen under difficult community conditions. There is, as in every other branch of medicine, no substitute for an adequate history and examination of the patient. Provided this is done, the diagnosis is abundantly clear in the majority of subjects. However, it must be noted that even when the emphasis of a study is on the diagnostic process and its refinement, spectacular errors can still be made clinically after a single examination.

Much is talked about the problem of distinguishing dementia from normal ageing and whether or not that distinction is aetiologically sensible. The majority view is that dementing conditions are disease entities, not on a continuum with normality. However, the pathological processes associated with dementia are certainly to be found in the brains of normal elderly people.

We have little idea what happens to the brain as human beings age. Studies examining the psychology of ageing have not always excluded cases of illness. In our studies, using crude measures of intellectual function on random samples of elderly interviewed in the community, we found no significant differences between two groups aged 65–74 and 75 and over, when those with mental illness were excluded. It would therefore seem unwise to assume too easily that abnormalities in the mental state of the elderly are due to normal ageing. Although most people are conscious of difficulties with memory as ageing occurs, such difficulties rarely cause problems with living or develop further without other clear evidence of disease. It is likely that in the normal elderly sudden changes of environment, stressful life events and physical illness may be associated with errors of memory and poor performance on cognitive testing, so that under these circumstances it may be difficult to obtain a true picture of the underlying mental state. On the whole, preconceptions of normal ageing should not be taken into consideration when assessing patients for dementia.

Errors in making the diagnosis of dementia, although probably not frequent, are of considerable importance, as the consequences for the patient, and relatives, could be considerable. In 1972 Marsden and Harrison reported that out of a total of 106 patients given a provisional diagnosis of presenile dementia at a major teaching hospital, 16 were later judged not to be demented. Similar findings were reported by Nott and Fleminger in 1975 who followed up 35 of 50 patients diagnosed as having presenile dementia, only to find that half of these appeared to have recovered from their dementia on re-examination. Bergmann in 1977, following up a group of elderly subjects described as having 'chronic brain failure', found approximately one-third had subsequently recovered. Ron et al in 1979, in a follow-up study of 51 patients with presenile dementia, found that in 16 the diagnosis had been inappropriate.

The above studies mainly concerned patients under the age of 65. However, Smith and Kiloh (1981) studying 200 patients diagnosed provisionally as dementing, found that 3.6% of a sub-sample of 55 aged over 65 years were suffering from functional illnesses or other organic brain syndromes, and that a further 3.8% had a treatable cause. In 1975 Copeland et al, confirmed that differences between the United States and United Kingdom national statistics for patients aged over 65 years, admitted to state and area mental hospitals, and diagnosed as having organic disorders, were due almost entirely to the excessive diagnosis of organic illness in the US hospitals. When these patients were re-examined three months later, many were found to have recovered, having followed a similar clinical course to those diagnosed as suffering from affective disorders. Ron et al, in their study, found that patients with apparent presenile dementia which failed to progress had been depressed at the time of the original assessment.

They were also more likely to have had a past history of depression than those patients who pursued a progressive downhill course. Our own interim follow-up of community samples of elderly persons with minor organic symptoms shows that most do not progress to dementia but tend to develop clear depressive illnesses some months later. These studies serve to underline the importance of keeping the diagnosis of dementia under constant review if there is uncertainty at the first examination.

The stages in the diagnosis of dementia will require the following distinctions to be made: (a) organic from functional conditions such as depression and schizophrenia, mainly by the relative severity of the symptoms of each condition, (b) chronic organic states from acute or subacute forms, usually on the time interval between onset and examination and the presence or absence of clouding of consciousness, (c) dementia from other chronic organic states, and (d) one type of dementia from another, by clinical course, physical examination and special investigations. However, it may not be possible to take the stages of diagnosis in this order.

THE CLINICAL EXAMINATION

The importance of an adequate history, mental state and physical examination cannot be overemphasized. In practice, the clinician will be undertaking the full assessment of the patient, of which diagnosis is only a small, if essential part.

History of the illness

The examination of the patient can take place in a variety of settings. That in the patient's own home is likely to yield the most information. It affords a ready appreciation of the patient's day-to-day living and the opportunity to observe the interaction between the patient and his or her relatives and neighbours. Relatives or neighbours are usually available to act as informants. An informant interview is a crucial part of the assessment because patients with cognitive disturbance cannot give an adequate history of their own illnesses. Where there is no informant so that the clinician must depend mainly on an examination of the mental state and such physical examination as may be possible, a full assessment will probably require hospital admission.

It is generally necessary to interview both the informant and the patient separately in order to avoid one helping or hindering the other. However, it is valuable also to see them together at some stage in order to observe their interaction. Gardner (1984) stresses the importance of the informant's interview and draws attention to a number of problems which may arise when interviewing at the patient's home. Not only do informants tend to answer mental state questions on behalf of the patient but, sometimes, in an effort to impress the doctor with the seriousness of the situation, they may deliberately attempt to muddle the patient.

The recent work of Herbst (1980) has drawn attention to the importance of deafness as a complication in the assessment of dementia. It is important to ensure that the patient is able to hear the questions before a failure to respond or seemingly irrelevant replies are assumed to be signs of organic illness.

It is not the intention in this chapter to give a detailed description of the history and examination of a psychiatric patient. An attempt will be made to highlight certain areas of importance and interest, particularly relevant to the elderly.

The length and type of onset will help to establish whether the illness is an acute or chronic organic state, or a functional psychiatric illness. Essentially, a change from normal behaviour is being sought. In the dementing, this change may progress quickly so that the patient not only mislays personal objects but also forgets major appointments and the names of close family and friends, leading eventually to disorientation in time and, later still, in space. In retrospect, it is possible to see that other more subtle changes have taken place such as blunting of emotions and narrowing of interests, a lack of warmth and response to affection.

A sudden onset of symptoms over several days will indicate enquiry about recent distressing life events, changes in medication and alcohol consumption, and the usual physical systems questions in order to exclude pneumonia, urinary infection and other common causes of delirium.

A gradual or insidious onset over several months with a smooth, inexorably deteriorating course will suggest a dementing process or a functional illness such as depression. A prolonged stepwise course, often with abrupt onset, with each step representing an acute worsening of the condition, followed by some variable amount of recovery, will suggest multi-infarct dementia. The sudden onset may be accompanied by paralysis, dysphasia, dyspraxia or other less obvious neurological signs. In the early stages of the illness, there may be almost complete return to normal behaviour before the next episode occurs. Later, residual deficits remain and the degree of improvement becomes less obvious. In the later stages, lucid periods and periods of confusion may occur during the daytime and should be inquired for, as should episodes of laughing or crying uncontrollably. Informants may give accounts of serious memory loss such as leaving the gas burning, forgetting to take the kettle off the boil, or wandering apparently aimlessly into the street or losing the way home. As always, people will tell more to the clinician who is prepared to listen.

In practice, multi-infarct dementia does not always show a stepwise deterioration, perhaps when the infarcts are small and multiple. The development of depression can sometimes show fluctuations in the severity of symptoms in response to adverse life events.

If the informant has known the patient for some years, it will be important to ask about a previous history not only of depression and schizophrenia but also of stroke, epileptic fits, diabetes mellitus, disorders of the thyroid, high blood pressure and any other severe physical illness. Particularly a history of arterial disease should be enquired for: angina pectoris, sudden blindness in one eye, myocardial infarction and intermittent claudication.

Unless the informant is a relative of the patient, it will be difficult to enquire about family history of mental illness or suicide, or other indicators of inherited functional illness. A relative may know about the subject's previous examination levels and scholastic ability. The opportunities for secondary education were limited at the turn of the century and, therefore, a failure to take examinations, or leaving school at the age of 14, was the rule rather than the exception. Nevertheless, the passing of examinations, attendance at a normal school, or holding a responsible job may indicate that the patient's mental state has recently deteriorate. Mental handicap may be mistaken for dementia.

Brain damage may sometimes be confused with dementia, and therefore a history of trauma to the head should be enquired for, so should a history of abusing alcohol, delirium tremens and other psychiatric complications of excessive alcohol intake. A proportion of dementias will have resulted from previous alcohol ingestion which has ceased to progress because alcohol is no longer being consumed. Rarer causes for progressive dementia, such as the punch drunk syndrome of boxers and Huntington's chorea with a family history, should be borne in mind, although they usually affect younger age groups.

MENTAL STATE

Only those points essential to the differential diagnosis of dementia will be discussed. It is the opinion of the author that the mental state should be undertaken in a formal standardized manner, and that in this respect it can be regarded as equivalent to the physical examination in general medicine. Of course, a physical examination is also important. Much of relevance to the mental state will have been obtained during the history-taking. Certainly, observing the patient when he or she is unaware of the examiner's purpose is most valuable. Although it is probably true that a skilled interviewer can ask anyone anything anywhere, those patients who have insight into their intellectual deterioration often find the examination of the cognitive areas particularly distressing. It is therefore helpful to start with simple enquiries of the kind that the patient expects a doctor to make. It is also important at this stage that the patient should be seen alone in order to avoid distraction and the interference of well-meaning informants.

The examiner should note the condition of the patient's house and rooms if the interview is taking place at the subject's home. Deterioration in paintwork and in the fabric of the dwelling will probably indicate that decline has been gradual. An untidy room with unwashed dishes, remnants of partially eaten meals, unmade beds, layers of dust and dirt, even the smell of incontinence and the presence of excreta in severe cases will all provide important clues to long-term deterioration. A home spotlessly kept by the patient would be powerful evidence against long-term decline.

A useful approach is to ask the patient to remember the doctor's name, pointing out that he or she will be asked to repeat it again in due course. This may be followed by questions such as, 'What year were you born? How old are you? Can you give me the exact address where you are living? and What is your telephone number?' Such questions are often sufficient to suggest the diagnosis and yet are not seen as threatening by the subject. The doctor should observe the patient's manner of speech, his or her ability to answer questions, the presence of perseveration and whether or not failing to answer questions or getting them wrong causes the patient anxiety. Some patients with insight into their illness may attempt to evade the questions or excuse themselves by such comments as, 'That sort of thing doesn't interest me any more'. It will then be appropriate to enquire if anything is worrying the patient. Allowing him or her to enlarge upon problems for some minutes gives the patient the impression that you are interested in what he or she has to say rather than merely applying tests. Severe cases of Alzheimer-type dementia often declare that they have no problems.

Emotions such as anxiety may now be enquired for. Patients with multi-infarct dementia are sometimes highly anxious, and this may present a problem with management. Following anxiety it is convenient to ask about depressive moods. Remember that at least one-third of elderly subjects with severe depression tend to deny feeling depressed, and a diagnosis must then be made on the presence of other important symptoms. Depression is not uncommonly associated with multi-infarct dementia and may represent a reaction to the knowledge of failing intellectual powers. Enquiry should be made about the frequency of crying, and particularly if the patient claims to be unable to cry whether or not they feel they would like to but cannot. The latter is often an important symptom of severe depression. Diurnal variation of mood should be enquired for, and a useful question is to ask how the patients views the future and how they expect it to work out for them. Elderly people do not have exciting plans for the future but tend to live from day to day. They are not usually pessimistic about the future unless they are suffering from depressive illness. Other symptoms which help to confirm the presence of depressive illness will be a recent loss of interest in usual activities, hobbies, housework and leisure activities, a loss of energy and a feeling of having enjoyed almost nothing in recent weeks. Usual questions on weight, appetite and sleep disturbance should be asked and help to disguise the psychiatric nature of the enquiry. If depressive mood is present, it will be essential to assess the degree of suicidal risk. Suicide is not uncommon in elderly subjects with depression, especially when associated with organic symptoms. Mood swings are also not uncommon in normal elderly people, and it is useful to ask whether the depressive mood lasts for longer than a few hours.

At this stage it is usually possible to enquire more about cognitive skills and memory. A large proportion of elderly people will complain about memory, but it rarely becomes a problem for them unless they are suffering from an added illness. It is often helpful to say, 'There are some questions I want to ask you. They may seem very simple to you, but we ask them of everybody. For example, can you tell me the day of the week today . . . the month . . . the year? Can you tell me the name of the Prime Minister? Who was his or her predecessor?' Although the use of the Prime Minister's name in an interview of this kind is often derided and its effectiveness as a test must, to some extent, depend upon the notoriety of the Prime Minister and the length of office, it still emerges consistently in studies as an important diagnostically discriminating question. Of course, like the month and the year, there are certain patients who will make accidental mistakes, but making two such mistakes is rare in normal persons. It may be helpful to enquire more about memory. In what way does this affect the elderly person? Do they tend to misplace objects, find difficulty in naming even close friends? Have they sometimes lost the way home or had difficulty doing activities which, up to recently, they had found simple and part of everyday life?

It will now be necessary to ask questions about spacial and personal orientation. Can the subject name the place he or she is in and the locality? Have they ever seen the doctor before and, in severe cases, can they name any close relatives or neighbours present? Simple arithmetical questions may be asked. Does the subject have difficulty calculating change when shopping? Sometimes the patient may be asked to say the weeks or the months of the year backwards. Certain patients with multi-infarct dementia have a patchy loss of cerebral function and may suffer from aphasia, agnosia or apraxia. Asking the subject to draw a cube or copy a simple design as used in the Mini-Mental State (Folstein et al, 1979) can be helpful. Such symptoms tend to occur before disorientation. The patient can be asked to name everyday objects such as a pencil, pen, button or coin, and say to what use they are generally put. It must be said that in the majority of cases, by the time the patient is brought to the attention of a doctor, often quite simple questions about age etc. are sufficient to make the intellectual changes clear. On a domiciliary visit it will rarely be necessary to assess intellectual function in detail. Such an examination can await admission or attendance at the hospital or day hospital.

It cannot be overemphasized that simple scores of intellectual deterioration such as those obtained by the Mini-Mental State and similar devices are no substitute for a full mental state examination. Such scores are often affected by other conditions such as acute organic states including drug overdosage and by significant levels of depression. They may be useful for assessing degrees of dementia once the diagnosis has been established by the usual methods.

If the intellectual deterioration seems to be slight compared with other complaints, then the examiner should not hesitate to enquire for possible delusions or hallucinations. Patients who have suffered from these for many years often learn to conceal them. They have sufficient insight to realize that those to whom they confess often laugh or dismiss their experiences out of hand. It may be necessary to start such enquiry gently with general questions about how they get on with others, their relatives or neighbours. Do they have good relationships with them? Are they particularly annoying in any way? Could they be deliberately trying to annoy or even harm the patient? 'Often when one is elderly, other people are unsympathetic or do not understand. Is that a problem?'

At this stage of the examination it should be reasonably clear whether or not an organic state exists and whether or not it is acute or chronic. It is usually also plain whether depressive symptoms are a minor part of the illness or are the overwhelming feature with organic symptoms secondary to the depressive state. A small proportion of patients will remain where the diagnosis is in serious doubt. These patients should be admitted to hospital for further investigations.

PHYSICAL EXAMINATION

A careful physical examination is essential if remedial causes of dementia are to be excluded. A general examination including skin, hair and tongue may reveal evidence of myxoedema or vitamin deficiency. Apraxia may suggest acute confusional state due to general infection or primary infection of the brain itself. Infections, of course, are often not accompanied by pyrexia in elderly people. On examination of the cardiovascular system the blood pressure, any evidence of congestive cardiac failure, arteriosclerosis, the condition of the carotid arteries and any intra cranial bruits should be noted. Focal signs in the central nervous system would suggest multi-infarct dementia, especially if bilateral or, if unilateral, conditions such as cerebral tumour or other space-occupying lesions. It is often difficult to detect visual field defects due to the patient's inability to cooperate. Examination of the optic fundi will usually, but not always, reveal raised intracanial pressure. Abnormalities of the pupils will raise suspicions of syphilis. Strabismus may occur in Wernicke's encephalopathy and nystagmus in some drug intoxications. Evidence of pseudobulbar palsy should point to a diagnosis of multi-infarct dementia. Evidence of peripheral neuropathy will suggest that alcohol may be the underlying aetiology of the dementia. Evidence of early incontinence and gait abnormalities would indicate the need for further investigation to exclude normal pressure hydrocephalus. Choreiform movements may be present in rare cases of Huntington's Chorea in this age group, myoclonic jerks may accompany Creutzfeldt-Jakob disease, and the characteristic movements of Parkinson's disease may be present.

DIFFERENTIAL DIAGNOSIS AND FURTHER SPECIAL INVESTIGATIONS

Certain investigations will be required in all cases of dementia. They will be so familiar that they will merely be listed: haemoglobin, full blood count, erythrocyte sedimentation rate, syphilitic serology, serum electrolytes, blood urea, serum protein and liver function tests. Routine urine testing will be required and a chest X-ray may reveal carcinoma of the lung. A skull X-ray may show erosion of the clinoid processes, suggesting raised intracranial pressure or pineal shift. A routine electroencephalogram is indicated and may show generalized or focal abnormality. In cases where cerebral embolism is suspected, an electrocardiogram would help to exclude myocardial infarction.

Other laboratory tests are usually undertaken routinely in many clinics: serum vitamin B_{12}, folate, protein-bound iodine and T4, serum cholesterol, calcium, phosphorus and blood sugar. Where drug overdosage is suspected, barbiturate and other drug levels may be assessed. In most cases, a brain scan is valuable for excluding focal disease. Computerized axial tomography, although now available in most large centres, is not usually part of the routine investigation. As many as 20% of investigations may be at variance with the clinical diagnosis. The CAT scan has not been fully evaluated as a diagnostic aid in dementia. Its significance is dealt with in Chapter 5. In a small minority of cases, cerebral syphilis, for example, where intracranial pressure or a cerebral tumour is not suspected, lumbar puncture may be diagnostic. On the whole, cerebral biopsy is best avoided except where deterioration is rapid and the clinical picture raises serious doubts about diagnosis.

POINTS IN THE DIFFERENTIAL DIAGNOSIS

After a careful history, mental state, physical examination and such special investigations as are indicated, the diagnosis will be clear in the large majority of cases.

The first stage requires the differentiation between organic and functional states. Disorientation, clouding of consciousness and perseveration are obvious distinguishing features rarely, if ever, present in depression. From our own experience the distinction between organic states and depression is not usually a difficult one to make, but may be almost impossible for a very small number of cases. Depression sometimes accompanies a primary diagnosis of dementia. It is then, generally, what is called reactive or neurotic depression or dysthymic mood. It is probably no more than the kind of depression which accompanies many unpleasant physical disorders or adverse life events. It should not present diagnostic difficulty if the history is carefully taken. It occasionally happens, however, that the symptoms of endogenous or psychotic depression or major affective disorder seem to coexist with dementia, and then the diagnosis is much less clear. When organic symtoms accompany primary depression, in our experience, they are rarely substantial and almost never progress to perseveration or disorientation. It is unlikely that by themselves they would warrant a diagnosis of dementia. In general the onset of depression tends to occur over weeks rather than months and may be sudden. The mood change precedes intellectual, particularly memory, deterioration, and the disabilities tend to be patchy rather than global. The patient is generally distressed but makes no attempt to make facile excuses for his or her failures. In dementia, the memory presents a problem from an early stage and is quickly accompanied by other intellectual changes. Emotional change is usually secondary and rarely develops depth. Disabilities tend to be global and not to cause distress: the patient either remains bland or indifferent to his or her errors or dismisses them with unrealistic excuses. This may not be the case in multi-infarct dementia, where some insight may be retained. Clearly, it is this condition with its variable, irregular lesions which lack the global nature of other forms of dementia that poses the greatest diagnostic problem. Sometimes the uncontrollable laughing or crying associated with pseudobulbar palsy confuses the picture, but patients may be able to indicate that they do not actually 'feel' these emotions at the time they display them.

The failure of intellectual function in primary depression may be due to an underlying lack of brain cell reserves, but it may also be due to the presence of retardation, so that the patient may respond to questions appropriately if given time. However, it must be remembered that studies have shown clinical recovery occurring from depressive illness before a corresponding improvement in the results of psychological tests of cognitive function. Blessed (1984) has shown that in a hospital-based study of dementia, 17 patients were sufficiently depressed to warrant antidepressant treatment. However, only six of these were found to have morphologically normal brains at necropsy. Three cases of depression not associated with clinical dementia showed mild Alzheimer's disease. The relationship between the two may therefore be more complex than has been suggested. This may be the reason why some cases remain so difficult to diagnose, and diagnosis made with some confidence may subsequently be proved incorrect. We have suggested that these cases should be given a double diagnosis of depression and dementia and treated as if they were the former.

Schizophrenia rarely presents a problem except in longstanding cases who have serious emotional deficits and other negative features. However, the intellectual deterioration is rarely sufficient to make living outside an institution impossible. Schneiderian first rank symptoms do occur in the elderly. These and other delusions and hallucinations may be prominent and out of proportion to the intellectual deterioration which rarely if ever reaches the stage of true disorientation.

Stage two, the distinction between chronic and acute organic states, is to be made on the length of history and the absence of clouding of consciousness and evidence of acute physical illness. Acute and chronic are ambiguous terms, but they are used here to imply those conditions which start relatively suddenly over a few days, in persons who have hitherto behaved normally, and those which usually start slowly and have a protracted history. One of the most important causes of acute organic states which must be excluded early is overdosage from drugs or alcohol. The elderly are often sensitive to drug therapy, and there is a lamentable tendency to add further drugs without considering what the patient is already taking. It is surprising how often a dramatic return to normality occurs when the patient is withdrawn from all drugs. All psychiatrists who have done domiciliary visits will have had the experience of being called to see a patient with dementia who turned out to have basal pneumonia which could have been excluded if the referring clinician had asked about the length of history from an informant or elicited that she was shopping for herself several days ago.

Stage three, the distinction between dementia and other chronic organic states and stage four, between remediable and non-remediable forms of dementia, may require admission to hospital or at least attendance at outpatients or day hospital.

Focal signs, if they are present, are, of course, important in suggesting local rather than general disease. They may occur, however, in multi-infarct dementia. Frontal lobe lesions may mimic dementia and may cause deterioration in personality leading to lack of cleanliness and social disinhibition. Such lesions, however, do not affect memory and other intellectual functions and should be readily distinguishable from dementia. Lesions of the temporal lobe causing severe abnormalities of speech and comprehension may simulate dementia when they occur in the dominant hemisphere. However, it should be noted that such lesions are generally unilateral and therefore do not usually affect memory. Focal seizures of temporal lobe type may be present, and a preceding aura is not uncommon. Disorientation and memory loss may be associated with the amnesic syndrome, but neither intellectual function nor personality tend to deteriorate to the same degree. Lesions of the parietal lobe produce a variety of characteristic syndromes but tend to be unilateral and to lack the global intellectual deterioration which would point to dementia as the underlying cause.

Brain tumours rarely simulate dementia unless they are infiltrating, produce raised intra cranial pressure, or are so vascular that they refuce the blood flow to other parts of the brain. They should be detected by the special investigations mentioned above.

Normal pressure hydrocephalus is characterized by the gradual onset of memory impairment, both physical and mental slowness, accompanied by early disorders of gait and incontinence of urine. Insight is said to be lost at an early stage. The appearance of incontinence, usually a late feature in most dementias, is not consistent with the general severity of the illness. There is no clinical evidence of raised intracranial pressure. Intrathecal injection of radio-iodinated human serum albumen has been used in attempts to visualize the CSF flow. The surgical establishment of a ventri-culo-atrial shunt may prove of considerable benefit in some patients. The diagnosis is suggested by the clinical picture and the history of previous subarachnoid haemorrhage, meningitis or head injury.

Other potentially remediable causes include subdural haematoma, which must always be borne in mind but should be clearly visible on brain scan, and various vitamin and metabolic disorders. Their status as causes of dementia is uncertain, but they are generally included in the list of inves-tigations, and any deficiencies corrected. Hypothyroidism is particular case in point, although true dementia with global loss of intellectual function is not common.

NON-REMEDIABLE CAUSES OF DEMENTIA

There remain a group of dementias for which specific curative treatment is not yet available. Particularly important is the distinction between multi-infarct dementia and other forms. A useful advance was made by Hachinski et al (1975), who devised an ischaemic score based on the clinical descrip-tions by Meyer Gross et al (1954). In a very selected sample, this score produced good discrimination between cases of senile dementia and multi-infarct dementia. Some further validation of this score has now been achieved by Harrison et al (1979). Roth (1981) has recently suggested some modifications to this scale. The Hachinski ischaemic score allots two points each if there is evidence of: abrupt onset, fluctuating course, history of stroke, focal neurological signs and focal neurological symptoms. One point is awarded for evidence of: stepwise deterioration, nocturnal confusion, relative preservation of personality, depression, somatic complaints, emotional incontinence, history of hypertension, and evidence of associated atherosclerosis. The possible total score is 18. Hachinski found in his small sample that a score of 7 or more was likely to select cases of multi-infarct dementia, while scores below 4 tended to nominate senile dementia of the Alzheimer type. The scale is fairly crude, and diagnostic errors are likely to occur. However, it ought to be possible from the results of further studies to define the items of the scale more exactly and to modify the weightings. (See also Chapter 12.)

Huntington's chorea is not a common condition in the elderly. When Huntington's chorea does present in later life, it is said to show fewer chor-eiform movements and more intention tremor than at earlier ages. Parkinson's disease may be associated with dementia, although the precise mechanism is debated. This dementia, if it exists, forms one of the group of subcortical dementias. It is supposed to be caused by a relative loss in the input from activating sensors below the cortex with a consequent decline of cortical function. If this is so, the cortex itself may remain intact in such cases, and the condition is therefore possibly amenable to drug therapy. The matter is confused by the fact that degenerative diseases like Alzheimer's disease and multi-infarct dementia cause extensive damage to the brain, including the extrapyramidal systems. It has now been shown that vascular diseases per se do not cause specific bilateral lesions of the basal ganglia or related structures which are the areas affected in Parkinson's disease.

Creutzfeldt-Jakob disease has caused much anxiety since its viral cause was established. The course is usually rapid over nine months or less, with multiple focal signs and myoclonic jerks. Epileptic fits are also not uncommon. In most cases the CSF is normal, but abnormalities of the EEG occur in nearly all cases, showing generalized slowing of activity with sharp waves and slow spike and wave formation progressing to regular slow triphasic bursts. There may be a history of recent neurological or opthalmic surgery.

THE DIAGNOSIS OF EARLY CASES OF DEMENTIA

At present, little is known about how to diagnose early cases of dementia. Until the results of longitudinal community studies are reported, little further advance will be made. Bergmann (1979) found that the majority of subjects who developed dementia during an average three-year follow-up of a community sample came from the original 'normal' fraction and had therefore not been detected initially. Of those whom they had designated early and mild cases, only one-third had developed dementia. These were subjects with a low score on memory and information tests who nevertheless coped with their environment and showed little other intellectual deterioration. Just over a further third turned out to be psychiatrically normal subjects of low IQ and social class at follow-up, and the rest remained of uncertain diagnostic status. The interim follow-up of our own longitudinal community study shows that the majority of those thought to be borderline cases of dementia at the original interview had progressed either to depressive illness or reverted to normality at follow-up some months later. No advice can be offered at this stage on the recognition of 'early cases' likely to advance to a full dementing picture.

OTHER ASSESSMENTS USED IN THE DIAGNOSIS OF DEMENTIA

A variety of short assessments such as the Mini-Mental State (Folstein et al, 1979) are sometimes used for the assessment and even the diagnosis of dementia, often naively interpreted. They are not diagnostic aids. The results of such tests may be affected by the presence of depression and, of course, acute confusional states. They may be helpful as part of a more wide-ranging assessment or as a method of assessing severity or change over time. The CAPE (Pattie & Gilleard, 1975) which incorporates the Stockton Geriatric Rating Scale and a cognitive section is widely used for the assessment of dementing patients in the UK. Again, it is not a diagnostic instrument but is a useful form of rapid assessment once the diagnosis has been made.

Psychological tests as diagnostic aids have proved disappointing. Cowan et al (1975) showed that a good diagnostic discrimination could be made on inpatients between depression and organic states, but that it was no better than that made by the psychiatrists using a standardized clinical examination. The results of our own studies have not yet demonstrated that psychological tests are superior to clinical judgment. They may, however, form a valuable baseline for assessing deterioration and produce supporting evidence for diagnosis. They have not yet proved themselves useful in the detection of early cases of dementia, perhaps, because most established tests have been developed on hospital inpatients.

THE DIAGNOSIS OF DEMENTIA FOR RESEARCH

Research in the psychiatry of old age has been bedevilled by lack of standardized techniques and diagnostic criteria. The recent introduction of DSM III (1980), although a major advance in standardizing the criteria for diagnosis, has been found difficult to apply in practice to dementia (see below). Because of this lack of standardization, Copeland et al (1976) developed the Geriatric Mental State schedule partly from the Present State Examination (Wing et al, 1974) and the Psychiatric Status Schedule (Spitzer et al, 1970). They incorporated a substantial proportion of additional sections. This method, already translated into six languages to meet the need of researchers in other countries, is now in use in a variety of studies. The interview has been developed into a complete GMS-AGECAT package including the original mental state, the History and Aetiology Schedule, Social Status Schedule, and the Physical Examination Schedule. A comprehensive computerized diagnostic system, AGECAT, has been developed (Copeland et al, 1986) and validated against psychiatric judgment on over 1600 patients and community residents. The method now provides a standardized diagnosis which includes the diagnosis of dementia, providing, for each subject, main diagnostic syndromes, a profile of symptom groups, level of certainty of being a psychiatric case and a list of principal symptoms. Thus each subject's psychiatric condition can be described in some detail in a standardized manner, and changes can be monitored over time. The results of longitudinal studies of dementia and other conditions using these measures should become available over the next few months. Such methods are, however, not yet adapted for clinical use, although work is proceeding in this direction.

INTERNATIONAL CRITERIA FOR THE DIAGNOSIS OF DEMENTIA

ICD-9 maintained the concept of delirium as both acute and reversible compared to dementia, considered chronic, progressive and generally irreversible. In DSM III the distinction centres on the state of consciousness. In delirium there is cognitive impairment and disorientation, but consciousness is clouded, while in dementia cognitive impairment occurs in a clear state of consciousness. DSM III has accepted that whether or not the condition is irreversible depends on the aetiology and as such does not enter into the definition. This would certainly seem an advance. Dementia after all is not a diagnosis but a syndrome with a number of aetiologies, some of which are reversible, some can be arrested, while others in our present state of knowledge inevitably progress.

The subdivision, 'dementias arising in the senium and presenium', aims to remove the emphasis of age, as both senile and presenile now become subclasses and not primary divisions. This was considered desirable owing to the lack of evidence for a neuropathological distinction between the two conditions. Both these primary degenerative dementias may then be classified according to the presence of delusions or depression. The substitution of multi-infarct dementia for arteriosclerotic dementia is in line with current thinking, although it seems to leave little room for other rare arteriopathic disorders.

The provision of diagnostic criteria for dementia is welcome. However, some of the criteria are left surprisingly vague, e.g. 'memory impairment'. It is well known that patients with depression are apt to complain of memory impairment, but it rarely presents severe problems in daily living. The interviewing psychiatrist's judgment of memory impairment may be associated with depression in the patient, but again this is unlikely to reach the severity found in most cases of dementia. It would be helpful to have specified here the type of memory impairment required for the criteria. Again, 'impaired judgment' is open to wide interpretation. Small but obvious impairments of judgment can occur in a variety of conditions in the elderly. Are these to be included, or only those which cause a problem in daily living?

In general, the criteria for dementia used by DSM III seem to be relatively imprecise. In our own studies we found it difficult to be confident that we had applied them consistently. The way in which DSM III links social performance with mental state items may also be considered a disadvantage as there are times, particularly for research, when it would be convenient to keep these independent.

The Research Diagnostic Criteria as published by Spitzer et al (1978) do not contain criteria for dementia. A system put forward by Gurland et al (1983) of pervasive and limited dementia again mixes social performance with mental state items but is more precise and has been shown to be reliable. On the whole, there is good agreement between the syndrome of pervasive dementia as applied in the US/UK Diagnostic Project and DSM III criteria applied to the same patients. The Diagnostic Project's concept of limited dementia will need much more extensive validation before its usefulness can be demonstrated.

Finally, there is still much work to be done in order to improve the criteria for dementia and for delineating the progress of the illnesses subsumed under this rubric. Although Reisberg et al (1982) have put forward a method for staging the conditions, it is not clear from the literature how this method was derived. It also appears to have been validated on small samples over a short follow-up period. If it is based on clinical observation, it will need to be more substantially validated before it can be accepted a useful for either clinical work or research. Much work is now proceeding on longitudinal studies, and it is hoped that the results of these will shortly help us to recognize dementia which is likely to progress, at a much earlier and potentially reversible stage in its evolution, than is at present possible.

REFERENCES

American Psychiatric Association 1980 Diagnostic and Statistical Manual of Mental Disorders (DSMIII) 3rd edn. American Psychiatric Association, Washington DC
Bergmann K 1977 Progress in chronic brain failure. Age and Ageing 6 (Suppl) 61–66
Bergmann K, Day D W K , Foster E M, McKenchie A A, Roth M, 1971 A follow-up study of randomly selected community residents to assess the effects of chronic brain syndrome and cerebrovascular disease. Proceedings of Fifth Congress of Psychiatry, Pt II, P 856–865
Blessed G 1984 Clinical features and neuropathological correlations of Alzheimer type disease, In: Kay D W K, Burrows G D (eds) Handbook of studies on psychiatry and old age Elsevier, Amsterdam
Copeland J R M 1978 Evaluation of diagnostic methods: an international comparison. In: Isacs A D Post F (eds) Studies in geriatric psychiatry. Wiley, Chichester, p 189–209
Copeland J R M, Kelleher M J, Gurland B J, Sharpe L et al 1975 Cross-national study of diagnosis of the mental disorders: a comparison of the diagnosis of elderly psychiatric patients admitted to mental hospitals serving Queens County in New York and the Old Borough of Camberwell, London. British Journal of Psychiatry 126: 11–20
Copeland J R M, Kelleher M J, Kellett J M, Gourlay A J, Gurland B J, Fleiss J L, Sharpe L 1976 A semi-structural clinical interview for the assessment of diagnosis and mental state in the elderly. The Geriatric Mental State Schedule 1. Development and reliability. Psychological Medicine 6: 439–449
Copeland J R M, Dewey M E, Griffiths-Jones H M (1986) Computerised psychiatric diagnostic system and case nomenclature for elderly subjects: GMS and AGECAT. Psychological Medicine 16: 89–100
Cowan D W, Copeland J R M, Kelleher M J, Kellet J M, Gourlay A J, Smith A, Barron G, De Gruchy J, Kuriansky J, Gurland B, Sharpe L, Stiller P, Simon S 1975 Cross-national study of the diagnosis of the mental disorders: a comparative psychometric assessment of elderly patients admitted to mental hospitals serving Queens County, New York and the former Borough of Camberwell, London. British Journal of Psychiatry 126: 560–570
Folstein M F, Folstein S E, McHugh P R 1975 Mini-mental state: a practical method for grading the cognitive state of patients for the clinician. Journal of Psychiatric Research 12: 189–198
Gardner A 1984 The assessment of dementia. In: Gaind R N, Fawzy F I, Hudson B L, Pasnau R O (eds) Current themes in psychiatry, vol 3. London, Macmillan

Gurland B J, Copeland J R M, Kelleher M J, Kuriansky J, Sharpe L, Dean L 1983 The mind and mood of ageing: the mental health problems of the community elderly in New York and London. Haworth Press, New York and Croom Helm, London

Hachinski V C, Iliff L D, Zilkha E, Du Boulay G H, McAllister V L, Marshall J, Russell R W R, Symon L 1975 Cerebral blood flow in dementia. Archives of Neurology 32: 632–637

Harrison M J G, Thomas D J, Du Boulay G H, Marshall J 1979 Multi-infarct dementia. Journal of Neurological Science 40: 97–103

Herbst K G, Humphrey C 1980 Hearing impairment and mental state in the elderly living at home. British Medical Journal 281: 903–905

Marsden C D, Harrison M J G 1972 Outcome of investigations of patients with pre-senile dementia. British Medical Journal 1: 249–252

Mayer-Gross W, Slater E, Roth M 1954 Clinical psychiatry. Cassell, London

Nott P N, Fleminger J J 1975 Pre-senile dementia: the difficulties of early diagnosis. Acta Psychiatrica Scandanavica 51: 210–217

Pattie A H, Gilleard C J 1975 A brief psychogeriatric assessment schedule — validation against psychatric diagnosis and discharge from hospital. British Journal of Psychiatry 127: 489–493

Reisberg B, Ferris S H, De Leon M J, Crook T 1982 The global deterioration scale for assessment of primary degenerative dementia. American Journal of Psychiatry 139: 9, 1136–1139

Ron M A, Toone B K, Garralda M E, Lishman W A 1979 Diagnostic accuracy in pre-senile dementia. British Journal of Psychiatry 134: 161–168

Roth M 1981 The diagnosis of dementia in late and middle life. In: Mortimer A J, Schuman L M (eds) Monographs in epidemiology and biostatistics. The epidemiology of dementia. Oxford University Press, New York p 24–61

Smith S J, Kiloh L G 1981 The investigation of dementia: results in 200 consecutive admissions. Lancet 1: 824–827

Spitzer R L, Endicott J, Fleiss J L, Cohen J 1970 Psychiatric status Schedule: a technique for evaluating psychopathology and impairment in role functioning. Archives of General Psychiarty 23: 41–55

Spitzer R L, Endicott J, Robins E 1978 Research diagnostic criteria. Archives of General Psychiatry 35: 773–782

Wing J K, Cooper J E Sartorius N 1974 The description and classification of psychiatric symptoms: an instruction manual for the PSE and Catego System. Cambridge University Press, Cambridge

Psychological assessment

INTRODUCTION

Definitions

Whalley (1981) defines the term dementia as a 'diffuse loss of mental functions' which results from organic brain disease. Three major deficits are associated with dementia: deterioration in the ability to register new memories; an impairment in the facility to reason so that a difficulty in making decisions occurs; and changes in feelings and conduct, several authors emphasizing the behavioural aspects of dementia (McHugh, 1975; Stoud & Jolly, 1981). The science of psychology is now paying attention not only to the measurement of cognitive functions in relation to the dementias but also of behavioural changes.

The earliest symptoms of dementia may pass unrecognized because they are so subtle that observers consider them to be just the normal signs of ageing. Relatively simple screening devices which will permit early detection of incipient dementia (Beaumont, 1982) are of great importance. Heston & White (1983) lay great stress on the exact diagnosis of the dementias because, with rapid progress in the brain sciences, more attention is being given to the illnesses of later life and their consequences, and some dementias have been found to be treatable.

To cover all the cognitive aspects of the elderly would require review and discussion of such topics as sensation and perception, attention and performance, learning and memory, and intelligence and problem solving. However, as the main purpose of this book is to consider all the aspects of dementia, only those areas of cognition relevant to that problem will be discussed.

Gerontology, lifespan development psychology and geriatric psychiatry

The psychological assessment of the elderly person presents a vast array of problems at the theoretical and technical levels. Psychologists studying in this area are working within the discipline of gerontology, which, as Bromley (1974) points out, is the scientific study of growing old. It has three main areas of study: the theoretical, which observes the conceptual systems that integrate and explain the observed facts about ageing; the methodological, where the development of suitable research instruments is examined in relation to these theories; and the applied, which is the prevention or amelioration of the adverse effects of ageing. Gerontology is also an interdisciplinary science incorporating the psychology of ageing with the biology, sociology and other components of ageing.

The psychology of ageing, according to Kausler (1982), contains three elements: experimental, psychometric and applied approaches, which to a certain extent correspond with the three aims of gerontology. Old age can also be considered from a lifespan developmental psychology stance, the senium being seen as an integrative or an age-segmented subject, influencing attitudes and the results obtained. Are there two forms of ageing, normal and abnormal (Miller, 1977)? And are the different forms of the dementias occurring in the elderly accelerated forms of normal ageing or systemic disorders with entirely different psychological consequences? (This area of study then incorporates the medical science of geriatrics.) If the dementias constitute abnormal ageing, then different theoretical propositions may be required from those concerned with normal ageing.

It is necessary to consider these areas in order to understand the manner in which the psychological assessment of the elderly person has developed. Because of diverse views there seems to have developed a situation of watertight compartments, with very little interaction between researchers in each particular area. Even in the mid-1980s the experimental and the psychometric literature contains few cross-references. This was pointed out by Kendrick (1982a), who could argue both as a clinical and an experimental psychologist, having researched both in human and animal psychology. His paper produced a dialogue in the clinical literature between experimental and clinical researchers (Kendrick, 1982a,b; Rabbitt, 1982a; Volans & Woods, 1983). The book by Wilson & Moffatt (1984) emphasizes the lack of communication between different professional groups and attempts to ease this situation with respect to the clinical management of memory problems. One of the main purposes of this chapter will be to integrate this literature further.

The development of the psychological assessment of the elderly

The psychological assessment of the elderly during the 1950s and 1960s saw what Miller (1977) has described as the 'alchemist's search for the philosopher's stone — a criticism reinforced by Marcer (1979) and Kendrick (1982a). Psychologists were looking for tests which would improve diagnostic precision, concentrating on, say, the right combination of Wechsler subtests, though little success was ever achieved. These techniques were largely irrelevant to the elderly both in content and in aim. There was a failure to appeciate that subject matter suitable for a 10-year-old may not be suitable for the 70-year-old. This flaw was probably part of the integrative approach of lifespan development psychology, an error arising from the Zeitgeist of the 1950s and 1960s.

Rabbitt (1982a) has taken the argument further. He claims that gerontologists have depended upon empirical techniques and functional models of cognitive performance, based upon the work of experimental psychologists studying young adults. This may have stifled original work because the models are all for steady-state systems, while gerontologists are very much concerned with changes in performance. He argues that there is still no single subsystem of process which allows for improvement with practice. As people practise, they not only become quicker but change the ways in which they carry out the tasks.

A significant feature of ageing is a dramatic increase in the differences between individuals in elderly populations. A small minority of elderly people may continue to perform as efficiently as most young people with whom they are being compared. However, the majority occupy various positions along a continuum of decrement. Rabbitt (1982b) argues that, to understand these increasing differences between individuals, models of change within and between people are required. Descriptions are urgently required of the ways in which people actively adjust their performance best to cope with changes in the task demand, and the ability to improve with practice, and new strategies to circumvent or minimize growing failures in efficiency. This increase in variance is opposed to the myth of the de-differentiation of elderly people. Kausler (1982) makes the point that the idea that people become more alike as they grow older, i.e. sexless and conservative (both politically and socially), translates into a negative stereotype of old age. Again this myth probably developed from a flaw in lifespan developmental psychology methodology in that there was a failure to distinguish between an age difference in behaviour and a true age change in behaviour (Cutler & Schmidhouser, 1975). Schaie in a number of papers discusses in great detail the problems of lifespan developmental psychology (1970, 1979, 1980).

The 1970s saw a move away from assessment to intervention (Woodruff, 1982). It was found that cohort differences accounted for much more of the behavioural variance in age-comparative studies than age change. While these findings further emphasized the problem of test ecology (Neisser, 1976) for the elderly, at the same time they indicated the hopeful finding of plasticity in the ageing process. This led to attempts to ameliorate deficits in performance and, in the clinical sphere, to the advent of reality orientation therapy (RO).

The 1970s also saw the recognition that, in the psychological assessment of the elderly, not only has the ecology of the subjects to be taken into account, but also some very important non-cognitive factors have to be considered. Marcer (1979) argues that a great deal of the research work with the elderly is concerned with memory problems, and ultimately most measures of memory depend upon the ability and the cooperation of the person to respond. Between them Botwinick (1978) and Marcer (1979) suggest that factors include mood, personality, the level of motivation, task relevance, over-cautiousness and generational differences. The general activity level of the person might also affect cognitive responding (Kendrick, 1975; Kendrick & Moyes, 1979; Thornton, 1984) and in general lifespan (Kendrick, 1984). From geriatric psychiatry came the impetus for differentiating between the cognitive responding of the depressed and the demented elderly (Kendrick, 1985), emphasizing that the subject's mood needs consideration in matters of psychological assessment.

The 1980s should see a coming together of all the strands so far indicated. Kendrick's (1982a) article concerning the integration of the experimental and clinical literature (entitled: Why assess the aged: a clinical psychologist's view) marks the direction which the psychological assessment of the elderly will take, arguing that with the advent of cognitive psychology the three rather disparate fields in the psychology of ageing can all be brought together under the unifying concepts of information processing, transmission and retrieval. This idea has been echoed by Gilleard (1984a) in reviewing the assessment of cognitive impairment in the elderly. (Kendrick also argued that the use of computers with the elderly was inappropriate because they did not belong to their ecology, but has since rescinded this argument (Kendrick, 1985).)

Memory has probably received more attention than any other topic from researchers into the ageing process, mainly because it is particularly important in the understanding of ageing. A recent book has been written solely about this topic (Poon et al, 1980) and other recent volumes have had a considerable number of chapters committed to this theme (Craik & Trehub, 1982; Kausler, 1982). The experimental literature shows a shift in theorizing from the multi-store models of memory in the 1960s and 1970s to a 'levels of processing' model. The multi-store model emphasized a distinction between storage structures and control operations. The locations of memory traces were considered to be the sensory, the short-term and the long-term stores. The control operations of these stores constituted such things as attention, rehearsal and organizational strategies. The sensory store was seen as a peripheral sensory system with a duration of less than one second. If the information was not attended to during this brief period, then it was forgotten. It is considered that there is a decline with age in the rate of information readout from the sensory store. The short-term or primary memory is of small capacity, with information being displaced if not released or transferred to long-term store. This system does not appear to decline much with age. Effectively, the long-term store seems to be of unlimited capacity and my be permanent. The encoding (storage) and retrieval of information are the basic processes involved in its operation. The accumulated experiences and knowledge of a lifetime stored here do not disintegrate with age unless there is a disease process.

A great deal of research has been carried out into the relationship between these various forms of store. Research, however, has moved on to consider the organization processes affecting storage and retrieval. There have been important results from the more recent work into the levels of processing framework (Craik & Lockhart, 1972; Craik & Bird, 1982; Perlmutter & Mitchell, 1982; Wilson & Moffatt, 1984), where memory is considered as a continuum of processing in which a hierarchy of stages is envisaged. This hierarchy is referred to as 'depth of processing'. This implies a greater emphasis on the semantic as opposed to the visual or auditory characteristics of the information to be processed or analysed. The outcome of this research has been to show that elderly people do not spontaneously use organization strategies as the young do. A number of studies of levels of processing have indicated that elderly subjects fail to process information as deeply as young people do, either in the encoding or the retrieval process. Elderly subjects show improvement when they are directed to process information where the semantic characteristics are emphasized. From such results a 'production deficiency' hypothesis has been generated, stating that elderly subjects are capable of depth processing but simply fail to do so in a particular situation (Perlmutter & Mitchell, 1982). Such results have important implications for the guidance of the elderly person (Wilson & Moffatt, 1984).

WHY ASSESS THE AGED?

Gilleard (1984a), in reviewing the assessment of cognitive impairment in the elderly, begins by stating that from the age of 60 and maybe before that there is an associated decline in many areas of cognitive performance. In particular there is an obvious speed loss on information processing, transmission and retrieval. He questions whether this is due to a pure ageing effect of the effect of historical and pathological forces exogenous to the ageing process, but although this may be of theoretical importance, he considers it 'tangential' in the clinical setting. This is a questionable assumption and it also represents the split between the experimental/theoretical and the psychometric and applied fields. From what has already been said it would seem obvious that not to consider the problem of normal and abnormal ageing in the clinical setting nor to consider the experimental literature on levels of processing in memory would stifle progress. If there is abnormal ageing, then different behavioural laws may operate which could have implications for clinical management. The results of the levels of processing studies have clear implications for the amelioration of memory difficulties.

The pros and cons

A primary aim of the psychological assessment of the elderly person is to relate varying degrees of cognitive deficit to the adaptability of that person

(Gilleard, 1984a). It should also be seen in the context of the aims of gerontology, at the theoretical, methodological and applied levels (Kendrick, 1982a). At the applied level the author has argued that assessment has implications for amelioration, if not prevention — for example, in the detection of early Alzheimer's disease, or the true significance of physical activity in the maintenance of cognitive status.

There are arguments against the psychological assessment of the elderly in the clinical setting. When the elderly person is clearly incapable of self-help and carrying out everyday activities, then psychological assessment may well be redundant. In this situation the person will probably be unable to cooperate and give responses to assessment techniques anyway, but other forms of assessment would be appropriate. Kendrick (1982a, 1985) has persistently argued that it is much more sensible to adopt a monitoring approach, by means of sequential assessment to signal significant changes in cognitive status. He has been criticized as not being psychological enough in his approach to the assessment of the elderly (Volans & Woods, 1983), but has been concerned with producing reliable and valid measures of cognitive status. As regards the diagnostic problems generated by geriatric psychiatry, Kendrick (1985) points out that diagnostic psychological tests are not valid unless they can clearly identify unequivocal cases; a theoretical approach may then help in developing methods in which these instruments can be useful in differential diagnosis.

Gilleard (1984a) also presents arguments against the non-assessment of the elderly. These are: reliable clinical information is not always obtainable from the patient, the patient's spouse, friends or relatives (Kuriansky et al, 1976); that in the present state of knowledge it is not possible to assume that measures of brain function or pathology correlate with present of future incompetence (Stefoski et al, 1976; Roberts & Caird, 1976; Nott & Fleminger, 1975); there is a lack of construct validity of purely clinical–behaviour information (Robertson & Malchick, 1968; Platt, 1980). There is also the problem of misdiagnosis: the mimicry of dementia by the functional disorders occurs with some frequency, resulting in an over-diagnosis of dementia (Marsden & Harrison, 1972; Post, 1975) with consequent implications for treatment and management. The recent resurgence of interest in the diagnosis of dementia and advance in the understanding of the development (Wilcock, 1984) and neurochemical aspects (Glen, 1979) of senile dementia of the Alzheimer type (SDAT) and the importance of recognizing symptoms early has made psychological assessment important. Behavioural and psychometric testing procedures need to be developed so that research studies in other fields can be appropriately assessed and compared (Smith et al, 1979).

(The need for the psychological assessment of the elderly is clearly evinced by the recent huge increase in the number of published articles by non-psychologist authors in the literature concerning this topic. Just a few of the many are: Arie, 1984; Barber, 1981; Coleman, 1984; Church &

Wattis, 1983; Davies et al, 1984; McCurren & Ganong, 1984; McKechnie & Corser, 1984; Poulton, 1984; Robertson, 1984; Wilkinson & Zissler, 1984).

HOW TO ASSESS THE AGED?

Reliability and validity

In psychometrics the problems of reliability and validity loom large in test construction. The reliability of a test is a measure of whether a score obtained from a test is accurate. Various forms of reliability are generally required in assessing the accuracy of an instrument. These are: test–retest reliability, that is whether the test gives the same score over different time intervals for each individual; split-half reliability, that is whether a test when suitably split in half has a high correlation between the two halves; interform reliability, that is where parallel (alternate) forms of a test must correlate equally well with an external criterion, as well as with each other, before they can be considered parallel. The validity of a test is the effectiveness with which it measures that which it is designed to measure. It is impossible to have a valid test that has low reliability, but you can have a very reliable measure that is not valid.

There are various forms of validity. Criterion-orientated or empirical validity involves the correlation of test scores with a predicted criterion. The magnitude of the correlation is an index of the validity of the test. This form of validation can also be classed as predictive or concurrent, the distinction depending upon whether the test scores are obtained before or simultaneously with some criterion measure.

Content validity is also referred to as validity by definition or logical validity. This form can also be subsumed under the general heading of face validity. It refers not to that which the test measures but that which it appears to measure. In general, content validity consists of showing that the test items represent the behavioural area of interest.

Construct validity is more difficult. This form of validity is necessary when some attribute or quality is to be measured for which there is no operational definition, or no valid criterion is available. There are several experimental methods of determining construct validity. *Group differences*: if two groups should theoretically differ on a specified construct, the investigation of this procedure constitutes a validational procedure. *Correlation* matrices; here tests measuring the same construct are expected to correlate positively with each other. *Studies of change over time*: for example, if a theoretical construct produces a prediction that there should be a difference in test scores after experimental intervention, then such an outcome would support construct validity. *Studies of internal structure*: once again predictions must be formulated according to an underlying theory — if the theory predicts high item intercorrelation, such correlations, if found, imply construct validity (Edmunds & Kendrick, 1979). *Factor analysis* is regarded as a construct validation technique. Construct validity is very important in the development of test for the elderly, especially in the areas of diagnosis and screening, for here, as Gilleard (1984a,b) points out, there is still a reliance on psychiatric diagnostic status as the principal source of concurrent validation.

The need for psychological assessment is apparent. Two main types of assessment will now be considered: cognitive, based mainly on psychometric procedures, and behavioural, which may be by means of behaviour rating scales or self-completed 'activities of daily living' (ADL) scales. A further method about to appear is that of computer-assisted techniques.

Cognitive assessment

The cognitive assessment of the elderly comprises:
1. diagnosing or screening for diffuse brain pathology
2. the test battery
3. the mental status questionnaire
4. the estimation of pre-morbid intellectual level.

Before evaluating these methods Gilleard (1984a), Kendrick (1982a) and Smith et al (1979) all agree that there are too many 'one-off' performance measures for the elderly. This stultifies attempts to compare research studies. Thorough examination of existing tests is now required to understand the factors contributing to the generation of impairment. This might in turn lead to more useful predictive judgments. It is not intended therefore to catalogue numerous tests but to review those for which a database has been reported.

Screening for diffuse brain damage

As already stated, a great deal of work has been carried out on memory. In the 1950s and 1960s, much of the work emanating from the Maudsley and Bethlem Royal Hospitals found memory impairment to be a source of variance in the cognitive performance of the elderly dementing or depressed person. From this developed the 'new word learning' technique from which such tests as the Inglis Paired Associate Learning Test (1965) were derived. The new learning impairment theory has also led to the study of the types of error that dementing people make, in contrast with depressed and the normal elderly person (Whitehead, 1973; Miller, 1977). Gibson (1981) in his examination of the Kendrick Object Learning Test (KOLT) (Kendrick, 1985) found that dementing subjects did not make significantly more perseveration errors over random ones than did depressed and normal subjects.

Other types of tests have been used in the detection of dementia, though in the main they have not been designed specifically for use with the elderly. These have been visual tests which require the subject to produce or recall visual images. This form of test has never supplanted the verbal learning ones, except for one, the KOLT, which will be dealt with in detail later.

The Kendrick Battery for the Detection of Dementia in the Elderly, KBDDE, (Gibson & Kendrick, 1979) is the product of a different theoretical and sophisticated statistical approach to the problem of screening for diffuse brain damage in the elderly. It is one of the few systems that takes into account the base-rates of the diagnostic categories. Its new title is the Kendrick Cognitive Tests for the Elderly, KCTE (Kendrick, 1985). There are both practical and theoretical reasons for this change in title. The KCTE in its present form consists of two tests: the Kendrick Object Learning Test, KOLT, and the Kendrick Digit Copying Test, KDCT. To these will be added, if appropriate reliability and validity studies warrant, decision-making and spatial tests. Both these latter tests will be used as screening instruments for the early detection of SDAT.

The development of the KCTE now spans 25 years (Gibson, 1979; Gibson, 1981; Gibson & Kendrick, 1979; Gibson et al, 1980; Kendrick, 1964; Kendrick, 1965; Kendrick, 1967; Kendrick, 1968; Kendrick, 1972; Kendrick, 1982a,b,c; Kendrick, 1985; Kendrick et al, 1979; Kendrick & Moyes, 1979; Kendrick et al, 1965; Kendrick & Post, 1967). The development of these tests charts the changes in style in cognitive assessment from the late 1950s to the early 1980s. They also represent the author's intent to take account of the inherent reliability and validity problems of psychometric tests.

Four categories of method of assessment are given in the introduction to this section, the first two being screening instruments and test batteries. The KCTE straddles these two categories. The new manual for the KCTE (Kendrick, 1985) clearly distinguishes between these two aspects of the tests, one of the main reasons for changing the title. As the KCTE was originally produced as battery, it will be discussed under the next heading.

Test batteries

It is only really in the late 1970s and early 1980s that attention has been turned to developing assessment procedures specifically designed for use with the elderly. Most test batteries are products of the integrative lifespan developmental methodology, and therefore their use with the elderly is now somewhat suspect. Further, the clinical psychologist's time is not spent these days on administering long test batteries, taxing for both the examinee and the administrator.

The problem of such lengthy instruments has been identified by Carson (1984) in trying to understand why the Halstead-Reitan Battery, HRB, (Golden et al, 1980; Russel et al, 1978) is not more wisely used in Great Britain by clinical psychologists. In the United States it is the most frequently used neuropsychological test battery. The battery was originally assembled to discriminate between subjects with known cerebral lesions form normal 'controls'. Research has shown that the Battery is highly effective in discriminating between the presence and absence of brain damage, and it also provides information on laterality, which lobe is predominantly affected and clues to the type of pathological process. The HRB samples a wide range of behaviours, from sensori-perceptual skills to complex cognitive ones. It was not specifically designed for use with the elderly. The Battery has little theoretical background and few changes have been made despite recent advances in our understanding of brain-behaviour relationships. It is very expensive, around: £1800, and takes a long time to administer. (This last criticism can also be levelled against the Luria-Nebraska Neuropsychological Battery (Golden, 1979). The HRB's Average Impairment Rating indicating severity of diffuse brain pathology has been compared with the diagnosis of brain damage from the KOLT. The congruence of the 'hit rate' between the two measures is impressive, indicating that as much information of this nature can be gained from a very short test as from a long test battery (Drinkwater, 1981). Similarly the pathognomic scale of the Luria-Nebraska Neuropsychological Battery has been found to agree with a brain damage diagnosis from the KDCT (Fish et al, 1982). However, such long test batteries are probably not efficient techniques for use with the elderly because poor attention and fatigue lose the subject's cooperation. Extended accounts of these two batteries can be found in the Handbook of Clinical Neuropsychology by Filskov & Boll (1981).

Other test battery approaches have largely been based upon the use of intelligence tests, 'the alchemist's search for the philosopher's stone'. A fairly exhaustive investigation was reported by Bolton et al (1966), showing that there was very little value in attempting to diagnose by this method. The Weschsler Memory Scale has been reviewed by Erikson and Scott (1977), with the conclusion that it is an unsatisfactory test. Although more recent work (Weingartner et al, 1981; Gilleard, 1980) showed that significant differences between nominated groups could be obtained, these differences were probably a function of the test's relationship with verbal learning ability. The Kendrick Cognitive Tests for the Elderly (previously known as the Kendrick Battery for the Detection of Dementia in the Elderly, Kendrick, 1985) are short, simple and easy to administer. The tests are the KOLT and the KDCT, and when used together and in a sequential testing programme they have been found to differentiate between elderly normal and dementing people to a high level of accuracy. They can be used for other assessment and differential diagnostic purposes. The KOLT is a test of recall of everday objects after a brief viewing period. The KDCT is a simple test of speed performance. The author claims that the tests can be used in the following ways: to screen for the presence of dementia (but not to distinguish between the various forms of the dementias); for the differential diagnosis between dementing, pseudodementing, depressive and normal modes of responding; and research. The KOLT is so designed that different types of scores can be obtained in order that levels of processing or types of error can be measured in relation to different diagnostic categories. The KDCT can be used to measure continuous processing of information. Both the KOLT and KDCT are highly reliable, and it can be shown that they are producing predictive, concurrent, content and construct validity.

The background to the tests of the KCTE is that they were designed to assess those cognitive abilities which appear to be most sensitive to age changes, as well as helping in diagnosis, namely sensory memory coupled with level of processing, and speed of processing and recording information. Not only is there empirical basis for the KCTE but Kendrick has also presented a theoretical framework for the tests (Kendrick, 1972; Kendrick, 1985; Kendrick & Moyes, 1979). The theory is based upon a two-arousal hypothesis (Routtenberg, 1968), Surwillow's (1970) timing of behaviour theory and Post's (1966) somatic approach to psychiatry. The theory gives rise to testable hypotheses concerning the manner in which dementing, depressed, pseudodementing and normal people should repond to the tests. A drug and an activity hypothesis are incorporated which allow the author to account for two forms of psueodementia: depressive and drug-induced. Kendrick has always insisted that the theory must be regarded as a 'weak' one; nevertheless it will be some time before it can be assessed as progressive or degenerating, in the sense of Lakatos as quoted by Eynsenck (1976). To date some predictions have been validated (Kendrick, 1985).

In reviewing the research carried out on the KOLT and the KDCT used individually and in concert, Kendrick (1985) comes to the following conclusions. The KDCT has been shown to have concurrent validity both for the dementing/non-dementing dichotomy, as well as for normal, affective and dementia differentiation (Cowan et al, 1975). Construct validity is being found in that the KDCT consistently correlates with the digit symbol sub-test of the Wechsler Adult Intelligence Scale and with measures of parieto-temporal dysfunction (Hendrickson et al, 1979; Jacoby & Levy, 1980a, 1980b; Naguib & Levy, 1982). Predictive validity has been shown in that low scores are associated with death in the dementing person within 30 months (Naguib & Levy, 1982). Considering the KOLT, Kendrick (1985) finds that it has good within, between and test–retest reliability for both the total score and the various subscores based upon the different types of item within the test. Concurrent validity is high for the test not only for the total score but also for the various types of items and the individual cards that make up the test. The test discriminates at the group mean level between demented, depressed, pseudodemented and normal people (Fish et al, 1983). The predictive validity of the test is now under review (Searle, 1984). The KOLT total score indicates severe diffuse brain pathology irrespective of age (Drinkwater, 1981), and the test used in sequential form differentiates between normal, depressed and dementing groups of elderly people (Gibson, 1981).

When the KOLT and the KDCT have been used together diagnostically, the battery has been found to be deficient in chronically institutionalized people (Gibson et al, 1980). In its screening ability it is highly effective (Kendrick, 1985). The overall conclusion concerning this instrument is that a solid database is being built up which allows it to be used both diagnostically and for research.

Mental status assessment devices

To a certain extent these instruments derive from procedures employed in the mental state examination in psychiatry. Aspects found to be particularly useful in the examination of the elderly are orientation for time or place and general information items. Hinton & Withers (1971) confirm these findings. Other tests such as serial sevens, recall of stories, digit span etc. have not been found to be particularly useful. In Gurland's (1980) review of some of the more common mental status screening instruments he found that all consisted of either orientation and information questions, or that this type of item composed the principal feature.

Pattie et al (1979) have found that this type of examination is predictive of hospitalization outcome in the psychiatric setting. Gilleard (1984), in reviewing the mental status screening instruments, concludes that they have coarse though evident value in assessing mental competence in the elderly. He also adds that most of them rely on diagnostic status as the main source of concurrent validation.

Gilleard is the co-author of the Clifton Assessment Procedures for the Elderly, CAPE, (Pattie & Gilleard, 1976). There is a short form of the CAPE known as the Survey Version (Pattie, 1981). Using the Survey Version, which is made up of the information/orientation test and a physical disability scale, it was found that in 400 subjects, 100 each living in the community, social services institutions, geriatric or mental wards and psychogeriatric wards over a two-year period, 55% remained at the same level of disability, 31% deteriorated and only 14% showed any improvement. These findings reinforced Gilleard's argument that little is known about the long-term stability or otherwise of performance deficits over differing lengths of time, in different settings with different groups of elderly people. He adds that only minimal changes are seen even where strenuous intervention efforts are made both at the cognitive and behavioural levels in the institutionalized dementing population. This type of finding will be considered in the next section. Copeland (Searle, 1984) is presently developing a dementia scale based upon the Geriatric Mental State Schedule (GMS) (Copeland et al, 1976). This is a prospective study. Amongst the psychological tests being used are the KOLT and KDCT. So far, encouraging interrelations have been found between both these tests and the dementia scale. This scale is being devised to assess levels of dementia — something that the KCTE is not known to do, though there are indications that both the dementia scale and the KCTE may be able to do this.

Some interelationships have already been found between the CAPE and the KCTE. Kendrick (1985) reports that preliminary results from an ongoing study show that the KOLT correlates positively and significantly with the Cognitive Assessment Scale, CAS, of the CAPE and significantly and negatively with the Behaviour Rating Scale, BRS, of the CAPE. The KDCT correlates similarly with these scales but only significantly in the case of the CAS.

The mental status screening tests reviewed by Gurland (1980) are: Orientation Scale for Geriatric Patients, OSGP (Berg & Stevenson, 1980); Mini-Mental State Examination, MMSE (Folstein et al, 1975); Abbreviated Mental Test, AMT (Hodgkinson, 1972); Orientation Test, OT (Irving et al, 1970); Tests of Mental Impairment, TMI (Issacs & Whalley, 1964); Mental Status Questionnaire, MSQ (Kahn et al, 1960); Kew Test (McDonald, 1969); Short Portable Mental Status Questionnaire, SPMSQ (Pfeiffer, 1975); and Roth and Hopkins Test, RH (Roth & Hopkins, 1953).

The mental status examination systems are open to all the problems described in the section on reliability and validity. The CAPE will probably generate a reasonable database in the near future.

The estimation of premorbid level of intelligence

In research work with the dementing person it is often important to try and establish the approximate intellectual level of the subject in order that appropriate comparisons can be made with people of the same level within other diagnostic categories. Two interesting variances of the vocabulary test have been found to be useful in this case.

Kendrick (1964) found that by using the score obtained from the synonym section of the Mill Hill Vocabulary Scale (Raven, 1958) and adding the appropriate 'expected' score for the definition section to obtain a total score which could be converted into an IQ equivalent gave an indication of premorbid level of intellectual function in dementing persons. It was found, when IQs derived in this manner were compared with those from the verbal scale of the WAIS, that the mean Mill Hill IQ was significantly higher than that for the WAIS in dementing subjects but that there were no significant differences between the two mean estimates for a matched group of depressed people.

A more recent device is the National Adult Reading Test (Nelson, 1982; Nelson & McKenna, 1975; Nelson & O'Connell, 1978). This test consists of irregular words where the pronunciation does not conform to regular rules. The ability to pronounce these words measures previous familiarity with them rather than current ability to analyse. However, the test is unreliable for previously low or high intellectual status subjects, nor has it been standardized on subjects over the age of 70 years. Both these techniques rely on previous familiarity with the language, which may be a diagnostic tool which has been neglected in dementia.

Behavioural changes

Not only is a diagnostic assessment of the pathology of the disabled/dementing person useful, but also the degree and type of disability. Therefore it is important to know not only what the person is capable of cognitively but physically and habitually as well.

The analysis of the behavioural field has lead to the notion of the area of activities of daily living assessment (ADL). This is one of three methods that are currently in use, the others being survey indices and global ratings of impairment. The behavioural analysis approach is that of the evaluation of 'functional status' or 'behavioural competence'.

One of the greatest problems with any of these types of analysis is that important discrepancies exist between self-report, observer report and performance-based report in assessing ADL function in the elderly (Kuriansky et al, 1976). As such, survey methods and global ratings have been subject to a great deal of unreliability.

Since the mid-1960s, measurement concerns have shifted from psychopathology to self-care impairment, and an increased interest in the scaling and construct validity of these devices. Factor analysis has been applied to many ADL scales, revealing that three consistent sources of disability emerge: physical diability or self-care impairment, cognitive function impairment, and social–emotional behaviour disturbance (Gilleard, 1984b). Gilleard has investigated 28 rating scales developed for use with the elderly. He found that there were wide ranges in the number of items used, with those containing few items giving a wide response format, whilst those containing many items generally used the forced-choice yes/no technique. Those scales with few items tended to focus on physical disability or self-care impairment, in contrast to those scales with many items which tended to contain more of the social interaction-disturbance and mood-related type. Scales that have been developed since 1970 appear to have a broader, more evenly spread set of items than those produced previously. However, Gilleard still notes a discrepancy between the ADL approach and that of the behaviour rating scale methodology. This division maintains the concept of a single construct of disability rather than a multidimensional one. Future developments in this area will probably focus on the interactions between biological/mechanical and social/environmental influences on measures of disability. Incompetence is not the constitutional right of the elderly, and matters can be altered by both positive and negative medical and environmental interventions. What might be the limits of these interventions is unknown. One such intervention is reality orientation (RO).

REALITY ORIENTATION

Reality orientation therapy was developed by Tualbee & Folson (1966) to counteract environmental understimulation in the institutionalized. It consists essentially of verbal, visual and tactile repetition to patients of the time, date, weather, names of others in the group, along with common courtesies, the use of money and the identification and use of common utensils. Today, in 1985, RO is in a state of crisis. Research indicates only marginal improvement in the functioning of patients where RO is the current form of treatment. Holden & Woods, 1982; Powell-Proctor & Miller, 1982; Hanley, 1984; and Greene, 1984, have all reviewed the current status of RO. One of RO's objectives is to improve cognitive and behavioural functioning, but it can also be seen as basically humanitarian in its concern for the way in which care is given to people with dementias. However, according to Hanley (1984), RO is in a conceptual dilemma. There appears to be no consensus as to what constitutes RO. It ranges from a board on a wall giving day, date and time, to 24-hour monitoring. Clear definitions of aims and procedures need to be developed. RO seems to be practical common sense, but it has failed to develop over the past 20 years scientifically. Much more evidence from empirical studies of memory, learning and behaviour both of an experimental and clinical nature need to be incorporated into RO procedures. This would give it greater scientific credibility and allow for future evaluation and development.

COMPUTERS AND THE ELDERLY

If psychologists are going to develop assessment techniques that are part of the elderly person's ecology, then within ten years the 65-year-old will be computer-aware. Kendrick (1982a) argued against the use of cumputers for the assessment of the elderly because they latter were not familiar with them. But since then there has been a huge increase in the computerization of the Western world.

Researchers working with computer-assisted assessment of the dementing elderly have found some problems. A meeting held in June 1983 at University College Hospital, London, of research workers in this field item-ized the following difficulties: Responses need to involve minimum physical effort, because of movement or muscular problems. Responses need to be accompanied by a 'clock' to maintain attention. Response pads should be mobile so that they can be attached to wheelchairs etc. Old people, being long-sighted, do not like to sit near the screen. The main problem identified with the demented was that they fail to grasp the relationship between the screen and the keyboard, so that extensive practice was required. It is prob-ably not appropriate to expect dementing subjects to be able to be tested by means of computer operations. If it takes so long to teach the person to respond, this defeats the whole exercise.

The use of computers for assessing the elderly will come about by using the equipment to monitor cognitive status long before any dementing process is behaviourally apparent. Computers will also be useful in simulating everyday activities such as supermarket shopping (Rabbitt, 1982a). Computers will allow the development of entirely new tests with accurate time measurements as well as response scoring and the rapid manipulation of data with constant references to databases.

Computer sound and graphics are now so good that the attention problems of the elderly person can be maintained by various procedures.

However, computer-assisted assessment techniques will be subject to the same standards of reliability and validity restraints as in all forms of psychometric work. This will take considerable time and effort to effect. It will also mean that when computer tests are developed, there should be manual versions developed as well, since computers do break down, programs will not load etc. It will mean too that a complete interrelationship between the computer and manual forms of the tests will have to be established.

CONCLUSIONS

In this chapter the development of the cognitive assessment movement in relation to the elderly with particular reference to the dementing has been discussed. The author has stressed that experimental, psychometric and applied fields have to a certain extent developed separately. It has also been emphasized that from the 1950s to the early 1970s the integrative lifespan developmental psychology research paradigm held sway. This paradigm has recently been opposed by the ecology of testing movement. This stresses that there are important differences in the type of intelligence and memory tests that are appropriate for each generation. To give the same intelligence tests throughout the lifespan is to disadvantage some generations. Because of this, many of the traditional psychological tests are inappropriate if applied to certain age cohorts. It is only now that specialized tests are being developed for the elderly, and too many ad hoc tests are being used. This has resulted in difficulties in comparing the outcomes of research studies, as researchers in other areas of gerontology have not been slow to point out (Smith et al, 1979).

Therefore there is now a great challenge to psychometrists to develop tests with adequate databases and take into account not only the experimental psychologists' findings but also those from other disciplines where brain–behaviour relationships are being discovered. Psychologists, including the author, have been criticized both at the theoretical and practical level for using global diagnostic categories such as 'diffuse brain damage'. Gilleard (1984b) presents a review of the evidence as to why global categories need to be more carefully researched. The author is aware that tests should be devised which could discriminate between the different dementias, especially between multi-infarct and SDAT.

In discussing why the elderly should be assessed, Kendrick (1982a) indicated four areas where research is urgently required. These were: the detection of early SDAT; the pseudodementing effects of the anticholinergic drugs; the significance of late-onset depression; and the relationship between physical activity, ageing and mental status. Professor Rabbitt, who debated these points in the literature (Rabbitt, 1982a), at the Age and Cognitive Performance Research Centre at Manchester University, is already researching with the collaboration of Professor Gray and his colleagues at the Institute of Psychiatry new techniques for assessing the cognitive status of the Alzheimer patient. If the elderly do become computer-aware, then there really is a magnificent opportunity to develop new methods of cognitive assessment for them. In the manual for the KCTE, Kendrick (1985) sets out a five-year plan for the computerization of the tests. However, the KDCT is not amenable to computerization because it relies for its effectiveness on the subject's well-practised ability to write numbers. It cannot be assumed that people will be universally adept with a Qwerty keyboard. Therefore a new test will have to be devised to substitute for the KDCT. Branconnier & De Vitt (1983) are also developing a similar system concerning the early detection of incipient Alzheimer's disease. Of the tests specifically designed for use with the elderly, both the KCTE and the CAPE are developing respectable databases. The KCTE is appearing in a variety of research projects, from survey work to heart operations and the effects of general anaesthetics.

Under the general heading of the transmission, meaning and retrieval of information there should be a gradual merging of the three areas of the psychology of ageing to produce a more coherent whole.

REFERENCES

Arie T 1981 Don't play the parcel game with the demented. Geriatric Medicine July/August: 9–11
Barber J H 1981 Screening and assessment: a challenge to GPs. Geriatric Medicine April: 39–45
Beaumont G 1982 Dementia and the general practitioner. Psychiatry in Practice 1:5
Berg S, Svensson T 1980 An orientation scale for geriatric patients. Age and Ageing 9: 215–219
Bolton N, Britton P G, Savage R D 1966 Some normative data on the WAIS and its indices in an aged population. Journal of Clinical Psychology 22: 183–188
Botwinick J 1978 Aging behavior: a comprehensive integration of research findings. Springer, New York
Branconnier RJ, De Vitt DR 1983 Early detection of incipient Alzheimer's disease: some methodological considerations on computerized diagnosis. In: Reisberg B (ed) Alzheimer's disease, the standard reference. Free Press, New York
Bromley D B 1974 The psychology of human ageing, 2nd edn. Penguin, Harmondsworth
Carson J 1984 Why is the Halstead Reitan Battery so unpopular with British clinical psychologists? Newsletter of the Divison of Clinical Psychology 46: 58–60
Church M, Wattis J P 1983 The importance of assessment. Geriatric Medicine November: 833–835

Coleman P G 1984 Assessing self esteem and its sources in elderly people. Ageing and Society 4: 117–135

Copeland J R M et al 1976 A semi-structured clinical interview for the assessment of diagnosis and mental state in the elderly

The Geriatric Mental State Schedule: 1 Development and reality. Psychological Medicine 6: 439–449

Cowan D W et al 1975 Cross-national study of diagnosis in the mental disorders: a comparative psychometric assessment of the elderly patients admitted to mental hospitals serving Queen's County, New York and the former Borough of Camberwell, London. British Journal of Psychiatry 126: 560–570

Craik F I M, Byrd M 1982 Aging and cognitive deficits: the role of attentional resources. In: Craik F I M, Trehub S (eds) Aging and cognitive processes. Plenum Press, New York

Craik F I M, Lockhart R S 1972 Levels of processing: a framework for memory research. Journal of Verbal Learning and Verbal Behavior 11: 671–684

Craik F I M, Trehub S (eds) 1982 Aging and cognitive processes. Plenum Press, New York

Cutler N E, Schmidhauser J R 1975 Age and political behaviour. In: Woodruff D S, Birren J E (eds) Aging: scientific perspectives and social issues. Van Nostrand, London

Davies A, Goldberg G B, Wilkinson I 1984 A methodology for manpower planning. Nursing Times 80: 44–46

Drinkwater J 1981 The Kendrick Battery and other neuro-psychological assessments in known cases of brain damage. Paper read at Kendrick Battery Workshop, University of Hull, Hull

Edmunds G, Kendrick D C 1980 The measurement of human aggressiveness. Ellis Horwood, Chichester

Erickson R S, Scott M L 1977 Clinical memory testing: a review. Psychological Bulletin 84: 1130–1149

Eysenck H J 1976 The measurement of personality. MTP, Lancaster

Filskov S, Boll T 1981 Handbook of clinical neuropsychology. Wiley, Chichester

Fish M, Marcus S, Hayslip B, Haynes J R 1982 Validity of the Kendrick Battery in differentiating organicity and depression in the institutionalized aged. Presented at the 90th Annual Convention of the American Psychological Association, Washington DC

Folstein M F, Goldstein S E, McHugh P R 1975 Mini-Mental State: a practical method for grading the cognitive state of patients for the clinician. Journal of Psychiatric Research 12: 189–198

Gibson A J 1979 Institutionalization: its effect on the cognitive status of long stay psychiatric patients who are elderly. Unpublished doctoral dissertation, University of Hull Library, Hull

Gibson A J 1981 A further analysis of memory loss in dementia and depression in the elderly. British Journal of Clinical Psychology 20: 179–185

Gibson A J, Kendrick D C 1979 The Kendrick battery for the detection of dementia in the elderly. NFER-Nelson, Windsor

Gibson A J, Moyes I C A, Kendrick D C 1980 Cognitive assessment of the elderly long-stay patient. British Journal of Psychiatry 137: 537–55

Gilleard C J 1980 Wechsler Memory Scale performance of elderly psychiatric patients. Journal of Clinical Psychology 36: 958–960

Gilleard C J 1984a Assessment of cognitive impairment in the elderly: a review. In: Hanley I, Hodge J (eds) Psychological approaches to the care of the elderly. Croom Helm, London

Gilleard C J 1984b Assessment of behavioural impairment in the elderly: a review. In: Hanley I, Hodge J (eds) Psychological approaches to the care of the elderly. Croom Helm, London

Glen A I M 1979 Choice of therapeutic agents in Alzheimer's disease. In: Glen A I M, Whalley L J (eds) Alzheimer's disease: early recognition of potentially reversible deficits. Churchill Livingstone, Edinburgh

Golden C 1979 Luria-Nebraska neuropsychological test battery. University of Nebraska Press, Omaha

Golden C, Osmon D, Moses J, Berg R 1980 Interpretation of the Halstead-Reitan neuropsychological test battery. A casebook approach. Grune & Stratton, New York

Greene J G 1984 the evaluation of reality orientation. In: Hanley I, Hodge J 1984 (eds) Psychological approaches to the care of the elderly. Croom Helm, London

Gurland B 1980 The assessment of mental health status of older adults. In Birren J E, Sloan R B (eds) Handbook of mental health and aging. McGraw-Hill, New York

Hanley I 1984 Theoretical and practical considerations in reality orientation therapy with the elderly. In: Hanley I, Hodge J 1984 (eds) Psychological approaches to the care of the elderly. Croom Helm, London

Hendrickson E, Levy R, Post F 1979 Average evoked responses in relation to cognitive and affective state of anxiety of elderly psychiatric patients. British Journal of Psychiatry 134: 494–501

Hetherington R 1965 A neologism learning test. Bulletin of the British Psychological Society 18: 21A–22A

Heston L L, White J A 1983 Dementia. Freeman, New York

Hinton J, Withers E 1971 The usefulness of the clinical tests of the sensorium. British Journal of Psychiatry 119: 9–18

Holden U P, Woods R 1982 Reality orientation. Churchill Livingstone, Edinburgh

Hodgkinson H M 1972 Evaluation of a mental test score for assessment of mental impairment in the elderly. Age and Ageing 1: 233–238

ınglis J 1959 A paired associate learning test for use with elderly psychiatric patients. Journal of Mental Science 105: 440–448

Irving G, Robinson R A, McAdam W 1970 The validity of some cognitive tests in the diagnosis of dementia. British Journal of Psychiatry 117: 149–156

Isaacs B, Walkey F A 1964 Measurement of mental impairment in geriatric practice. Gerontologia Clinica 6: 114–123

Jacoby R J, Levy R 1980a Computed tomography in the elderly. 2. Senile dementia diagnosis and functional impairment. British Journal of Psychiatry 136: 256–269

Jacoby R J, Levy R 1980b Computed tomography in the elderly. 3. Affective disorder. British Journal of Psychiatry 136: 270–275

Kahn R L, Goldfarb A l, Pollack M, Gerber I E 1960 Brief objective measures for the determination of mental status in the aged. American Journal of Psychiatry 117: 326–328

Kausler D H 1982 Experimental psychology and human aging. Wiley, New York

Kendrick D C 1964 The assessment of premorbid level of intelligence in elderly patients suffering from diffuse brain pathology. Psychological Reports 15: 188

Kendrick D C 1965 Speed and learning in the diagnosis of diffuse brain damage in elderly subjects. British Journal of Social and Clinical Psychology 4: 141–148

Kendrick D C 1967 A cross-validation study of the SLT and DCT in screening for diffuse brain pathology in elderly patients. British Journal of Medical Psychology 40: 173–178

Kendrick D C 1968 The problem of differentiating dementia from normal ageing and depression. In: Clarke P R F (ed) The nature and consequences of brain lesions in children. British Psychological Society, London

Kendrick D C 1972 The Kendrick battery of tests: theoretical assumptions and clinical uses. British Journal of Social and Clinical Psychology 11: 373–386

Kendrick D C 1975 Activity and ageing. New Behaviour 1: 256–258

Kendrick D C 1982a Why assess the aged? : a clinical psychologist's view. British Journal of Clinical Psychology 21: 47–54

Kendrick D C 1982b Psychometrics and neurological models: a reply to Dr Rabbitt. British Journal of Clinical Psychology 21: 61–62

Kendrick D C 1982c Administrative and interpretive problems with the Kendrick Battery for the Detection of Dementia in the Elderly. British Journal of Clinical Psychology 21: 149–150

Kendrick D C 1984 Open-field behaviour, growth rate and life span in the black-hooded rat. Mechanisms of Ageing and Development 26: 265–275

Kendrick D C 1985 The Kendrick cognitive tests for the elderly. NFER-Nelson, Windsor

Kendrick D C, Moyes I C A 1979 Activity, depression, medication and performance on the revised Kendrick Battery. British Journal of Social and Clinical Psychology 18: 341–350

Kendrick D C, Post F 1967 Differences in cognitive status between healthy, psychiatrically ill and diffusely brain-damaged elderly subjects. British Journal of Psychiatry 113: 75–81

Kendrick D C, Gibson A J, Moyes I C A 1979 The revised Kendrick Battery: clinical studies. British Journal of Social and Clinical Psychology 18: 329–339

Kendrick D C, Parboosingh R C, Post F 1965 A synonym learning test for use with elderly psychiatric patients: a validation study. British Journal of Social and Clinical Psychology 4: 63–71

Kuriansky J B, Gurland B J, Fleiss J L 1976 The assessment of self-care capacity in geriatric psychiatric patients by objective and subjective methods. Journal of Clinical Psychology 32: 95–102

Marcer D 1979 Measuring memory change in Alzheimer's disease. In: Glen A I M, Whalley L J (eds) Alzheimer's disease: early recognition of potentially reversible deficits. Churchill Livingstone, Edinburgh

McCurran C A, Ganong L H 1984 Assessing cognitive functioning in the elderly with the 'Inventory of Piaget's Developmental Tasks'. Journal of Advanced Nursing 9: 449–456

McDonald C 1969 Clinical heterogeneity in senile dementia. British Journal of Psychiatry 115: 267–271

McHugh P 1975 Dementia. In: Beeson P B, McDermott W (eds) Textbook of medicine, 14th edn. Saunders, Philadelphia

McKechnie A A, Corser C M 1984 The role of psychogeriatric assessment units in a comprehensive psychiatric service. Health Bulletin 42: 25–29

Marsden C D, Harrison M J G, 1982 Outcome of investigation of patients with presenile dementia. British Journal of Medicine 2: 249–252

Miller E 1977 Abnormal ageing: the psychology of presenile dementia. Wiley, Chichester

Naguib M, Levy R 1982 Prediction of outcome in senile dementia — a computed tomography study. British Journal of Psychiatry 140: 263–267

Nelson H E 1982 The National Adult Reading Test. NFER-Nelson, Windsor

Nelson H E, McKenna P 1975 The use of current reading disability in the assessment of dementia. British Journal of Social and Clinical Psychology 14: 259–267

Nelson H E, O'Connell A 1978 Dementia: the estimation of premorbid intelligence levels using the New Adult Reading Test. Cortex 14: 234–244

Neisser U 1976 Cognition and reality. Freeman, San Franciso

Nott P N, Fleminger J J 1975 Presenile dementia: the difficulties of an early diagnosis. Acta Psychiatrica Scandinavica 51: 210–217

Pattie A H 1981 A survey version of the Clifton Assessment Procedures for the Elderly (CAPE). British Journal of Clinical Psychology 20: 173–180

Pattie A H, Gilleard C J 1979 Manual for the Clifton Assessment Procedures for the Elderly. Hodder & Stoughton Educational, Sevenoaks

Pattie A H, Gilleard C J, Bell J 1979 The relationship of the intellectual and behavioural competence of the elderly and future needs from community, residential and hospital services. Report to the Yorkshire Regional Health Authority

Perlmutter M, Mitchell D B 1982 The appearance and disappearance of age differences in adult memory. In: Craig F I M, Trehub S (eds) Aging and cognitive processes. Plenum Press, New York

Pfeiffer E 1975 A short portable mental status questionnaire for the assessment of organic brain deficit in elderly patients. Journal of the American Geriatrics Society 23: 433–441

Platt S 1980 On establishing the validity of objective data: can we rely on cross-interview agreement. Psychological Medicine 10: 573–581

Poon L W, Fozard J L, Cermak L S, Arenberg D, Thompson L W 1980 New directions in memory and aging. Erlbaum, Hollsdale, New Jersey

Post F 1966 Somatic and psychic factors in the treatment of elderly psychiatric patients. Journal of Psychosomatic Research 10: 13–18

Post F 1975 Dementia, depression and pseudodementia. In: Benson D F, Blumer D (eds) Psychiatric aspects of neurological disease. Grune & Stratton, New York

Poulton K 1984 A measure of independence. Nursing Times 80 August: 32–35

Powell-Procter L, Miller E 1982 Reality orientation: a critical appraisal. British Journal of Psychiatry 140: 457–463

Rabbitt P 1982a How to assess the aged? An experimental psychologist's view. Some comments on Dr Kendrick's paper. British Journal of Clinical Psychology 21: 55–60

Rabbitt P 1982b How do old people know what to do next? In: Craik F I M, Trehub S (eds) Aging and cognitive processes. Plenum Press, New York

Raven J C 1958 Guide to using the Mill Hill Vocabulary Scale with the Progressive Metrices. Lewis, London

Roberts M A, Caird F T 1976 Computerised tomography and intellectual impairment in the elderly. Journal of Neurology, Neurosurgery and Psychiatry 39: 986–989
Robertson C 1984 Screening for health. Nursing Times 80 August: 44–45
Robertson R J, Malchik D L 1968 The reliability of global ratings versus specific ratings. Journal of Clinical Psychology 23: 256–258
Roth M, Hopkins B 1953 Psychological test performance in patients over sixty. Journal of Mental Science 99: 439–450
Routtenberg A 1968 The two-arousal hypothesis: reticular formation and limbic system. Psychological Review 75: 51–80
Russell E W 1975 A multiple scoring method for the assessment of complex memory functions. Journal of Consulting and Clinical Psychology 43: 800–809
Russell E W, Neuringer C, Goldstein G 1970 Assessment of brain damage. A neuropsychological key approach. Wiley, New York
Schaie K W 1970 A reinterpretation of age-related changes in cognitive structure and functioning. In: Goulet G R, Baltes P B (eds) Life-span developmental psychology: research and theory. Academic Press, New York
Schaie K W 1979 The primary mental abilities in adulthood: an exploration in the development of psychometric intelligence. In: Baltes P B, Brim O G (eds) Life-span development and behaviour. Academic Press, New York
Schaie K W 1980 Intelligence and problem solving. In:Birren J E, Sloane R B (eds) Handbook of mental health and aging. Prentice-Hall, Englewood Cliffs, New Jersey
Searle R T 1984 A community based follow-up of some suspected cases of early dementia: an interim report. Bulletin of the British Psychological Society 37: A20–A21
Smith C M, Swash M, Exton-Smith A N 1979 Effects of cholinergic drugs on memory in Alzheimer's disease. In: Glen A I M, Whalley L J (eds) Alzheimer's disease: early recognition of potentially reversible deficits. Churchill Livingstone, Edinburgh
Stefoski D, Bergen D, Fox J, Morrell F, Huckman M, Ramsey R 1976 Correlation between diffuse EEG abnormalities and cerebal atrophy in senile dementia. Journal of Neurology, Neurosurgery and Psychiatry 39: 751–755
Stout I, Jolley D 1981 The dementia syndrome: how to recognise it. Geriatric Medicine February: 15–18
Surwillo W W 1970 Timing of behavior in senescence and the role of the central nervous system. In: Talland G A (ed) Human aging and behavior. Academic Press, New York
Taulbee L R, Folsom J C 1966 Reality orientation for geriatric patients. Hospital and Community Psychiatry 17: 133–135
Thornton E W 1984 Exercise and ageing: an uproven relationship. University of Liverpool Press, Liverpool
Voland P J, Woods R T 1983 Why do we assess the aged? British Journal of Clinical Psychology 22: 213–214
Walton D 1958 The diagnosis and predictive accuracy of the Modified Word Learning Test in psychiatric patients over 65. Journal of Mental Science 104: 1119–1122
Weingartner H, Kaye W, Smallberg S A, Ebert M H, Gillin J C, Sitaram N 1981 Memory failures in progressive idiopathic dementia. Journal of Abnormal Psychology 90: 187–196
Whalley L J 1981 Differential diagnosis and management of dementia. Geriatric Medicine 11 January: 179–186
Whitehead A 1973 Verbal learning and memory in depressives. British Journal of Psychiatry 123: 203–208
Wilcock G 1984 Research into Alzheimer's disease is bearing fruit. Geriatric Medicine 14 July/August: 12–15
Wilkinson I, Zissler L M 1984 Standardised assessments for the elderly: clinical applications. Nursing Times 80 January: 36–37
Wilson, B A, Moffatt, N (eds) 1984 Clinical management of memory problems. Croom Helm, Beckenham
Woodruff D S 1982 Advances in the psychophysiology of aging. In: Craik F I M, Trehub S (eds) Aging and cognitive processes. Plenum Press, New York

Electrophysiological and brain imaging investigations

Electrophysiological and brain imaging techniques used in the study and evaluation of dementia include:
1. Electroencephalography
2. Cortical evoked potentials
3. X-ray computerized tomography
4. Positron emission tomography
5. Single photon emission tomography
6. Nuclear magnetic resonance imaging

ELECTROENCEPHALOGRAPHY (EEG)

EEG is a measure of cortical activity and, as such, should be useful in the diagnosis of dementia and in categorizing the clinical subgroup. However, there are difficulties in interpreting the results of EEG findings, particularly in separating ageing factors and the effects of drugs and concomitant physical illness, particularly cardiovascular or metabolic. Furthermore, conventional techniques do not readily lend themselves to quantification

Changes take place in the EEG during the process of maturation which stabilize during adult life only to give way to further effects with advancing age (Davis, 1941). The alpha rhythm in young adults has a mean frequency of 10–10.5 Hz. This declines with age to 9–9.5 Hz at age 70 and 8.5–9 Hz at 80 years (Katz & Horowitz, 1982). The decrease in frequency is prominent in dementia, when a decline to less than 7 Hz is common. The posterior dominant alpha frequency declines by 0.08 Hz per year of age over 60 (Wang & Busse, 1969).

Changes in beta rhythm have been more inconsistently reported. Although the frequency is much the same in the young as in the elderly (Mundy-Castle, 1951), the amplitude is greater in the latter. Computer frequency analysis (Roubicek, 1977) allows separation of this frequency band into its two components — those less than 30 Hz and those greater. The former decreases with a decline in alpha frequency, but the latter does not.

Diffuse and focal slow activity (theta and delta) increase with age. These changes correlate with reduction in cognitive functions and reduction in lifespan (Muller & Schwartz, 1978), and are greatest in the more severe cases. Slight changes in EEG activity may occur in those with normal intellectual functions. Intermittent focal theta and delta activity occurs over the temporal regions, particularly the left, in elderly persons (Kooi et al, 1964). Such changes are not the invariable consequences of ageing being seen in only 17% of normal 70-year-olds and occupying only 1% of the EEG recording (Katz & Horowitz, 1982)

With increasing age, total sleep falls, particularly in stages 3 and 4, and this is reflected in EEG changes. Decreases in REM sleep correlate with cognitive and memory decline (Kahn & Fisher, 1969), and are particularly noted in the demented (Johannesson et al, 1977).

EEG may be of value in distinguishing dementia from pseudo-dementia due to functional disorders and in separating those due to focal lesions from the diffuse types. Serial EEGs are more helpful than a single recording, particularly if a record is available early on in the illness. In general, EEG abnormality correlates well with severity of dementia (Johannesson et al, 1977) as measured in psychometric tests, but poorly with degree of cortical atrophy as measured by X-ray computerized tomography (Kaszniak et al, 1979).

During the early stages of Alzheimer's disease the EEG may be normal or may show minimal slowing of the alpha rhythm. If focal cognitive deficits are present, this may be reflected in focal or lateralized slowing on EEG, which is mild or intermittent. More continuous slowing should cause the diagnosis to be questioned. As the disease progresses, generalized slowing appears and bursts of bilateral synchronous frontal temporal delta activity, worsening during drowsiness, occur. The preservation of the alpha rhythm in the presence of often moderate or severe background abnormalities would require the diagnosis of Alzheimer's disease to be questioned. The greater the slowing, the more rapid the disease course (Swain, 1959). The EEG in Pick's disease remains normal or near normal, even in advanced cases.

The relationship between EEG slowing and decreased cerebral blood flow has given contradictory results. Multi-infarct dementia gives rise to focal or bilateral independent slowing on the EEG with preservation of the alpha rhythm.

Creutzfeldt-Jakob disease, in its early stages, shows mild excessive generalized slowing, more marked over one hemisphere, or focal. With progression, repetitive sharp waves at 0.5–1 s intervals, initially unilateral but eventually becoming bilateral and synchronous, occur (Au et al, 1980). Repetitive sharp waves are occassionally seen in Binswanger's subcortical encephalophy (White, 1979) and Alzheimer's disease (Watson, 1979). These sharp waves do not occur with the regular rate characteristic of Creutzfeldt-Jakob, and in any case serial EEG should help resolve any uncertainty.

Most EEG studies in Parkinson's disease show non-specific slow wave abnormalities in as many as 40% of patients (Sirakov & Rezan, 1963). The commonest finding is decrease in frequency of the posterior dominant rhythm below 8 Hz. This should be distinguished from the tremor artefact sometimes seen in this region.

Although mild EEG abnormalities are not unusual in older patients with Huntington's chorea, these are generally present in the more advanced cases and are of no value in identifying prodromal phases of the disease. In cases with established dementia there is overall reduction in voltage to less than $10\mu V$ in about one-third of cases (Scott et al, 1972).

EVOKED POTENTIALS (EPs)

Event-related potentials or evoked potentials are changes in brain electrical activity following a specific event such as a sensory stimulus or a movement. These are not ordinarily visible in the EEG but may be extracted from the EEG record by a procedure known as averaging. The electrical changes in EEG activity following a given event are added together, and temporal components separated longitudinally using digital computer methods. Several types of EPs are present:
1. Sensory EPs elicited by sensory stimuli
2. Long latency potentials associated more with meaning than the physical properties of the stimulus
3. Motor potentials associated with movement
4. Contingent negative variation (CNV)

Prolongation of latency of the cortical evoked response and lower amplitude of response occur in the elderly when a sensory stimulus is applied (Levy et al, 1971). The delays are central in location, as impairment of peripheral sensory nerve conduction does not occur in senile dementia. Similar delays are found in the visual evoked response.

Transmission time (interval between peaks I and V) of auditory evoked response is prolonged in Alzheimer's disease compared with control subjects (Harkins, 1981). These changes are not age-related, and suggest brain-stem pathology in these patients. Increasing stimulus strength enchances the amplitude of the auditory evoked potential and shortens the latencies of both short and long latency components. When further information is added irregularly and the subject is asked to respond to these, the positive and negative elements of the long latency undergo changes and a new phenomenom appears at an interval of 300–350 ms — the P_{300} wave (Sutton et al, 1965). The latency of P_{300} increases with age and even more with dementia. The P_{300} wave appears when a subject perceives and carries out a congnitive process in response to an occasional stimulus of which he or she is warned beforehand. Inattention, stress and fatigue may alter the P_{300}. P_{300} latencies correctly classified 80% of a group of demented patients and gave only 5% false positive results (Goodin et al, 1978). The P_{300} latency increases in dementia to a much greater degree than do the earlier responses, in relation to ageing, suggesting that the effects of ageing and dementia on the two components are different. Some studies have, however, failed to confirm these findings (Slaets & Fortgens, 1984). Early visual evoked potential amplitudes are greater and latencies after 100 ms increased in elderly demented compared with age-matched controls (Vissen et al, 1976).

If an individual is given a warning stimulus followed by a second stimulus which requires a response, a negative potential can be recorded from the vertex. The negative potential that appears between the first stimulus and response is called the contingent negative variation (CNV) (Walter et al, 1964). These may be influenced by the cognitive set of the individual. Apart from these factors, ageing and dementia contribute by virtue of delaying reaction times or prolonging decision-making.

X-RAY COMPUTERIZED TOMOGRAPHY

This technique can be used in a number of ways to evaluate dementia:
1. Diagnosis of gross morphological lesions: infarcts, tumors, haematomata
2. Evaluating cerebral atrophy by:
   a. Assessing size of cortical sulci
   b. Various linear measures of increase in size of ventricles, e.g. width between frontal horns of lateral ventricles, 3rd ventricular width at the level of the caudate nucleus
   c. Area ratios, e.g. ventricular brain ratio
   d. Volume measures of cerebrospinal fluid spaces (ventricular, subarachnoid)
   e. Region of interest measures of altered X-ray density

The value of X-ray CT in diagnosing gross pathological changes involving the brain is undisputed. Of 500 consecutive cases of dementia investigated, most showed cerebral atrophy or infarction. Eighty-two were normal and 42 revealed tumours, In all, 10% had a treatable lesion and 5% had no other sign or symptoms (Bradshaw et al, 1983). Important treatable causes include normal pressure hydrocephalus (Rudick & Joynt, 1980) with its characteristic features. The presence of 'hypernormal' CT scans in isodense subdural haematomas which show small ventricles and minimal sulci should be particularly noted (Jacobson & Farmer, 1979). Some chronic subdural haematomata may appear as calcified lesions (Debois & Lombaert, 1980). The presence of cerebellar atrophy in the elderly independent of cerebral atrophy and without clinical signs has been observed (Koller et al, 1981).

Ventricular size has been shown to increase with age in both normals and those with a dementing process (Barron et al, 1976; Ford & White, 1981). Although the extent of the age variation in normals has been shown to differ (Jacoby, 1980a), patients with dementia show more atrophy than non-demented persons of equivalent age (Fox et al, 1975; Jacoby et al, 1980b), but there is overlap, with some non-dementing patients showing consider-able cerebral atrophy. Cortical atrophy and ventricular dilatation correlate with each other in controls, but not in dements. This tends to suggest that the atrophy process in ageing and dementia may be different. In controls, cognitive decline correlates with cortical atrophy, but in dements it corre-lates with ventricular dilatation. The digit symbol test correlates most highly with ventricular measures and latency of auditory evoked potential (Hendrickson et al, 1979). On the other hand, there is an inverse relation-ship between cortical atrophy and the presence of delusions in dements (Jacoby et al, 1980b). The age-related increase in cortical sulci in normals over the age of 60 is not present in dements, who tend to show higher values in all age groups (Kohlmeyer & Shamena, 1983). Differences between the groups only reached significance in those aged 60–69. This same study gave further conformation of the findings that the atrophy change of dements were predominantly identified by increased ventricular dimensions by showing that, although both 3rd ventricular diameter and Huckman number increased with age, significant values were only obtained in the demented group. The ventricular index and scella media index are unchanged with age in both the controls and dements. They furthermore found that the strongest age correlation was in the size of the lateral ventricles and that this was confined to the demented group. Using a composite measure of cerebral atrophy derived from ventricular and sulcal widths, Wilson et al (1982) did not find any correlation between degree of atrophy and degree of dementia determined psychometrically; however, using ventricular size only, a positive correlation was found (Gado et al, 1983).

The usefulness of measures of cerebral atrophy in assisting with the diagnosis of individual early cases is limited by the absence of a clear-cut difference from normals, particularly when age-related factors have been taken into account. This problem may be partly resolved, especially in presenile groups, by serial scans at intervals of approximately 2 years. Markedly increased ventricular size, particularly of the lateral ventricles, occurs in the dementia group (Brukman & Langen, 1984) by comparison with the normals and separates those changes due to normal ageing and the dementia process. Volumetric measures of ventricular size and sulcal size can be carried out by an algorithm summation of the numbers of pixels with a pre-defined CSF range in selected brain scan sections, correcting for brain size. On this basis, cognitive deficit is correlated with ventricular size (George et al, 1983). This technique is presumed to be more accurate than linear and area measures, which have given variable results.

In multi-infarct dementia, specific lesions may be seen. These include low-density white-matter lesion subcortical lacunar infarcts and cortical infarcts (Rosenberg et al, 1979; Loizon et al, 1981).

Dementia is associated with histopathological changes in various regions of the brain. These tend to be most marked in frontal and temporal lobes.

Such changes are not seen on visual examination of the scans but may be identified by numerical measures of X-ray density of the tissues. X-ray CT numbers or Hounsfield units may be obtained for various regions of interest. Patients with senile dementia had significantly reduced Hounsfield units in the frontal and medial temporal lobes and head of the caudate nucleus of both sides. These differences were not related to age or to the size of the ventricles (Bondareff et al, 1981). Although reductions in CT numbers were also found by Naeser et al (1980) in patients with presenile dementia, Wilson et al (1982) found no difference in a group of senile dements. Gado (1983) found no differences in density measures of pure grey or white matter samples between senile dements and controls, but there was loss of discriminability between these two tissues. Correlations between some density measures and psychometric test results were reported. This technique suffers from the problems of instrument variation, and patient variation in the X-ray penetration of extracerebral tissues. This limits its use in assessing individual cases, and may account for some of the discrepant findings.

POSITRON EMISSION TOMOGRAPHY (PET)

PET is a method of imaging the distribution of a pharmaceutical in the body. Certain cyclotron produced radionuclides decay by emitting positrons (positively charged electrons). Each positron decays rapidly into a pair of gamma-rays which travel in diametrically opposite directions. The pharmaceutical or substrate to be studied is labelled with a chemically appropriate positron emitter before being administered to the patient. The gamma-rays are detected as they emerge from the patient, and by identifying pairs of gamma-rays a three-dimensional tomographic image showing the distribution of the radiopharmaceutical can be built up.

The technique is of particular interest as many biologically interesting elements have positron emitting isotopes. For example, regional cerebral blood flow (rCBF) can be measured by inhalation of the positron emitting ^{15}O in the form $C^{15}O_2$. Inhalation of this gas at a constant rate results in the ^{15}O being transferred to circulating water ($H_2{}^{15}O$). This labelled water diffuses into the brain, and the balance between diffusion into and diffusion out of the brain and the rapid radioactive decay of the ^{15}O allows rCBF to be estimated. This test can be followed by one involving the inhalation of $^{15}O_2$. $^{15}O_2$ will label metabolically produced water. By taking the ratio of the ^{15}O distribution image to the $C^{15}O_2$ image, an image showing the regional extraction ratio of oxygen (OER) can be formed.

With increasing age both CBF and cerebral metabolic rate of oxygen ($CMRO_2$) decline, the latter to a lesser extent. There is increased oxygen extraction compensating for the fall in CBF and maintaining the $CMRO_2$ at higher levels than would be possible if $CMRO_2$ and CBF fell in parallel (Frackowiack et al, 1984). In dementia, CBF and $CMRO_2$ both decline.

This decline is greater in the more severe cases. OER is, however, maintained at the same level as in normal subjects. In both degenerative and vascular dementias, CBF and $CMRO_2$ fall but OER is maintained. Presumably, in vascular cases the O_2 requirements of metabolically active tissue are satisfied in the presence of declining blood supply by increasing the level of oxygen extraction, and in the degenerative cases reduction in metabolic requirements of ailing neuroses means that lower blood flow adequately meets the O_2 demand (Frackowiack et al, 1981). This supports the view (Hachinski et al, 1974) that chronic global cerebral ischaemia is not a major mechanism of dementia and therefore merely increasing CBF would not improve cerebral functioning. The coupling of blood flow and O_2 utilisation suggests that techniques of measuring regional CBF alone are probably a reliable way of looking at cerebral function.

Falls occur in regional (r) CBF and $rCMRO_2$ in grey (30%) and white matter (23%). These correlate with severity but not type of dementia and occur irrespective of the presence of lacunar infarction (Frackowiack et al, 1981).

In early dementia the greatest decline in $rCMRO_2$ occurred in the degenerative type and in the parietal regions predominantly, with regional decline also in frontal and temporal areas. In advanced cases decline occurred in all regions and in both dementia types. Patients with the Binswanger's type showed the lowest $rCMRO_2$ for white matter of either the vascular or degenerative groups.

The other method of measuring regional metabolic activity in brain tissue utilizes the labelling of 2-deoxyglucose with short half-life positron emitters (^{18}F or ^{11}C). This substance undergoes a single biochemical reaction, the first step (phosphorylation) of the hexokinase pathway. The total amount of the radioactive product formed and the specific activity of the precursor at the enzyme site can be determined (Sokoloff & Smith, 1983). From this data and using a correction factor for the difference in kinetic behaviour of deoxyglucose and glucose, the net rate of glucose phosphorylation measured (in vivo) is the net rate of the entire glycolytic pathway.

Imaging regional changes in cerebral glucose utilization with ^{18}fluorodeoxyglucose has shown (Kuhl et al, 1984) that the mean cerebral metabolic rate for glucose declines at a faster rate with advancing age than $CMRO_2$, taking into account effects of enlarged ventricles. Patients with Alzheimer's disease show markedly depressed glucose metabolism in the cerebral cortex averaging 30% in comparison with controls. The areas of most profound reduction are the posterior parietal lobes and adjoining areas of the posterior temporal and anterior occipital cortex.

Duration of illness but not age correlated with average cortical metabolism. In both patients and control subjects, there is a correlation between cortical glucose utilization and measures of general cognitive function, e.g. IQ. In individual patients with Alzheimer's disease there is a close relationship between principal psychometric deficit and major hypometabolic focus, e.g. language difficulties — left parasylvian region; visuo-spatial difficulties — right posterior parietal; dyscalculia — left angular gyrus; personality changes — frontal lobes. Glucose metabolism was also reduced in the basal ganglia but to a lesser extent (Chase et al, 1984).

In Parkinson's disease (Kuhl et al, 1984) global cerebral glucose utilization was reduced by about 20% compared with controls, but regional distribution was not distinguishable from that of the normal subject nor was there a relationship with clinical factors — duration, stage or severity of the disease — nor was any selective reduction in CMR glucose detected in the striatum.

In Huntington's chorea (Kuhl et al, 1984) local glucose utilization was depressed in the caudate and putamen regardless of disease duration or presence of caudate atrophy. Even in early cases the caudate is hypometabolic with respect to the rest of the brain. The mean cortical metabolic rate for glucose is normal in most patients with Huntington's chorea and correlates with neither duration of the disease nor severity of the dementia. This contrasts with the findings in Alzheimer's disease.

Protein synthesis has been studied using ^{11}C-methionine as a tracer. In Alzheimer's disease there is reduction in protein metabolism in the frontal cortex, and this is greatest in severe cases. These metabolic changes precede changes as identified by X-ray CT (Bustany et al, 1983).

Rapid advances are taking place in imaging functional events occurring in response to ageing and dementia. This will no doubt be further expanded by imaging changes in specific neurotransmitter systems, and will provide a more direct means of testing existing neurochemical hypotheses of aetiology.

SINGLE PHOTON EMISSION TOMOGRAPHY (SPET)

PET imaging techniques give useful information but unfortunately require expensive equipment and are time-consuming. Imaging of rCBF can supply information of diagnostic potential in the dementias.

There are three general methods of rCBF imaging. The first uses $C^{15}O_2$ inhalation and positron emission tomography and is described above. The second involves measuring the rate at which the brain saturates (or desaturates) an inert diffusible tracer presented to the cerebral tissue at constant concentrations. From these measures the mean transit time of the tracer across tissue can be calculated, and hence CBF. ^{133}Xe inhalation has been used for this purpose (Obrist et al, 1967). Because its low energy emission reduces its sensitivity, and since the technique requires the measurement of temporal variation in activity, a number of technical problems are encountered and image quality is usually poor.

A more useful and practicable approach utilizes a tracer which is trapped in its first pass through the brain (Sapirstein, 1958). The fraction of cardiac output retained in the brain reflects CBF. ^{99}Tc labelled microspheres have

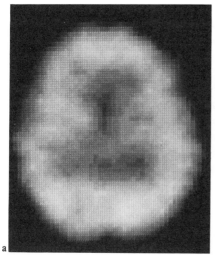

a

Fig. 5.1 (a) Normal IMP brain images of an elderly subject — transverse section at mid-ventricular level. Ventricles and white matter appear as central low uptake areas

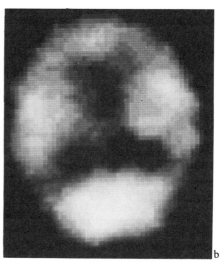

b

Fig. 5.1 (b) Section through same level as above in patient with Alzheimer's disease. Both parietal areas show very low uptake, and the frontal areas show reduced uptake

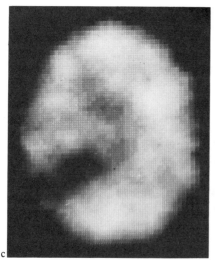

c

Fig. 5.1 (c) Multi-infarct dementia following three cerebrovascular accidents. Reduced uptake is seen in left cerebral grey, both parietal and frontal

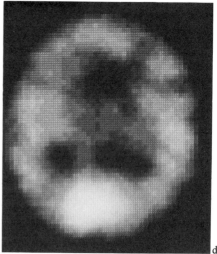

d

Fig. 5.1 (d) Multi-infarct dementia of Binswanger's type showing general reduction of uptake in both cerebral hemispheres. Note the absence of a disproportionate parietal reduction

been used (Verhas et al, 1976), but the resulting capillary occlusion results in risk, especially in those with vascular disease. ^{13}N, a positron emitter in the form of ^{13}NH$_3$, is trapped in the cerebral glutamate pool (Phelps et al, 1977) and is a suitable tracer for use in this way but requires positron imaging.

More recently, (Winchell et al, 1980), a gamma-ray emitter which is completly removed on first pass through the brain has become available. N-isopropyl ^{123}iodo amphetamine (IMP) localizes in cerebral tissue because it is lipophilic, has a high brain blood ratio and a slow washout from cerebral tissue. ^{123}I has a half-life of 13 hours. The net uptake of material remains constant during the first 24 hours, and quantitation of the uptake gives values for CBF which fall within the expected normal range. The stability of the uptake pattern allows ample time for tomography to be carried out. The value of this simple and practical imaging technique in the investigation of patients with cerebrovascular accidents, tumours and epilepsy has been demonstrated (Ell et al, 1983). There are early indications (Gemmell et al, 1984) that this technique demonstrates the reduced rCBF in the posterior parietal and frontal regions of patients with Alzheimer's disease (Fig. 5.1). The consistently reduced regional uptake of this and other tracers (^{18}FDG and ^{11}C methionine already discussed) and the correspondence with regions of neuronal degeneration (Brun & Englund 1981) may, assuming an intact blood — brain barrier, allow these tracers to act as non-specific indicators of impaired neuronal function (Friedland et al, 1985). It is of interest that this pattern of deficit has been described in the rCMRO$_2$ images (Frackowiack et al, 1981) and in the ^{18}FDG images (Kuhl et al, 1984) of patients with Alzheimer's disease. rCBF in multi-infarct dementia shows a patchy reduction, and in Huntington's chorea with dementia the CBF is normal, again in keeping with the ^{18}FDG findings (Kuhl et al, 1984).

This technique of rCBF imaging as a diagnostic instrument may have greater practical application by virtue of its non-invasive nature and relatively low cost by comparison with other dynamic imaging techniques.

NUCLEAR MAGNETIC RESONANCE (NMR)

The notion of constructing images based on the behaviour of protons in response to magnetic influences (Damadian, 1974; Lauterbur, 1973) has developed (Mallard et al, 1980) to the current status of a clinical imaging technique of great value. Protons (hydrogen nuclei) are spinning charged particles. When placed in a static magnetic field generated by large electromagnets, they align themselves in the direction of that field. If the magnetization is momentarily tilted away from the direction of the original field by application of a radio frequency pulse (RF), the angle at which the protons spin (precess) alters and then gradually recovers (relaxes). A variety of RF pulse sequences have been used. The 'spin echo' technique (Hahn, 1950) involves a one-second sequence of 90° RF pulses with 180° RF pulses at varying intervals after the first RF pulse. The 'spin-warp' technique (Johnson et al, 1981) employing a 2-second sequence of 90° pulses at one-second intervals with a 180° pulse at a varying time (tau, usually 200ms) before alternate 90° pulses. Signals are detected following the applications of these RF pulses. The decay characteristics of these signals reflect the relaxation behaviour of the protons as they return to their previous position. These signals are detected by the same coils that provide RF pulses. The frequency at which protons precess depends on the magnetic field strength. To achieve spatial discrimination, a magnetic field gradient is employed across the object to be imaged. Small differences in precession frequency generated by this allow position coding of individual voxels imaged.

The pulse sequence employed in spin-warp imaging allows a variety of data to be collected. Proton density (PD) is a measure of the concentration of mobile protons in the imaged tissue. The intensity of the signal resulting from the 90° pulse can be related to the concentration of mobile protons. Relaxation data obtained in the spin warp imaging system are derived from the recovery characteristics of the protons following inversion to 180°. The ratio of signal at the 180° pulse followed by that at 90° allow the spin lattice relaxation characteristics to be calculated. The 90° pulse follows the 180° pulse at a time interval (tau) which can be varied, but in the dementia studies was fixed at 200 ms. At this interval the degree of relaxation of the protons would vary from tissue to tissue and with pathological processes within the tissue. The image constructed based on data collected at this 90° pulse (following the 180° pulse) is called the inversion recovery (IR) image. The image based on the calculated time taken for the protons to return to their previous resting state is the spin lattice relaxation time (T_1). For each pixel the T_1 is the average value for that volume of tissue. Images can be constructed based on T_1 data (Mallard et al, 1980). From spin echo sequences the faster relaxation properties of the protons following 90°–180° RF pulse sequences give transverse relaxation (T_2) data from which images may be constructed.

Relaxation times T_1 and T_2 reflect the state of water in the tissue imaged. Water is observed in two states — 'free' and 'bound' by virtue of its relationship to larger molecular structures (Mathur-de-Vere, 1979). The contrast in T_1 image of soft tissues depends both on the variation in the proportions of free to bound water and the difference between the T_1 values of water in these states. At low magnetic field strengths this difference can be considerable, the T_1 of free water being much longer than bound. Thus a small change in percentage of free water may give a large change in T_1. In brain, for instance, T_1 of grey matter is longer than white, giving definitions between these two tissues on T_1 images. T_1 in white matter may be prolonged by a variety of pathological lesions, e.g. demyelinization, tumours or infarcts. The water content of grey and white matter, however, is very similar and this is reflected by their similar proton density measures. Distinction on PD images does not therefore occur.

NMR imaging has the further advantage of being able to display images three-dimensionally, giving transverse, coronal and saggital views without the requirement of separate patient positioning for each. Furthermore, the absence of ionizing radiation allows repeated exposure of the same individual to be carried out with safety. The fact that the technique does not rely on penetration of structures with external radiation sources means that bony objects do not distort the image, as for example occurs in posterior fossa displays on X-ray CT. On the other hand, metallic objects, for example foreign bodies or surgical clips, destroy the image and in the case of high field strength systems may dislodge surgical clips, especially those recently applied (Lancet Editorial, 1985; Smith, 1985). Other handicaps are the long imaging times (4 minutes per section), and the fact that the patient is in a confined space sometimes causes a problem to those who are claustrophobic. As in all imaging techniques, significant head movement introduces artefacts.

Images based on T_1, IR, PD data can be displayed and a variety of pathological processes identified. Table 5.1 summarizes the characteristics of these lesions (Cherryman 1985a; Cherryman, 1985b; Smith et al, 1984; Bryan et al, 1983).

Table 5.1 NMR image characteristics and lesion pathology

Pathology of lesion	Image characteristics		
	T ms	PD units	IR image intensity
Demyelinzation	Increased	No change	Increased
Astrocytoma	Increased mainly Occasionally reduced or same	No change or reduced	Increased
Meningioma	Increased (occasionally reduced	No change	Increased
Recent infarct	Increased	No change	Increased
Old infarct cystic	Increased	Reduced	Increased
Old infarct gliosis	Falls to about normal level	Increased	—
Subdural haematoma — acute	Reduced	Increased	—
— chronic	Increased	Reduced	
Periventricular white matter change	Increased	No change	Increased

Periventricular white matter change may occur in normals over age 65 years (Bradley et al, 1984a). However, such lesions at multiple sites including punctate foci at a distance from the ventricles are found in association with cognitive loss (Brant-Zawadzki et al, 1984). Periventricular abnormalities may also be found in multiple sclerosis, subcortical arteriosclerotic encephalopathy (Binswanger's disease), post-radiation changes and

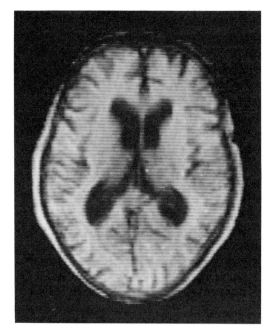

Fig. 5.2 (a) PD image of patient with Alzheimer's disease showing dilated ventricular system and increased sulcal size

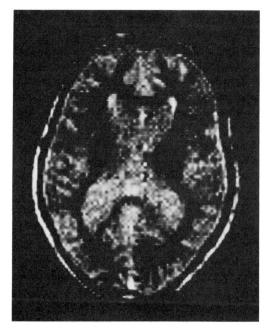

Fig. 5.2 (b) IR image of above section showing increased signal intensity over frontal horns of lateral ventricles.

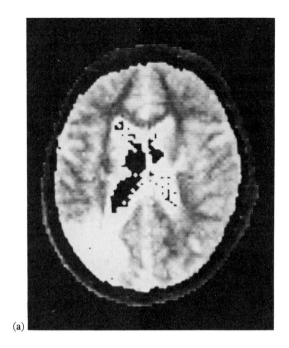

(a)

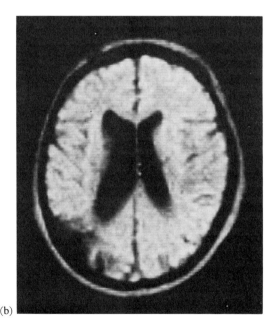

(b)

Fig. 5.3 T_1 (a) and PD (b) images of a patient with MID showing high T_1 and low PD areas in the left parietal and right frontal areas, sites of old infarction

various forms of hydrocephalus. These disorders cannot merely be distinguished on the basis of the periventricular white matter abnormalities, although it is suggested (Bradley et al, 1984b) that in normal pressure hydrocephalus the border is smooth. Atrophy of the head of the caudate nucleus has been identified in Huntington's chorea, and the possible value of this in identifying early cases has been suggested (Bydder & Steiner, 1982). Cortical atrophy is, however, the only feature of Creutzfeldt-Jakob disease (Kovanen et al, 1985). Figures 5.2 to 5.5 illustrate some of the image characteristics present in the dementias.

Numerical T_1 measures might provide information when visual lesions are not present. Changes in T_1 and PD of cerebral white matter have been suggested (Besson et al, 1983) to be useful in separating Alzheimer's type dementia from multi-infarct dementia, and furthermore (Besson et al, 1985) these changes (in T_1) seem to be greater in the more severe cases. There is also the suggestion that the regional T_1 changes may occur in areas where functional deficits (identified by psychometric tests) are present. Furthermore, there is increased T_1 in the basal ganglia of patients with Parkinson's disease and in the cerebral white matter of those with and without dementia (Besson et al, 1985). The significance of T_1 changes in these circumstances is unknown but may be due to glial proliferation or be secondary to altered neuronal membrane characteristics influencing the free:bound water ratio.

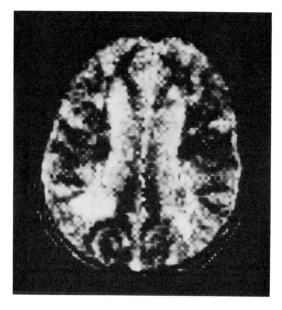

Fig. 5.4 IR image of patient with multi-infarct dementia (Binswanger's type) showing marked increased signal in the periventricular areas anterior, superior and posterior to the lateral ventricles

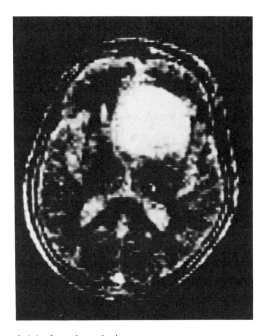

Fig. 5.5 IR image of right frontal meningioma

CONCLUSIONS

Electrophysiological and brain imaging studies are of assistance in the differentiation of degenerative dementias and vascular dementias from dementia due to gross cerebral lesions. The more recent imaging techniques are sophisticated and expensive to administer and clearly unsuitable for routine investigation. However, in younger patients they may be of assistance in making a firm diagnosis, although even with these techniques doubt may exist in individual cases. Their potential benefits rest in the attempts to throw more light on the biological nature of this major clinical and social problem. Methods of separating objectively the types of dementia, e.g. Alzheimer's type dementia and multi-infarct dementia, may add greater meaning to therapeutic trials involving these patients with their diseases.

REFERENCES

Au W J, Gabor A J, Vijayan N Markand O N 1980 Periodic lateralized epleptiform complexes in Creutzfeldt-Jakob disease. Neurology 30: 611–617
Barron S A, Jacobs L, Kinkel W R 1976 Changes in size of normal lateral ventricles during ageing determined by computerized tomography. Neurology 26: 1011–1013
Besson J A O, Corrigan F M, Foreman E I, Ashcroft G W, Eastwood L M, Smith F W, 1983 Differentiating senile dementia of Alzheimer's type and multi-infarct dementia by proton NMR imaging. Lancet 11:789
Besson J A O, Corrigan F M, Foreman E I, Eastwood L M, Smith F W Ashcroft G W,

1985a Nuclear magnetic resonace NMR: imaging in dementia. British Journal of Psychiatry 146: 31–35

Besson J A O, Mutch W J, Downie A W, et al 1985b T_1 changes in Idiopathic Parkinson's disease. In: Hopf M-A, Bydder G M (ed) Magnetic resonance imaging and spectroscopy. Rotoprint S A, Geneva, p: 151–156

Bondareff W, Baldy R, Levy R 1981 Quantitative computed tomography in senile dementia. Archives of General Psychiatry 38: 1365–1368

Bradshaw R, Thomson J L G, Campbell M J, 1983 Computed tomography in the investigation of dementia. British Medical Journal 286: 277–280

Bradley W G, Waluch V, Brant-Zawadzki M 1984a Patchy periventricular white matter lesions in the elderly: a common observation during NMR imaging. Non Invasive Medical Imaging 1: (1)35–41

Bradley W G, Waluch V, Wycoff R R, Yadley R A 1984b Differential diagnosis of periventricular abnormalities in MRI of the brain. Proceedings of the Society of Magnetic Resonance in Medicine, 3rd Annual Meeting New York, 82

Brant-Zawadzki M, Fein G, Van Dyke C 1984 MRI of the ageing brain: Patchy white matter lesions and dementia. Precedings of the Society of Magnetic Resonance in Medicine 1984 3rd Annual Meeting New York, 92

Brukman S D, Langen J W 1984 Changes in brain ventricular size with repeated CAT scans in suspected Alzheimer's disease. American Journal of Psychiatry 141: 81–83

Brun A, Englund E 1981 Regional pattern of degeneration in Alzheimer's disease: neuronal loss and histopathological grading. Histopathology 5: 549–564

Bustany P, Henry J F, Sargent T, et al 1983 Local brain protein metabolism in dementia and schizophrenia: in vivo studies with ^{11}C methionine and positron emission tomography. In: Heiss W-D, Phelps M E, Springer Verlag, (eds) Positron emission tomography of the brain. p: 208–211

Bydder G M, Steiner R E 1982 NMR imaging of the brain. Neuroradiology 23: 231–240

Chase T N, Foster N L, Fedio P, Brooks R, Mansi L, Di Chiro G 1984 Regional cortical dysfunction in Alzheimer's disease as determined by positron emission tomography Annals of Neurology 15 Suppl 170–174

Cherryman G R 1985a Magnetic resonance imaging in the diagnosis of cerebro-vascular pathology. In: Hopf M-A, Bydder G M, (ed) Magnetic Resonance Imaging and Spectroscopy, Rotoprint S A, Gevena: 157–164

Cherryman G R 1985b Nuclear magnetic resonance imaging in the detection and diagnosis of cerebro-vascular disease: Proceedings of the 4th Beaune conference on "New brain imaging techniques in cerebro-vascular disease" Libby, (in press)

Damadian R 1974 Appratus and method for detecting cancer in tissue. U S Patent 3789832 1974 (filed March 1972)

Davis P A, 1941 The electroencephalogram in old age. Diseases of the Nervous System 2:77

Debois V, Lombaert A 1980 Calcified chronic subdural haematomata. Surgical Neurology 14: 455–458

Editoral 1985 Safety of NMR. lancet i: 913–914

Ell P, Lui D, Callum I, Jarritt P A, Donaghy M, Harrison M J G 1983 Cerebral blood flow studies with [123]iodine labelled amines. Lancet i: 1348–1352

Friedland R P, Brun A, Budinger T F 1985 Pathological and positron emission tomographic correlations in Alzheimer's disease. Lancet i:228

Feinberg I, Koresko R L, Heller N 1967 EEG sleep patterns as a function of normal and pathological ageing in man. Journal of Psychiatric Research 5: 107–144

Ford C V, Winter J 1981 Computerised axial tomograms and dementia in elderly patients. Journal of Gerontology 36: 164–169

Fox J H, Huckman M S, Topel J L 1975 The use of computerised tomography in senile dementia. Journal of Neurology, Neurosurgery and Psychiatry 38: 948–953

Frackowiack R S J, Pozzilli C, Legg N J, du Boulay G H, Marshall J, Lenzi G L, Jones T 1981 Regional cerebral oxygen supply and utilization in dementia. Brain 104: 753–778

Frackowiack R S J, Wise R J S, Gibbs J M, Jones T 1984 Positron emission tomographic studies in ageing and cerebrovascular disease at Hammersmith Hospital. Annals of Neurology 15: Suppl 112–118

Gado M, Danziger W L, Chi D, Hughes C P, Coben L A 1983a Brain parenchymal density measurements by CT in demented subjects and normal controls. Radiology 147: 703–710

Gado M, Patel J, Hughes C P 1983b Brain atrophy in dementia judged by CT scan ranking. American Journal of Neuroradiology 4: 499–500

Gemmell H G, Sharp P F, Evans N T S, Besson J A O, Lyall D, Smith F W 1984 Single photon emission tomography with ^{123}I isopropylamphetamines in Alzheimer's disease and multi-infarct dementia. Lancet 11:1348

George A E, De Leon M J, Rosenbloom S, Ferris S H, Gentes C, Emmerich M, Kricheff I 1983 Ventricular volume and cognitive deficit: a computed tomographic study. Radiology 149: 493–498

Goodin D S, Squires K, Starr A 1978 Long latency of event related components of the auditory evoked potential in dementia. Brain 101: 635–648

Hackinski V, Lasser N A, Marshall J 1974 Multi-infarct dementia: A cause of mental deterioration in the elderly. Lancet 11: 207–209

Hahn E L 1950 Spin echos. Physics Review 80: 580–594

Harkins S W 1981 The effects of presenile dementia of the Alzheimer's type on brain stem transmission time. International Journal of Neurosciences 15: 165–170

Hendrickson E, Levy R, Post F 1979 Average evoked potentials in relation to cognitive and affective state in elderly psychiatric patients. British Journal of Psychiatry 134: 494–501

Jacobson P L, Farmer T W 1979 The "hypernormal" CT scan in dementia: Bilateral isodense subdural haematomas" Neurology 29: 1522–1524

Jacoby R J, Levy R, Dawson J M 1980a Computed tomography in the elderly. 1. Normal population. British Journal of Psychiatry 136: 249–255

Jacoby R J, Levy R, Dawson J M, 1980b Computed tomography in the elderly (2) Senile dementia: diagnosis and functional impairment. British Journal of Psychiatry 136: 256–269

Johannesson G, Hagberg B, Gustafson L, Ingvar D H 1977a EEG and cognitive impairment in presenile dementia. Acta Neurologica Scandinavica 59: 225–240

Johannesson G, Brun A, Gustafson L Ingvar D H 1977b The EEG in presenile dementia related to cerebral blood flow and autopsy findings. Acta Neurologica Scandinavica 56: 89–103

Johnson G, Hutchinson J M S, Eastwood L M S 1981 Instrumentation for NMR spin warp imaging. Journal of Physics E: Scientific Instruments 15: 74–79

Kahn E, Fisher C 1969 The sleep characteristics of the normal aged male. Journal of Nervous and Mental Diseases 148: 477–494

Kaszniak A W, Garron D C, Fox J H, Bergen D, Huckman M 1979 Cerebral atrophy EEG slowing, age, education and cognitive functioning in suspected dementia. Neurology 29: 1273–1279

Katz R I, Horowitz G R 1982 The septuagenarian EEG: studies in a selected normal geriatric population. Journal of the American Geriatric Society 3: 273–275

Kavonen J, Erkinjunti T, Iivanainen M, et al 1985 Cerebral NMR and CT imaging in Creutzfeldt-Jakob disease. Journal of Computed Axial Tomography 9: (1)125–128

Kohlmeyer K Shamena A R 1983 Computed tomographic assessment of CSF spaces in the brain of demented and non-demented patients over 60 years. American Journal of Neuroradiology 4: 706–707

Koller W C, Glatt S L, Fox J H, Kaszniak W, Wilson R S, Huckman M S 1981 Cerebellar atrophy: relationship to ageing and cerebral atrophy. Neurology 31: 1486–1488

Kooi K A, Guvener A M, Tupper C J, Bagchi B K 1964 The electroencephalographic patterns of temporal regions in normal adults. Neurology 14: 1029–1035

Kuhl D E, Metter J, Riege W H, Hawkins R A 1984 The effect of normal ageing on patterns of local cerebral glucose utilization. Annals of Neurology 15:Supplement 133–137

Kuhl D E, Metter J, Riege W H, Markham C H, 1984 Patterns of cerebral glucose utilization in Parkinson's disease and Huntington's disease. Annals of Neurology 15: Supplement 119–125

Lauterbur P C 1973 Image formation by induced local interaction: examples employing nuclear magnetic resonance. Nature 242: 190–191

Levy R, Isaacs A, Behrman J 1971 Neurophysiological correlates of senile dementia: 11 The somatosensory evoked response. Psychological Medicine 1: 159–165

Loizon L A, Kendall B E, Marshall J 1981 Subcortical arteriosclerotic encephalopathy: a clinical and radiological investigation. Journal of Neurology, Neurosurgery and Psychiatry 44: 294–304

Mallard J R, Hutchison J M S, Edelstein W A, Ling C R, Foster M A, Johnson G 1980 In vivo NMR imaging in medicine: the Aberdeen approach both physcial and biological. Philosophical Transactions of the Royal Society of London B 289: 519–533

Mathur-de-Vre 1979 The NMR studies of water in biological systems. Progress in Biophysics and Molecular Biology 35: 103–134

Muller H F, Schwartz G 1978 Electroencephalogram and atrophy findings in geropsychiatry. Journal of Gerontology 33: 504–513

Mundy-Castle A C 1951 Theta and beta rhythm in the electroencephalograms of normal adults. Electroencephalography and Clinical Neurophysiology 3: 477–486

Naeser M A, Gebhardt C, Levine H H 1980 Decreased computerised tomography numbers in patients with presenile dementia 1980. Archives of Neurology 37: 401–409

Obrist W D, Thompson H K, King C H, Wang H S 1967 Determination of regional cerebral Blood flow by inhalation of ^{133}xenon. Circulation Research 20: 124–135

Phelps M E, Hoffman E J, Rayband C 1977 Factors which affect cerebral uptake and retention of $^{13}NH_3$. Stroke 8: 694–702

Roubicek 1977 The electroencephalogram in the middle aged and elderly. Journal of the American Geriatric Society 25: 145–152

Rosenberg G A, Kernfeld M, Stooring J, Bichnell J M 1979 Subcortical arteriosclerotic encephalopathy (Binswanger): computed tomography. Neurology 29: 1102–1106

Sapirstein L A 1958 Regional blood flow by fractional distribution of indicators. American Journal of Physiology 193: 161–168

Scott D F, Heathfield W G, Toone B, Margerison J H 1972 The EEG in Huntington's chorea: a clinical and neuropathological study. Journal of Neurology, Neurosurgery and Psychiatry 35: 97–102

Sirakov A A, Mezan I S 1963 EEG findings in Parkinsonism. Electroencephalography and Clinical Neurophysiology 15: 321–322

Slaets J, Fortgens C 1984 On the value of P_{300} event related potentials in the differential diagnosis of dementia. British Journal of Psychiatry 145: 648–652

Smith F W, 1985 Safety of NMR. Lancet i:1108

Smith F W, Cherryman G R, Besson J A O, Pitt M, Macdonald A F, Hutchison J M S 1984 Is proton imaging more useful than xray CT in the diagnosis of intracranial pathology? Review of 500 cases. Magnetic Resonance Imaging 2:235

Stigsby B, Johnneson G, Ingvar D 1981 Regional EEG analysis and regional cerebral blood flow in Alsheimer's and Pick's disease. Electroencephalography and Clinical Neurophysiology 51: 537–547

Sutton S, Braren M, Zubin J John E R 1965 Evoked potential correlates of stimulus uncertainty. Science 150: 1187–1188

Swain J M 1959 Electroencephalographic abnormalities in presenile atrophy. Neurology 9: 722–727

Verhas M, Schoutens A, Demol O, Patte M, Rokossky M, Struyven J, Capen A 1976 Use of ^{99}m Tc labelled albumin micro spheres in cerebral vascular diseases. Journal of Nuclear Medicine 17: 170–174

Visser S L, Stam F C, Van Tilburg W, Op Den Velde W, Blom J L, De Rijke W 1976 Visual evoked response in senile and presenile dementia. Electroencephalography and Clinical Neurophysiology 40: 385–392

Walter W G, Cooper R, Aldridge V J, McCallum W C, Winter A L 1964 Contingent negative variation: an electrical sign of sensorimotor association and expectancy in human brain. Nature 203: 380–384

Wang H S, Busse E W 1969 EEG of healthy old persons — a longitudinal study. I Dominant background activity and occipital rhythm. Journal of Gerontology 24: 419–426

Watson C P 1979 Clinical similarity of Alzheimer's and Creutzfeldt-Jakob disease. Annals of Neurology 6: 368–369

White J C 1979 Periodic EEG activity in subcortical arteriosclerotic encephalopathy (Binswanger's type). Archives of Neurology 36: 485–489

Wilson R S, Fox J H, Huckman M S, Bacon L D, Lobick J J 1982 Computed tomography in dementia. Neurology 32: 1054–1057

Winchell H S, Horst W D, Braun L 1980 N-iso propyl ^{123}1 p-iodo amphetamine: single pass brain uptake and washout; binding to brain synaptosomes and localization in dog and monkey brain. Journal of Nuclear Medicine 21: 947–952

Alzheimer's disease: aetiology

INTRODUCTION

We live at a time of unprecedented human longevity, a time when disability, dependency and rates of institutional care among the aged threaten to overwhelm the most generous forecasts of health care funding for the aged. Although reassuring evidence of reduced morbidity and mortality arising from cardiac and cerebral vascular disease is emerging in Western society, organic mental impairment, notably due to dementia of the Alzheimer type, is the major single pathology associated with demand for institutional care. Comaish (1976) offered a crude formula to calculate relative priorities for research spending on various medical problems. The prevalence at any one time, P, is multipled by S, the severity of the disease on an arbitrary scale of O to 10, and divided by C, the 'curability' (also on a scale of O to 10) to arrive at a relative figure. Under this system of calculating priorities for research, chronic renal failure merits 1×10^4 in research monies, multiple sclerosis would merit 2×10^5, but the dementing illnesses are deserving of 13×10^5 research units. Fundamental research into the dementias has, in recent years, been accorded priority status by national research funding bodies. As an example, in 1984, the National Institutes of Health in the United States of America allocated US$40 million for research into the dementing illnesses of later life.

Research output centring on the aetiology of Alzheimer's disease (AD) accelerates rapidly, with weekly referencing journals such as Current Contents (Life Sciences) invariably citing significant publications under the heading of Alzheimer's disease. Despite such activity, debate continues, stressing the need to refine techniques of diagnosis in order better to establish the presence of this major form of dementia during life.

While some scientists consider that the varied symptoms at different ages of onset point to subsets of disease sharing a common neurological pathway, most believe that a single disease entity is responsible for the degenerative changes that characterize dementia of the Alzheimer type. This unitarian view has gained ground steadily with the identification of electron microscopic pathology and neurotransmitted alterations without evidence of significant qualitative differences.

AETIOLOGY

Despite considerable progress in the past decade in defining the neuro-chemical and structural pathology of AD, the aetiological factor(s) that give rise to these findings remain(s) unknown. Major hypotheses can be conveniently grouped under the following headings:
1. genetic
2. immunological
3. toxic
4. transmissible agent
5. nerve survival/growth factors

1. Genetic factors

A genetic basis for some cases of AD was first discussed in the English literature by Gillespie (1933). Since then more than 30 published reports of familial incidence have appeared consistent with autosomal dominant inheritance (Wheelan, 1959; Feldman et al, 1963; Landy & Bain, 1970; Wright & Whalley, 1984), with a recent case report describing AD in a mother and identical twin sons, all dying below the age of 50 years (Sharman et al, 1979). Kallman & Sander (1949) reported high concord-ance rates among both monozygotic and dizygotic twins. With one twin affected, the risk for the identical twin was 43%; for the non-identical 8% compared to a 6.5% risk for non-twin siblings.

There are fewer population studies, the limitations and conclusions of which are well reviewed by Pratt (1970). The most painstaking of these studies by Larsson et al (1963) and Constantinidis et al (1962) disagree on the risk of AD among the first-degree relatives of victims. Larsson and co-workers found the morbidity risk for senile dementia among the siblings of those with this disorder to be four times the risk in the general popu-lation. This study favoured a single autosomal dominant gene with low penetrance, a view that cannot be excluded, since single-gene disorders with no selective disadvantage can reach a high population prevalence. Pratt (1970), however, concluded that a polygenic inheritance pattern more likely operated in AD with only 10–15% of cases of AD revealing positive heredity in their family background, while the remaining (majority) of cases present as sporadic in type. Thus, though uncommon, true familial cases do occur and appear to deviate by showing a dominant inheritance pattern.

In the population study by Larsson et al (1963), if age at onset had been used as a basis for distinguishing between those with presenile and senile dementia, seven out of the 51 relatives with 'senile dementia' had an esti-mated age of onset before 65 years, therefore coming into the 'presenile' category. This figure gives a 10–20-fold higher morbidity risk for presenile onset AD in relatives (1.6%) compared with the general population (about 0.1% for presenile onset AD). Similarly, using age at onset, the morbidity risk for senile onset AD (65 years and over) in the relatives is found to be 10.6%, less than the four-fold increase in risk reported in Larsson's study. The study by Constantinidis et al (1962) suggested a genetic overlap between presenile and senile forms of AD.

Heston & Mastri (1977) avoided the uncertainties of large population studies by noting morbidity from AD in the relatives of 30 autopsied probands with histologically confirmed AD. The age of onset of AD in the probands was before 65 years of age. AD was found in 22 secondary cases (six being confirmed by autopsy). The heritability of AD in these 22 relatives with early-onset disease (before 65 years) was more marked than for those relatives with later onset AD.

In a recent review, Wright and Whalley (1984) estimated heritabilities on the basis of ages of onset in secondary cases detected in the Swedish studies (Sjogren et al, 1952; Larsson et al, 1963) and that of Heston and Mastri (1977). Results show the highest heritability estimates are found for early-onset illness in the relatives of early-onset probands. Clinical observations suggest early-onset AD is associated with increased severity (Roth, 1978).

More intriguing are unconfirmed reports that relatives of probands with histologically confirmed AD show excess morbidity from Down's syndrome and haematological malignancy (Heston 1977), a genetic defect expressed through disorganization of cell microtubules being postulated for this association. Birth order and maternal age do not appear to be risk factors in AD (Knesevich et al, 1982; Corkin et al, 1983).

The link between Down's syndrome and AD assumes prominence from the observation that persons with Down's syndrome, surviving to age 35 years, predictably and precociously develop a dementing illness with clinical and neuropathological features closely resembling AD (Burger & Vogel, 1973; Ellis et al, 1974). Conversely Heyman (1983) noted, in a study of 1200 families of patients with AD, that the incidence of Down's syndrome was three times that expected in the general population. The significance of this link remains obscure.

Chromosomal abnormalities have been reported in cases of AD (Nielsen, 1968; Bergener & Tungklaass, 1970; Cook et al, 1978) but not confirmed by others (Mark & Brun, 1973; Brun et al, 1978; Sulkava et al, 1979). However, an increase in the spontaneous occurrence of chromosomal aneuploidy (gain or loss of a chromosome) is known to occur in somatic cells with age (Schneider, 1978).

Immunological factors

2. There is reason to believe that brain changes noted in AD may be a reflection of immunological disturbances. Strongest evidence for this view is the presence of senile plaques containing amyloid fibrils rich in immuno-

globulin G (Ishii & Haga, 1976). Johnson et al (1981) have produced evidence that plaque and vessel amyloid may share a common antigen with neurofibrillary tangles. More recent reports by Glenner & Wong (1984) of the purification and characterization of cerebrovascular amyloid protein reveal this protein to have no homology with any protein sequenced to date, pointing its derivation from a unique serum precursor which may provide a diagnostic test for Alzheimer's disease.

More controversial is the occurrence of brain reactive antibodies noted in the serum of AD patients by Nandy (1978). An absence of brain antibodies in senile dementia was previously reported by Whittingham et al (1970). The crudity of such initial attempts to detect circulating anti-neuronal antibodies is emphasized by the recent observation of Ihara et al (1983) that antibodies raised in rabbits to highly enriched pair-helical filament (PHF) fractions, specifically labels PHF and not neurofilaments nor other cytoskeletal protein in brain sections. The availability of such externally raised antibodies that specifically recognize PHF in human brain tissue will allow immuno-affinity purification of PHF in AD and other human neurofibrillary diseases.

Studies of serum immunoglobulins and complement levels have produced results showing minor or no variation from age-matched controls, not strongly supporting the existence of an underlying immune disturbance (Henschke et al, 1979; Cohen & Eisdorfer, 1980; Miller et al, 1981; Pentland et al, 1982). Peripheral lymphocyte responsiveness to mitogenic stimuli shows no consistent change from age-matched controls (Henschke et al, 1979; Miller et al, 1981). Several studies fail to show histocompatibility antigens varying from the expected distribution in general populations (Henschke et al, 1978; Whalley et al, 1980; Reed et al, 1983). Thus despite the rapid advance in research methods in immunology, no worthwhile clue to any immune mechanism of pathogenesis presently exists in AD.

3. Toxic factors

The agent most often proposed as a possible aetiological agent is aluminium. A type of neurofibrillary tangle has been produced in laboratory animals, notably cats, by the intracranial injection of aluminium salts (Klatzo et al, 1965), but electron microscopy has shown that the experimental lesion consists of aggregates of 10 nm neurofilamentous structures rather than the helically wound filaments found in AD that cross one another every 80 nm.

Interest in aluminium as a possible aetiological agent was initially raises by Crapper et al (1976) reporting raised brain aluminium levels in patients with AD. Subsequent analyses by McDermott et al (1977) failed to confirm this finding. The disparity between the mean ages of controls (47 years) and demented subjects (68 years), in the study by Crapper, was offered as an explanation for the positive finding in the latter study. Brain aluminium concentrations in the study by McDermott et al (1979) were found to increase steadily with age, thus accounting for the positive result rather than the disease under study. Monkeys injected in the subarachnoid space with aluminium chloride solution reveal neurological sequelae, but no neurofibrillary degeneration is noted at autopsy (Wisniewski et al, 1977). Furthermore, brain aluminium concentrations in dialysis encephalopathy commonly exceed those found in AD by a factor of five, without neurofibrillary degeneration being evident on microscopy of brain tissue (Burks et al, 1976).

Increased iron levels have not been found in cortical samples in AD (Hallgren & Sourander, 1980). Speculation in the possible role of zinc in brain metabolic activity and dementia has been recently advanced by Burnet (1981). Although lipofuscin, a yellow insoluble pigment, increases inside neuronal perikarya as a function of age, no evidence of cell toxicity has been established, nor has increased content in dementia been noted (Mann & Sinclair, 1978). Nikaido et al (1972) demonstrated that formalin fixed plaques contain abnormal quantities of silicon, but that whole brain tissue in AD does not have levels higher than control brains.

4. Transmissible agents

Demonstration that kuru and Creutzfeldt-Jakob disease are each due to a transmissible virus (Gajdusek, 1977) has stimulated the hypothesis that a transmissible, slow or unconventional virus may play a role in the pathogenesis of AD. Kuru and Creutzfeldt-Jakob disease (occurring in humans), scrapie (sheep and goats) and transmissible mink encephalopathy are grouped histologically by the occurrence of vacuolation within the cytoplasm of axonal and dendritic processes of neurons and astrocytes. Viruses causing each have been maintained in vitro in cell cultures and transmitted to laboratory animals with resultant neuropathological lesions identical to those seen in the initial host. Traub and co- workers (1977) reported that in two out of six attempts they induced spongiform (vacuolation) change in primate brains injected with extracts from human brains affected by familial AD. Over thirty attempts to induce such brain changes with tissue from cases of sporadic AD failed. Cross-infection, arising from laboratory equipment contaminated with concurrently held material from cases of Creutzfeldt-Jakob disease (CJD), is the likely explanation for these two instances of 'transmitted' AD.

Further stimulus to the search for a transmissible agent came from a report by de Boni & Crapper (1978) that inoculating tissue cultures of human fetal cortex with cell-free extracts of AD brain induced the formation of paired helical filaments in the cultured fetal neurones. This result remains to be confirmed by other laboratories.

More recently, in this trail of enquiry, the scrapie agent has moved to centre stage. This agent causes a degenerative disorder of the central nervous system in sheep and goats. A study by Hadlow et al (1980) suggested that there may be similarities between the scrapie agent and CJD. Goats inoculated with brain tissue from demented patients dying of CJD developed a neurological disorder 3 to 4 years after inoculation. Experimental CJD in goats is indistinguishable both clinically and neuropathologically from natural scrapie in sheep. The finding that rapid disease induction was possible in hamster brains permitted purification and characterization of the scrapie agent.

Prusiner (1982), noting the scrapie agent contains a protein that is required for infectivity, coined the term 'prion' to denote a small proteinaceous infectious particle. This, unlike viruses, plasmids and viroids, is resistant to inactivation by most procedures that modify nucleic acids. This agent was found by Prusiner to have a molecular weight of less than 50 000 and to contain little or no DNA or RNA. Further work in this area has led to a possible link with AD. In extensively purified fractions of scrapie — infected hamster brain, a protease resistant protein (designated PrP), when subjected to electron microscopy reveals rod-shaped, fibre-like particles 10 to 20 nm in diameter and 100 to 200 nm in length (Prusiner et al, 1983). Arrays of such prion rods when stained with congo red dye show green birefringence under polarized light microscopy, similar to the amyloid found in the senile plaques of AD. This is the first suggestive evidence associating slow viral or prion diseases with AD.

Speculation can be advanced that amyloid might be a prime mover of the disease rather than a product of it. The development of prion-specific monoclonal antibodies should in time allow exploration of the putative relationship between prions and AD. Such ultrastructural links between scrapie and AD have been recently reviewed by Somerville (1985) who on weighing the available evidence concludes that amyloid in AD is of conventional origin — namely that it derives by partial degradation of a host protein, as occurs in all other forms of amyloidosis.

5. Nerve survival/growth factors

With the recognition of several nerve growth factors which promote nerve survival of autonomic and sensory nerves in the periphery (Honegger, 1983) it can be reasonably assumed that similar trophic agents exist in the central nervous system. The regulation of the expression of nerve growth factor genes is currently being defined, and may prove relevant in the understanding of central nervous system 'degenerative' diseases — notably those like AD in which defined populations of neurones are found to be affected (Whitehouse et al, 1980; Bondareff et al, 1982). The role of nerve growth factor is conceived as stimulating enzymatic reactions leading to neuronal differentiation (e.g. microtubule assembly) or to regulate the de novo synthesis of crucial proteins at the transcriptional level as has been shown in cultured animal neurons (Greene & Rubenstein, 1981).

The limitations of all the above conceptual models are clearly evident. Public interest in the progress of research into AD will ensure an increase in both research effort and funding. Wurtman (1985), providing a recent review of the disease for the popular science magazine, Scientific American, likened the many sets of data on AD to the tale of six blind men who, on contacting an elephant, reported it to be a wall, spear, snake, tree, fan or rope, depending on their direction of contact. In time, contributions in all areas may permit the essential nature of this distressing disorder to be revealed.

REFERENCES

Bergener M, Jungklaas F K 1970 Genetische Befund bei Morbus Alzheimer und seniler Demenz. Gerontology Clinics 12: 71–75

Bondareff W, Mountjoy C Q, Roth M 1982 Loss of neurons of origin of the adrenergic projection to cerebral cortex (nucleus locus ceruleus) in senile dementia. Neurology 32: 164–168

Brun A, Gustafson L, Mitelman F 1978 Normal chromosome banding patterns in Alzheimer's disease. Gerontology 24: 369–373

Burger P C, Vogel S 1973 The development of the pathologic changes of Alzheimer's disease and senile dementia in patients with Down's syndrome. American Journal of Pathology 73: 457–476

Burks J S, Alfrey A C, Huddlestone J, Norenberg M D S, Lewin E 1976 A fatal encephalopathy in chronic haemodialysis patients. Lancet 1: 764–768

Burnet F M 1981 A possible role of zinc in the pathology of dementia. Lancet 1: 186–188

Cohen D, Eisdorfer C 1980 Serum immunoglobulins and cognitive status in the elderly. 1. A population study. British Journal of Psychiatry 136: 33–39

Comaish J S 1976 How to set priorities in medicine. Lancet 2: 512–514

Constantinidis J, Garrone D, de Ajuriaquerra J 1962 L'hérédité de démenés de l'age avancé. L'Encephale 4: 301–344

Cook R H, Ward B, Austin J H, Robinson A 1978 Familial Alzheimer disease: its relation to cytogenetic abnormality and transmissible dementia. Neurology (Minneap.) 28:353

Corkin S, Growdon J H, Rasmussen S L 1983 Parental age as a risk factor in Alzheimer's disease. Annals of Neurology 13: 674–676

Crapper D R, Krishnan S S, Quittkat S 1976 Aluminium, neurofibrillary degeneration and Alzheimer's disease. Brain 99: 67–80

De Boni U, Crapper D R 1978 Paired helical filaments of the Alzheimer type in cultured neurones. Nature 271: 566–568

Ellis W G, McCulloch J R, Corley J 1974 Presenile dementia in Down's syndrome: ultrastructural identity with Alzheimer's disease. Neurology 24: 101–106

Feldman R G, Chandler K A, Levy L L et al 1963 Familial Alzheimer's disease. Neurology (Minneap.) 13: 811–824

Gajdusek D C 1977 Unconventional viruses and the origin and disappearance of kuru. Science 197: 943–960

Gillespie R D 1933 Discussion on the mental and physical symptoms of the presenile dementias. Proceedings of the Royal Society of Medicine 26: 1080–1084

Glenner G G, Wong C W 1984 Alzheimer's disease. Initial report of the purification and characterization of a novel cerebrovascular amyloid protein. Biochemical and Biophysical Research Communications 120: 885–890

Greene L A, Rubenstein A 1981 Regulation of acetylcholinesterase activity by nerve growth factor. Role of transcription and dissociation from effects on proliferation and neurite outgrowth. Journal of Biological Chemistry 256: 6363–6367

Hadlow W J, Prusiner S B, Kennedy R C, Race R E 1980 Brain tissue from persons dying of Creutzfeldt-Jakob disease causes scrapie-like encephalopathy in goats. Annals of Neurology 8: 628

Hallgren B, Sourander P 1960 The non-haemin iron in the cerebral cortex in Alzheimer's disease. Journal of Neurochemistry 5: 307–310

Henschke P J, Bell D A, Cape R D T 1978 Alzheimer's disease and HLA. Tissue Antigens 12: 132–135

Henschke P J, Bell D A, Cape R D T 1979 Immunologic indices in Alzheimer dementia. Journal of Clinical and Experimental Gerontology 1: 23–37

Heyman A, Wilkinson W E, Hurwitz B J, Schmechel D, Sigmon A H, Weinberg T et al 1983 Alzheimer's disease: genetic aspects and associated clinical disorders. Annals of Neurology 14: 507–515

Honegger P 1983 Nerve growth factor — sensitive brain neurons in culture. Monographs in Neural Science 9: 36–42

Ihara Y, Abraham C, Selkoe D J 1983 Antibodies to paired helical filaments in Alzheimer's disease do not recognize normal brain proteins. Nature 304: 727–730

Ishii T, Hagas 1976 Immuno-electron microscopic localization of immuno-globulins in amyloid fibrils of senile plaques. Acta Neuropathologica (Berlin) 36: 243–249

Johnson A B, Cohen S A, Said S I, Terry R D 1981 Neuritic plaque amyloid, microangiopathy and Alzheimer neurofibrillary tangles: do they share a common antigen? Journal of Neuropathology and Experimental Neurology 40: 310

Kallman R J, Sander G 1949 Twin studies of senescence. American Journal of Psychiatry 106: 29–36

Klatzo I, Wisniewski H M, Streicher E 1965 Experimental production of neurofibrillary degeneration. 1. Light microscopic observations. Journal of Neuropathology and Experimental Neurology 24: 187

Knesevich J W, La Barge E, Martin R L, Danziger W L, Berg L 1982 Birth order and maternal age effect in dementia of the Alzheimer type. Psychiatry Research 7: 345–350

Landy P J, Bain B J 1970 Alzheimer's disease in siblings. Medical Journal of Australia 2: 832–834

Larsson T, Sjogren T, Jacobson G 1963 Senile dementia, a clinical, sociomedical and genetic study. Acta Psychiatrica Scandinavica (Suppl 167): 1–257

Mann D M A, Sinclair K G A 1978 The quantitative assessment of lipofuscin pigment, cytoplasmic RNA and nucleolar volume in senile dementia. Neuropathology and Applied Neurobiology 4: 129–135

Mark J, Brun A 1973 Chromosomal deviations in Alzheimer's disease. Gerontologia Clinica 15: 253–258

Miller A E, Neighbour P A, Katzmann R, Aronson M, Lipkowitz R 1981 Immunological studies in senile dementia of the Alzheimer type: evidence for enhanced suppressor cell activity. Annals of Neurology 10: 506–510

McDermott J R, Smith I A, Iqbal K, Wisniewski M D 1979 Brain aluminium in aging and Alzheimer's disease. Neurology 29: 809–814

Nandy K 1978 Brain reactive antibodies in aging and senile dementia. In: Terry R D, Katzmann R, Bick K L (eds) Alzheimer's disease: senile dementia and related disorders. Raven Press, New York

Nielsen J 1968 Chromosomes in senile dementia. British Journal of Psychiatry 114: 303–309

Nikaido T, Austin J, Trueb L, Rinehart R 1972 Studies in aging in the brain. II Microchemical analyses of the nervous system in Alzheimer's patients. Archives of Neurology 27: 549–554

Pentland B, Christie J E, Watson K C, Yap P L 1982 Immunologic parameters in Alzheimer's pre-senile dementia. Acta Psychiatrica Scandinavica 65: 375–379

Pratt R T C 1970 The genetics of Alzheimer's disease. In: Wolstenholme G E W, O'Connor U (eds) CIBA Foundation Symposium. Churchill Livingstone, Edinburgh, p 137

Prusiner S B 1982 Novel proteinaceous infectious particles cause scrapie. Science 216: 136–144

Prusiner S B, McKinley M P, Bowman K A et al 1983 Scrapie prions aggregate to form amyloid-like birefringent rods. Cell 35: 57–62

Reed E, Thompson D, Mayeaux R, Suciu-Foca N 1983 HLA antigens in Alzheimer's disease. Tissue Antigens 21: 164–167

Roth M 1978 Diagnosis of senile and related forms of dementia. In: Katzmann R, Terry R D, Bick K L (eds) Alzheimer's disease: senile dementia and related disorders. Raven Press, New York

Schneider L 1978 Cytogenetics of aging. In: Schneider E L (ed) The genetics of aging. Plenum Press, New York

Sharman M G, Watt D C, Janota I, Carrasco L H 1979 Case report. Alzheimer's disease in a mother and identical twin sons. Psychological Medicine 9: 771–774

Somerville R A 1985 Ultrastructural links between scrapie and Alzheimer's disease. Lancet 1: 504–506

Sjogren T, Shogren J, Lindgren A G H 1952 Morbus Alzheimer and morbus Pick. A genetic, clinical and pathoanatomical study. Acta Psychiatrica Scandinavica Suppl 82: 1–52

Sulkava R, Rossi L, Knuutila S 1979 No elevated sister chromatid exchange in Alzheimer's disease. Acta Neurologica Scandinavica 59: 156–159

Traub R, Gajdusek D C, Gibbs C J Jr 1977 Transmissible virus dementia: the relation of transmissible spongiform encephalopathy to Creutzfeldt-Jakob disease. In: Smith W L, Kinsbourne M (eds) Aging and dementia. Spectrum, New York, p 91–172

Whalley L J, Urbaniak S J, Darg C, Peutherer J F, Christie J E 1980 Histocompatibility antigens and antibodies to viral and other antigens in Alzheimer pre-senile dementia. Acta Psychiatrica Scandinavica 61: 1–7

Wheelan L 1959 Familial Alzheimer's disease. Annals of Human Genetics 23: 300–310

Whitehouse P J, Price D L, Clark A W, Coyle J T, De Long M R 1981 Alzheimer's disease: evidence for selective loss of cholinergic neurons in the nucleus basalis. Annals of Neurology 10: 122–126

Whittingham S, Lennon V, Mackay I R, Davies G V, Davies B 1970 Absence of brain antibodies in senile dementia. British Journal of Psychiatry 116: 447–448

Wisniewski H M, Korthals J K, Kopellof L M et al 1977 Neurotoxicity of aluminium. In: Roizin L, Shiraki H, Groevic N (eds) Neurotoxicology. Raven Press, New York, p 313–315

Wright A F, Whalley L J 1984 Genetics: aging and dementia. British Journal of Psychiatry 145: 20–38

Wurtman R J 1985 Alzheimer's disease. Scientific American 252: 48–56

Alzheimer's disease: neuropathology

THE DEVELOPMENT OF THE PRESENT CONCEPT

The cognitive impairment in Alzheimer's disease results from a cortical abnormality associated with degeneration of the ascending cholinergic systems and other neuronal groups. The steps in the development of this concept were: the recognition of loss of brain tissue in mental disease characterized by loss of weight and reduced thickness of the cortex (Wilks, 1864); the identification of the major histological changes in the cortex, most notably by Alzheimer (1907), and the correlation of these with intellectual impairment (Blessed et al, 1968; Wilcock & Esiri, 1982); the final step was the identification of the selective degeneration of the cholinergic system and other subcortical neuronal groups and correlation of these changes with the cortical pathology and dementia (Perry et al, 1978).

The morbid anatomical study of the brain has shown the importance of neuritic (senile) plaques and, more importantly, neurofibrillary tangles to loss of intellectual function. In addition, it is becoming apparent that the pathology in the cortex is orientated to the columnar structure of the cortex rather than the laminar, suggesting an association between the cortical vertical columnar loss and the subcortical neuronal loss by degeneration of intercommunicating tracts. There is initially a slow progression of reduced protein synthesis associated with nuclear abnormalities, reduction of the dendritic pattern of the neurone and later loss of the larger neurones. The typical histological appearances are seen late in the course of the disease. Study of the brains of mildly demented Parkinsonian patients who do not have Alzheimer's changes in the cortex indicates that the dementia is associated with a cholinergic deficit. This suggests that the severe dementia seen in Alzheimer's disease results from a combination of cortical pathology most prominently in the frontal lobe, destruction of the hippocampus and degeneration of the subcortical nuclei. Why the cholinergic system should be so selectively damaged, be it because of metabolic or structural vulnerability, remains to be determined.

Histological study has suggested several areas of research to determine the possible aetiology. The identification of increased levels of aluminium

118

in the brain of these patients and its possible relationship to the development of neurofibrillary degeneration in experimental animals has directed research towards a possible toxic agent. Neurohistochemical study indicates that protein metabolism is abnormal, and this can be correlated with the increased amount of neurofilament present in the brain; however, why it accumulates at either poles of a cell and its relation to the neuritic plaque is uncertain. Transmission experiments have not supported the hypothesis that it has an infectious aetiology, despite some histological similarity to other transmissible degenerative diseases linked under the heading of spongiform encephalopathy.

THE RELATIONSHIP OF ALZHEIMER'S DISEASE TO NORMAL AGEING

Many of the features — both macroscopic and microscopic — of normal ageing are seen in Alzheimer's disease. It is only with more modern technology and innovation that it has been possible to quantify these changes and understand the shared and independent areas of these two processes. The major area of innovation has been the measurement of the volume of the brain with respect to the skull, using a simple balloon technique (Davis & Wright, 1977). The introduction of the brain scanner has allowed the normal volume of the ventricles to be measured. In addition, computer-assisted technology has allowed large numbers of cells to be counted and their contents assessed histochemically. Biochemical studies have identified neurotransmitter deficits, and the development of monoclonal antibodies will allow the deficit to be identified microscopically.

With age there is a progressive reduction of brain weight and volume (Dekaban & Sadowsky, 1978). This starts at the age of 20 and is most marked after the age of 50. The loss is probably exponential rather than linear (Davis & Wright, 1977). The loss of cortical tissue is most marked in the parasagittal frontal and parietal cortex and lateral frontal and temporal lobes rather than the occipital poles. The ventricles also increase in size in intellectually normal aged individuals and may be marked in 10% of cases. Initially the cortical tissue loss is less than the white matter (Corsellis, 1962, 1976a). This secondary loss of white matter may reflect loss of cortical neurones with secondary loss of myelinated axons.

One of the major problems in the study of Alzheimer's disease has been to establish if there is loss of neurones in the brain and, if so, how significant it is. The major difficulty was initially technical. There are a large number of neurones to be counted and many variables, including shrinkage of the brain, to be accounted for. However, the most recent studies indicate that there is a small but significant loss of neurones from the cortex in the normal aged individuals (Brody, 1953; Terry, 1980). The loss of cortical neurones with age is most marked in layers 2 and 4 of the cortex (Brody, 1955, 1970; Colon, 1972) in the frontal pole, precentral gyrus area striata and cingulate gyrus, and similar findings have been reported for the cerebellar Purkinje neurones (Hall et al, 1975). The numbers of neurones in the brain stem nuclei, however, are stable.

One of the easily observed changes in neurones with age is the linear accumulation of lipofuscin. It is widely found in neuronal groups, with few exceptions. It is thought to be formed from the gradual transformation of lysosomes (Sekhon & Maxwell, 1974). Several biological molecules including rough endoplasmic reticulum and mitochondria form crosspolymers which are hydrolytically indigestible and accumulate. The quantity of lipofuscin is most marked in several neuronal groups — the inferior olivary nuclei and lateral geniculate body (Scholtz & Brown, 1978). This material is probably the accumulation of cellular biproducts reflecting the functional activity of the cell. There is no evidence that it is deleterious to the cell.

There is a progressive loss of dendritic spines in the pyramidal nerve cells affecting the entire neurone throughout life. This is most marked in the third layer pyramidal cell of the prefrontal and superior temporal cortex. (Scheibel & Scheibel, 1975). Initially there is a progressive globular swelling of the cell body with lumps on the dendritic processes. The basilar dendrites are lost first, and then the branches, till finally there is a knobbly apical dendrite with few branches. These authors speculated that these changes are secondary to Alzheimer's neurofibrillary degeneration. However, the latter is uncommon in intellectually normal aged individuals.

The other major histological abnormalities of Alzheimer's disease, neuritic plaques, are commonly seen in intellectually normal individuals. Neuritic plaques, composed of abnormal nerve cell processes, many of which are presynaptic terminals containing degenerating mitochondria, glial cells and amyloid, are present in large numbers in the cortex of intellectually normal individuals. They are seen before Alzheimer's neurofibrillary tangles in the third decade and increase rapidly in number in the fifth and sixth decades. Initially they are composed of distended neurites with small numbers of glial processes. In the fully developed stage there is a central amyloid core, while finally the lesion is composed of a central core of amyloid surrounded by glial cells (Terry & Wisniewski, 1970).

Neuritic plaques, unlike Alzheimer's neurofibrillary tangles, can be found in large numbers in intellectually normal individuals (Tomlinson et al, 1970; Tomlinson & Henderson, 1976). In the latter authors' opinion, neurofibrillary tangles are never found in large numbers in intellectually normal individuals. When they are present, the number of neuritic plaques can be correlated with the degree of dementia early in the course of the illness. Similarly, granulovacuolar degeneration and Hirano bodies can be observed in intellectually normal individuals but are restricted to the pyramidal cells of Sommer's sector and the adjacent subiculum of the temporal lobe.

Atherosclerotic changes are commonly seen in the large intracranial vessels at autopsy in intellectually normal individuals. The small vessels show increasing tortuosity, spiralling and coiling. The relationship of these changes to loss of brain tissue and neurones is not clear. Studies of cerebral circulation and metabolism indicated that there is a slight metabolic diminution with age (Lassen et al, 1960). These abnormalities are common to individuals living in high altitudes without evidence of abnormally rapid ageing.

Amyloid deposition in both small and large vessels is a common finding of both the intracranial and extracranial vessels (Wright et al, 1969). The finding of amyloid within intracranial vessels is commonly associated with amyloid-containing neuritic plaques. Rarely are vessels involved without the presence of plaques. Thus all the macroscopic and microscopic changes described in normal aged individuals are common to Alzheimer's disease. The problem for future research is why they occur in such large numbers in Alzheimer's disease.

MACROSCOPIC PATHOLOGY IN ALZHEIMER'S DISEASE

A major macroscopic observation of the brain from a demented patient with Alzheimer's disease is loss of weight. However, this finding is variable, and

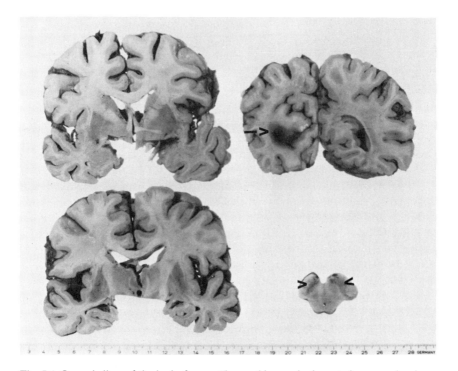

Fig. 7.1 Coronal slices of the brain from a 65-year-old severely demented woman showing atrophy of the temporal lobes and haemorrhage into the occipital lobe (arrow). There is associated Parkinsonism, with pallor of the substantia nigra (arrows)

patients with grossly reduced intellectual function can have normal brain weights (Terry, 1980) The widening of the sulci and narrowing of the gyri reflect the loss of cortical tissue and this is most pronounced in the temporal lobes (Fig. 7.1). There is no objective evidence of thinning of the cortex (Terry, 1980). Preliminary work indicates that the cortex is shortened (Duyckaerts et al, 1985) rather than thinned, which suggests there is a reduction in the number of vertical cortical columns and not a selective lesion in a specific layer. This observation supports other reports of micro-

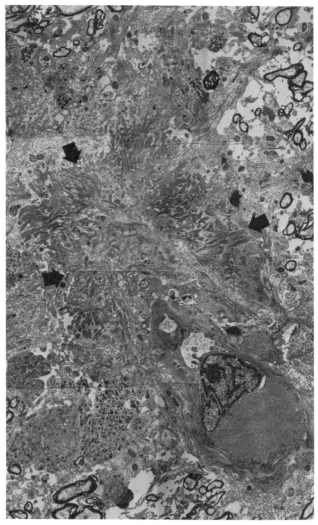

Fig. 7.2 Cerebral cortex in Alzheimer's disease to show congophilic angiopathy. Note the outward extension of amyloid bundles (arrows) from the walls of a blood vessel obliquely sectioned, and abnormally swollen processes in the left lower corner. E. M. mag. × 3122. (Courtesy of Dr Luis H. Carrasco)

scopic studies which suggest that the cortical damage is columnar (Pearson et al, 1985). In addition, the ventricles are commonly grossly enlarged, which reflects the myelin loss from the hemispheres. This occurs at a later stage than the cortical loss and is probably secondary to loss of the large motor neurones.

Intracerebral haemorrhages are rarely seen as a terminal event (Fig. 7.1). However, they can complicate congophilic angiopathy when the vessels are severely weakened by amyloid deposition (Fig. 7.2). Similarly, cerebral infarction occurs because of associated atherosclerosis and hypertension with occlusion of large vessels secondary to emboli.

MICROSCOPIC PATHOLOGY IN ALZHEIMER'S DISEASE

Neurones

Neuronal pathology

The dementia in Alzheimer's disease is associated with the loss of a small but significant number of large cortical neurones (Terry et al, 1981). Loss of cortical function can result from the loss of neurones but equally from loss of dendritic branching of neurones. The loss of dendrites from the pyramidal cells in the neocortex is a more marked feature and significantly in excess of that seen in normal aged individuals. The basilar and horizontal dendrites are particularly vulnerable and are important because they represent the receptors of the satellite cells of layers 2 and 4 and are involved in intracortical circuts, particularly the more subtle modulating inhibitory component of cortical activity (Scheibel & Scheibel, 1975). The loss of the dendritic arborization in association with intraneuronal fibrillary tangles has suggested that the latter interferes with cellular metabolism and transport, resulting in the dying back of the distal portion of the axon. The loss of the dendritic tree occurs in normal aged individuals without large numbers of neurofibrillary tangles, but the latter may be an additional factor late in the course of the disease.

It has been suggested that the accumulation of lipofuscin is excessive in Alzheimer's disease and that this leads to accelerated ageing (Torack, 1978); however, quantitative studies (Mann & Sinclair, 1978) have not confirmed this. In a series of blind patients the amount of lipofuscin was found to be less than that of normally-sighted controls, suggesting that the accumulation of this material is related to neuronal function (Scholtz & Brown, 1978). The same study included a group of Alzheimer patients, who showed amounts between the blind and control subjects, which suggests that the accumulation of lipofuscin is not a necessary association of dementia.

The neuronal pathology may be secondary to the effect of aluminium or a virus on the nucleus of the neurons. Aluminium is found in increased amounts in neuronal nuclei of Alzheimer brains, (Crapper et al, 1973, 1980). Experimentally there is an increased amount of neurofilaments in animals exposed to aluminium. In tissue culture aluminium increases the total amount of protein present as neurofilaments while reducing the amount of ribosomal RNA (Miller & Levine, 1974; Mann et al, 1981). Cytoplasmic RNA and nucleolar volume have been used as markers for protein synthesis and shown to be reduced in autopsy (Scholtz et al, 1981; Mann & Yates, 1982) and biopsy material (Mann et al, 1981). It is postulated that this is secondary to alteration in DNA-directed messenger RNA and occurs before the accumulation of neurofilaments. (Mann & Yates, 1982). Inclusion bodies have been described in the nuclei of neurones of patients with Alzheimer's disease (Troper et al, 1980), supporting the idea that a primary nuclear abnormality might be the cause of the disruption of protein synthesis.

Neurofibrillary tangles

Neurofibrillary tangles (see Figs. 7.3, 7.4) — first described by Alzheimer nearly 80 years ago (Wilkins & Brody, 1969) — have stood the test of time as one of the more important markers of this disease, both diagnostically and in relation to intellectual function. 'One or several fibres stood out due to their extraordinary thickness and impregnability. At a later stage, many fibrils appeared situated side by side and altered in the same way. Then they merged into dense bundles and reached the surface of the cell. Finally, the nucleus and the cell disintegrated and only a dense bundle of fibrils indicated the site where a ganglion cell had been.' Even more important, the initial description by Alzheimer gives an impression of a progressive

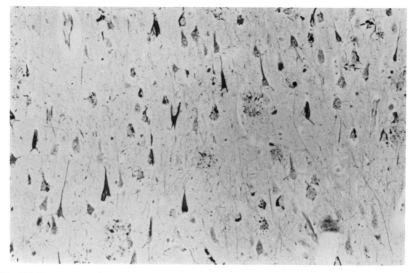

Fig. 7.3 Low-power photomicrograph of the hippocampus in Alzheimer's disease, showing large numbers of neuritic plaques and neurofibrillary tangles. (Modified palmgren × 75)

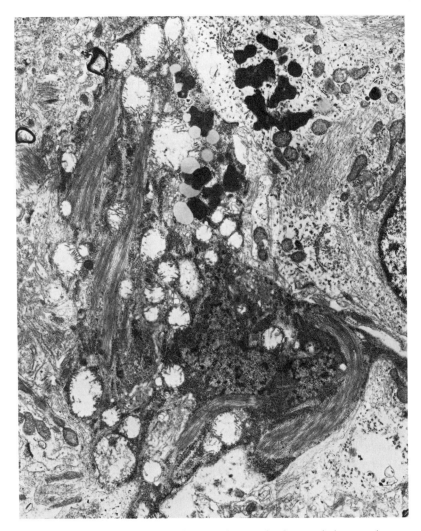

Fig. 7.4 Severe intracytoplasmic neurofibrillary degeneration in a cortical neuron in Alzheimer's disease. E. M. mag. × 66 000. (Courtesy of Dr Luis H. Carrasco)

accumulation of neurofilaments which alter in their staining reaction to silver to merge into dense bundles filling the cell. This raises the question of the origin, mode of development and nature of the densely argyrophilic fibrillary mass we commonly see in Alzheimer's disease.

Neurofilaments are one of the three major structural proteins which make up the cytoskeleton. They are also called intermediate filaments because they are intermediate in diameter (7–11 nm) between the smaller microfilament (6 nm) and the large microtubules (25 nm). Neurofilaments are linear structures composed of three subunits of 68 000, 160 000 and 200 000 daltons molecular weight (Schlaepfer, 1978). These polypeptides appear to be antigenically related and are physically arrahged with the 68 000 dalton unit in the central core and the 200 000 unit placed peripherally (Willard & Simon, 1981). In addition to these three major fibrous systems a fourth class of filament with a diameter of 2–3 nm has recently been described (Schliwa & van Blerkom, 1981); these filaments appear to function as 'linkers' between various fibres. These linker molecules have a specific capacity to associate with constituents of the intermediate filaments along with the 200 000 dalton unit of the neurofilament. Once formed, the neurofilaments move distally within the axon in the slow component of axoplasmic movement at a rate of 1 mm per day.

Neurofilaments can exist either as a structural organelle or as dispersed subunits in the cytoplasm. However, the aggregation and dispersion of the subunits is profoundly affected by ionic conditions of the cytoplasm and by certain agents such as colchicine and vinblastine (Weisenberg & Timasheff, 1970).

The development of the neurofibrillary tangles can be presented as either an abnormality of the synthesis of the fibrous protein subunits previously described or of the cell environment that affects subunit aggregation. The resulting abnormal filament interferes with cytoplasmic flow, particularly in the axons and dendrites, causing dilatation and degeneration of the synapses. It is the degeneration of these synapses which forms the neuritic plaque.

The alternative concept is that the proliferation of the filaments is a reaction to injury of the terminal synapses and axons. The potential damaging agent would interfere with axonal flow following dispersion of microtubules. Microtubules can be disrupted experimentally by elevation of serum calcium and vincristine, causing the accumulation of filament aggregates (Wisniewski et al, 1964). This accumulation is associated with increased production of fibrous protein, a well recognised event following distant injury after axon section and in association with vincristine neuropathy (Shelanski & Wisniewski, 1969). In this concept the neuritic plaque would be the initial lesion, a concept supported by the observation that these plaques are more common in non-demented people (Tomlinson et al, 1968).

Aluminium salts can also cause the accumulation of neurofilaments (Klatzo et al, 1965) which have many of the microscopic features of those seen in Alzheimer's disease; however, they are composed of 10 nm filaments and are not paired. They also lack birefringence and do not stain with congo red (Wisniewski, 1979) as the neurofibrillary tangles of Alzheimer's disease do. Increased amounts of aluminium have been found in neurones of Alzheimer's disease bound to DNA (Crapper et al, 1976). In neuroblastoma cells exposed to aluminium there was a reduction of ribosomal RNA and the level of the protein acetylcholinesterase was depressed (Miller & Levine, 1974). Thus aluminium, while not producing the typical neurofibrillary tangles of Alzheimer's disease, may have a role in their formation.

The composition of neurofibrillary tangles is still a matter of debate. Electron-microscopic examination of the tangles shows continuity of neurofilaments with neurofibrillary tangles (Oyanagi, 1974). These tangles are highly insoluble, which has made biochemical analysis and the development of antibodies particularly difficult. Fractioned enriched paired helical filaments have in addition a polypeptide molecule of about 50 000 daltons (Iqbal et al, 1974, 1975) possibly related to tubulin. Microtubules may also contribute to neurofibrillary tangles, as antisera to microtubules react with tangles and the putative tangle protein. However, this may be a serological artefact (Wisniewski & Iqbal, 1980). Thus it is not possible to say if the tangles in demented and non-demented subjects are the same or whether other parts of the cytoskeleton are involved in their development.

The microscopical study of neurones characterizes them as paired filaments each about 10 nm in diameter with periodic twists about every 80 nm, (Wisniewski et al, 1976). Neurofibrillary tangles fill the neuronal body and displace the organelles without disrupting them and are best seen using the silver impregnation techniques in the pyramidal cells of the hippocampal region (Figs 7.3 and 7.4). They occur in neurones elsewhere in the cerebral cortex and in the brain stem. Their appearance is dictated by the shape of the cell, and they tend to wind around the nucleus extending into the axon hillock.

Neurofibrillary tangles are not confined to Alzheimer's disease but may also be seen in the substantia nigra in post-encephalitic Parkinsonism, in the amyotrophic lateral sclerosis Parkinsonism dementia complex found on the island of Guam and in progressive supranuclear palsy. In addition they are found in Down's syndrome, tuberous sclerosis, subacute sclerosing panencephalitis and in boxers (Corsellis et al, 1973). In progressive supranuclear palsy (Steele-Richardson-Olszewski syndrome) where tangles are found mainly in the brain stem including the oculomotor nuclei, neurones may exist and function for a long time with tangles because there is no evidence from the examination of the third nerves or of the external ocular muscles of denervation (Behrman et al, 1969).

The number of tangle-bearing neurones in the neocortex correlates relatively highly with the degree of dementia as assessed on most tests irrespective of patient age (Wilcock & Esiri, 1982). Their presence points to a disorder of large cortical neurones and is in keeping with the finding of Terry et al (1981) of a specific reduction of large cortical neurones in Alzheimer's disease. The tangle-bearing neurones are found in the upper and lower layers of the cortex, with the relative sparing of the middle layer, 4. There seems to be a columnar arrangement of the neurones most affected, with sparing of other columns (Pearson et al, 1985). This observation correlates well with the observation of shortening of the cortex, which also suggests there is loss of vertical columns in Alzheimer's disease (Duyckaerts et al, 1985). In addition the reduction in CAT activity and not vasoactive intestinal peptide (VIP) activity in the cortex suggests that the CAT neurones not co-localized with VIP are selectively lost, while those co-localized are spared.

Neuritic plaques

The first complete description of the neuritic plaques (Figs 7.3 and 7.5) was made by Fuller (1911), but their importance in relation to dementia was not recognized until the studies of Tomlinson et al (1970). During this time the plaques' name has been changed from senile to neuritic, as the importance of their neuritic origin was recognized.

The neuritic plaque is composed of 9 nm extracellular amyloid filaments, thickened neurites representing distended dendrites and small axons dilated by masses of filaments, dense bodies and mitochondria. There are two glial elements: one directly related to the amyloid and considered to be of microglial origin and producing the amyloid, and a second fibrous astrocyte, possibly a reactive cell. The plaques may measure up to 200 μm or more in diameter, their borders are ill-defined and they are larger than the largest neurones.

The amyloid seen in the centre of the plaque is extracellular and histologically identical to that seen in systemic amyloid. It shares the birefringence seen in the neurofibrillary tangles on congo red staining and has a common β-pleated structure. Histochemically it contains less tryptophan and tyrosine than perivascular amyloid, which suggests that local factors may be important in its production (Powers & Spicer, 1977). Prealbumin has been observed in one report as a common constituent of vascular and plaque amyloid and neurofibrillary tangles, indicating that all three share a common antigen (Shirahama et al, 1982).

Plaques may develop in the absence of amyloid (Kidd, 1965), and so the latter is unlikely to be the initiating factor in plaque formation. The presence of amyloid in the plaque has been used to suggest that antibody–antigen complexes form locally. The inconstant relationship of plaques to blood vessels suggests an exogenous factor, e.g. immune complexes may be important in their aetiology. On leaking from a blood vessel into the perivascular space, the antibody antigen complexes may be catabolized by phagocytes and converted to amyloid by lysosomes (Wisniewski et al, 1975).

Amyloid commonly seen in the vessels of these patients may allow agents toxic to neurones to leak into the brain and activate an enzyme which converts neurofilaments to the tangles. It has also been suggested that amyloid is an aggregate of an unconventional infective agent which contains neither RNA or DNA — the prion (Prusiner et al, 1983).

The other important component of the neuritic plaque is the thickened neurites. These are seen early in the course of plaque formation (Fig. 7.5). The initiating factor may be an agent interfering with axonal flow. The accumulation of mitochondria and other organelles reflects the altered

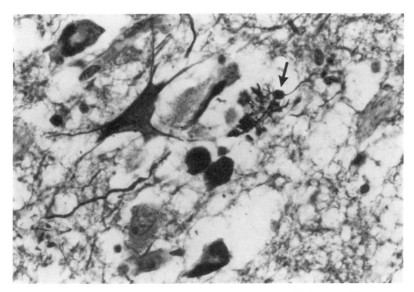

Fig. 7.5 Microphotograph of the hippocampus in a patient with Alzheimer's disease showing distended neuritic terminals around an axon. (Modified Palmgren × 150).

axonal flow. The maturation of the plaque depends on the release of amyloid and the astrocytic reaction. The changes in the glial cells follow those in the neurites. This is shown biochemically by the increased activity in Cathepin A, a marker for brain macrophages (Bowen et al, 1977) which are present in considerable numbers in Alzheimer's disease.

Plaques can be induced experimentally without amyloid formation in animals treated with aluminium (Wisniewski & Terry 1968) when the cortex is undercut. However, neuritic plaques have been described in association with amyloid in mice infected with the infectious agent for scrapie (Wisniewski et al, 1979).

Hirano bodies

These bodies (Fig. 7.6) were initially described by Hirano et al (1968) in cases of the Parkinsonism-dementia complex which occurs on the island of Guam. They are seen with increasing age in the hippocampus of adults without neurological disease and may be present in the hippocampus of Alzheimer's disease in large numbers. Usually they are immediately adjacent to the hippocampal pyramidal neurones but may be found away from neurones. They appear as paracrystalline, ovoid or spheroid bodies and are brightly eosinophilic on light-microscopic examination. Electron microscope examination shows them to be sheets of membrane-bound ribosomal particles derived from partially degraded rough endoplasmic reticulum (O'Brien et al, 1980).

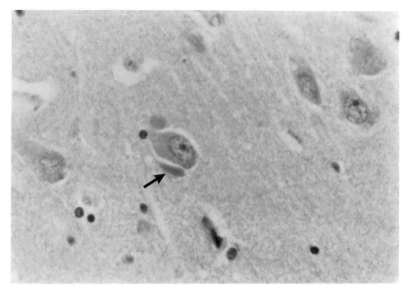

Fig. 7.6 Microphotograph of the hippocampus in a patient with Alzheimer's disease showing a crysalline Hirano body (H&E × 188)

Granulovacuolar degeneration

These are membrane-bound cytoplasmic bodies 3–5 μm in diameter containing an irregular electron-dense core surrounded by electron-lucent material (Fig. 7.7). One or more may be present in a neuron, and when large numbers are present the cell becomes distorted. They may be present

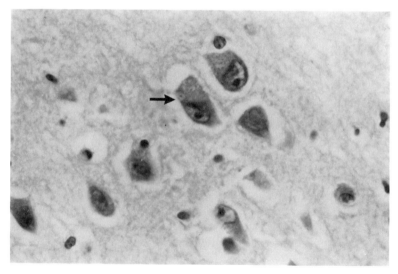

Fig. 7.7 Microphotograph of the hippocampus in a patient with Alzheimer's disease showing granulovascular degeneration (H&E × 188)

in individuals who are intellectually normal over the age of 65 and in a variety of neurological conditions. They are most characteristically seen in the pyramidal cells in the hippocampus.

CEREBROVASCULAR AMYLOID

The term amyloid was devised by Virchow (1860) to describe abnormal tissue aggregates that had staining properties similar to starch. The incidence of amyloid deposition in vessels increases progressively with old age and is accompanied by a loss of T-cell function with age in animals. (Rodney et al, 1971) and humans (Behan & Behan, 1979). Amyloid may be found predominantly in the meningeal vessels and cerebral vessels in normal aged individuals. The term congophilic angiopathy is applied when amyloid is deposited within cerebral arterioles, capillaries and vessels (Scholz, 1938). The amyloid, besides being present within vessels, may radially extend into the brain substance (Fig. 7.2). In this instance the angiopathy, if associated with intellectual impairment with absence of other pathology in the brain, constitutes an aetiologically unique form of dementia (Torack, 1978).

Cerebrovascular amyloid is one of the commonest findings in Alzheimer's disease (Mandybur, 1975). The amyloid usually begins to collect in the muscular layer and extends peripherally, replacing the adventitia. The amyloidogenic protein in the blood may be converted in the vessels, allowing other proteins to leak into the brain which in turn initiate the development of neurofibrillary tangles (Glenner et al, 1981).

Amyloid, both in vessels and plaques, shares several major physiochemical properties with neurofibrillary tangles. It has a fibrillar structure and shares a β-pleated configuration which is birefringent on congo red staining. In addition, the prion, a protein particle which does not contain RNA or DNA and is the infectious agent in scrapie (McKinley et al, 1983), has a similar staining reaction to congo red (Prusiner, 1984). Prusiner et al (1983) suggested that amyloid may be the infectious particle in Alzheimer's disease. The histopathological features of Alzheimer's disease are only partially similar to those of Creutzfeldt-Jakob disease, where a transmissible virus-like agent is thought to cause the disease. In the latter entity the cortex has a spongiform appearance with a marked astrocytic reaction which is not commonly seen in Alzheimer's disease. In addition the neuritic plaques and neurofibrillary tangles are not in evidence to the same extent.

SUBCORTICAL PATHOLOGY

One of the major observations in the study of the brains of patients with Alzheimer's disease has been the identification of pathology in subcortical nuclei. These nuclei are in the basal forebrain (medial septal nucleus, diagonal band of Broca and nucleus of Meynert), locus caeruleus and the raphe complex of the pons and brain stem. The study of these areas was initiated by the realization that the cortex in patients with Alzheimer's disease, which has reduced amounts of the biosynthetic enzyme for acetylcholine — choline acetyl transferase (CAT) — has few if any intrinsic CAT neurons and so there is dysfunction of the ascending pathways to the cortex. The origin of the ascending CAT projection to the cortex is in the nucleus of Meynert, and that of the hippocampal projection is in the septum. The loss of cortical dopamine-β-hydroxylase activity and noradrenaline is associated with loss of cells from the locus caeruleus (Bondareff et al, 1981). The dorsal raphe nucleus projects serotonin (5HT) to the neocortex. In Alzheimer's disease it shows marked neurofibrillary tangle formation. Which is the primary pathology, the cortical degeneration with secondary pathology in these nuclei, or vice versa, has yet to be decided. The readily apparent cortical pathology suggests that the cortex is the initial area damaged, and the common anatomy of the subcortical nuclei suggests that they may be destroyed because they are selectively vulnerable. These observations do not exclude the possibility that other neuronal groups are involved.

These subcortical nuclei have an additional feature in common besides the cortical projection: they all contain a large number of cells with a nonspecialized isodendritic pattern of extensive intermingling with other neurones which form a continuous isodendritic core extending from the spinal cord to the basal forebrain. Because of this microscopic feature they have been grouped under the heading of the isodendritic core. The neurones in this group are similar to what was called the reticular formation. The pathology of these nuclei is, firstly, neuronal loss. This is uniform throughout the nuclei and correlated with reduction in nucleolar volume, suggesting that there is a progressive reduction in protein synthesis leading to cell death (Mann et al, 1984). In the locus caeruleus the neuronal loss is not closely correlated with the clinical or pathological features of dementia (Tomlinson et al, 1981). Also in the nucleus of Meynert, neuronal loss in elderly patients is greater than in demented cases of Alzheimer's disease (Perry et al, 1983). The dementia in both Parkinson's disease and Alzheimer's disease is related to cortical cholinergic defects and to loss of neurones in the nucleus of Meynert. These abnormalities are no greater in the latter despite the more severe dementia. This suggests that the cognitive impairment in Alzheimer's disease originates from a primary cortical abnormality with secondary changes in the ascending cholinergic system. This supports the concept that the cognitive impairment is not necessarily a function of neuronal loss in this disease, but does not exclude the possiblity that other functional defects are also present, as the intellectual impairment correlates more closely with cortical neurochemistry than changes in the subcortical nuclei. The common pathology suggests that neurones in the isodendritic core are selectively vulnerable to this disease process.

The amygdala

The amygdala may play an important role in the pathogenesis of Alzheimer's disease because many of its functions — emotion motivation and memory — are disturbed in Alzheimer's disease. Bilateral lesions of the amygdala in animals produce striking abnormalities of behaviour and affect (Dicks et al, 1969). The amygdala, like the other subcortical areas involved in Alzheimer's disease, has extensive, direct and reciprocal connections with the frontal cortex (Nauta, 1961).

In Alzheimer's disease there is a 70% decrease in the absolute number of neurones (Hertzog & Kemper, 1980). The degeneration is selective, affecting the medial nucleus and the medial portion of the central nucleus. These parts of the amygdala are composed predominantly of fusiform isodendritic cells similar to those in the other subcortical areas involved in Alzheimer's disease.

PRESENILE AND SENILE FORMS OF ALZHEIMER'S DISEASE

There are no good neuropathological grounds for separating these two clinical groups (Corsellis, 1976b). In general terms the brains of the patients with the presenile forms tend to be more shrunken, often less than 1000 g, and the histological features of neuritic plaque and neurofibrillary tangle formation more severe and widespread. Atrophy is not a constant feature in extreme old age, and the major histological feature is the large number of neuritic plaques rather than the presence of tangles. Similarly, neuronal loss from the nucleus basalis of Meynert and locus caeruleus is greater in the presenile form. In the senile form, neuronal loss approached that of the age and sex matched controls (Mann et al, 1984).

FAMILIAL ALZHEIMER'S DISEASE

A family history of Alzheimer's disease has often been reported (Tomlinson & Corsellis, 1984) and up to one-third of cases may have a family history of pyschiatric illness.

Neuropathological study of the brains of familial cases shows that the histological and quantitative pathology is the same as in the spontaneous cases.

COMPLICATED ALZHEIMER'S DISEASE

Atherosclerosis of the intracranial muscular arteries is a common observation in aged individuals in our developed society and may be observed in patients with Alzheimer's disease. In general, patients in the presenile group are free of atherosclerosis, which is usually attributed to the poor state of nutrition during the terminal phase of the illness (Tomlinson &

Corsellis, 1984). Individuals of more advanced years are likely to have a similar distribution of atherosclerosis to age and sex matched controls. It is not uncommon to see the effects of atherosclerosis and hypertensive small vessel disease in the white matter and cortex of patients with Alzheimer's disease. Cerebral infarction may cause progression of the dementia in a patient with Alzheimer's disease, particularly if it results in destruction of an important area.

Occasionally, rapid progression of the disease or unusual symptoms may develop when the disease process is accelerated by trauma and the development of a subdural haematoma. Subdural haematoma can occur with minimal trauma in patients with gross cerebral atrophy when the subdural veins are readily torn. The subdural haematoma may be difficult to recognize in an individual who is partially demented. Similarly, individuals with severe vascular disease secondary to congophilic angiopathy can have secondary haemorrhage (Fig. 7.1). Should a demented individual have a myocardial infarct and suffer profound hypotension, it is possible for boundary zone lesions to cause progression of the brain damage.

RELATIONSHIP BETWEEN PARKINSONISM AND ALZHEIMER'S DISEASE

Patients with Parkinsonism can present with a cognitive defect of varying severity. Where the dementia is severe, neuropathological study shows all the features of Alzheimer's disease, and the two diseases appear to coexist. There is also a group of patients with Parkinsonism who have mild dementia and do not show the pathology of Alzheimer's disease in the cortex. In this group there is a markedly reduced CAT level (Perry et al, 1983). Study of the nucleus basalis of Meynert shows neuronal loss (Whitehouse et al, 1983).

Study of the subcortical regions known to be pathologically involved in Alzheimer's disease and Parkinsonism suggests that there are areas of involvement common to the two disorders. In both diseases the locus caeruleus, Meynert nucleus and dorsal raphe nucleus, all of which project to the cortex, there is neuronal loss which is more extensive in Parkinsonism than Alzheimer's disease. This suggests that the neurone number lost is not important to the dementia's severity.

CONCLUSION

Does the pathology of the cortex explain the dementia in Alzheimer's disease? Since the correlation of the dementia score and the number of neuritic plaques (Blessed et al, 1968), critical evaluation of this work has lead to doubt of the relevance of neuritic plaques to the dementia. This is because of a lack of homogeneity in the demented patient in the latter study (Ball, 1984). Additional work indicated that the correlation of dementia with neurofibrillary tangles is more impressive (Wilcock & Esiri, 1982). The cognitive impairment in Alzheimer's disease can also be correlated with the cholinergic deficit in the cortex and changes in the ascending cholinergic system. Preliminary macroscopic and histological study of the distribution of these tangles in the cortex indicated that they have a columnar arrangement. This suggests that one subset of neurones is involved in the disease process.

Comparison of the pathology in the less severely demented Parkinsonism without Alzheimer's disease with the severely demented Alzheimer's disease patients suggests that the more severe dementia in the latter group may be explained by the cortical pathology. The pathology of the secondary effect of the subcortical pathology on the cortex in the less severely demented cases of Parkinsonism has yet to be described.

At present there is no absolute pathological criterion for the diagnosis of Alzheimer's disease. Alzheimer patients may have a brain of normal weight with minimal cortical pathology, and intellectually normal individuals may have large numbers of neuritic plaques with significant numbers of neurofibrillary tangles. Future study must separate the latter group from Alzheimer's disease, both by quantifying the pathological features they share and by studying the pathological process as the disease develops. Neurones not involved in the Alzheimer's disease process have minor cellular changes which suggest that plaques and tangles represent the end stage of the disease process.

The study of the aetiology of Alzheimer's disease is primarily the search for an environmental agent which, after interacting with the genetic background of the individual, produces the disease. The identification of the agent has been slowed by the lack of an experimental model. The neurofibrillary degeneration produced by aluminium toxicity is not the same as the neurofibrillary tangles seen in Alzheimer's disease. Small amounts of silicon have been identified in plaques, which may also be significant.

Alzheimer's disease appears to lack transmissibility to animals, which may mean that those used are not permissive hosts. In one transmission experiment, where a disease developed in the monkey similar to Creutzfeldt-Jakob disease, there is doubt about the labelling of the specimens during preparation. The possible infective agent is the prion which may be similar to that seen in scrapie in sheep.

Besides study of the brains of patients, the rest of the host must be examined. Of particular relevance is the immune system and the role of the T-cell in the disease process and its relevance to the development of amyloid.

REFERENCES

Ball M J 1984 The morphological basis of dementia in Parkinson's disease. Canadian Journal of Neurological Sciences 11 Supp: 180–181
Behan P O, Behan W M H 1979 possible immunological factors in Alzheimer's disease. In:

Glen A I M, Whalley L J (eds) Alzheimer's disease: early recognition of potentially reversible deficits. Churchill Livingstone, Edinburgh

Behrman S, Carroll J D, Janota I, Matthews W B 1969 Progressive supranuclear palsy. Clinicopathological study of four cases. Brain 92: 663–678

Blessed G, Tomlinson B E, Roth M 1968 The association between quantitative measures of dementia and of senile changes in the cerebral grey matter of elderly subjects. British Journal of Psychiatry 114: 791–811

Bondareff W, Mountjoy C Q, Roth M 1981 Selective loss of neurones of origin of adrenergic projection to cerebral cortex (nucleus locus caeruleus in senile dementia). Lancet 1: 783–784

Bowen D M, Smith C B, White P, et al 1977 Chemical pathology of the organic dementias II. Quantitative estimation of cellular changes in post mortem brains. Brain 100: 427–453

Brody H 1955 Organisation of the cerebral cortex III. A study of ageing in the human cerebral cortex. Journal of Comparative Neurology 102: 511–536

Brody H 1970 Structural changes in the ageing nervous system. Interdisciplinary Topics in Gerontology 7: 9–21

Colon E J 1972 The elderly brain. A quantitative analysis of the cerebral cortex in two cases. Psychiatria, Neurolgia and Neurochirurgia (AMST) 75: 261–270

Corsellis J A N 1962 Mental illness and the ageing brain. Oxford University Press, London

Corsellis J A N 1976a Some observations on the Purkinje cell population and on brain volume in human ageing. In: Neurobiology of ageing, Terry R D, Gersham S (eds) Vol 3, Raven Press, New York

Corsellis J A N 1976b Ageing and the dementias. In: Blackwood W, Corselles J A N (eds) Greenfields neuropathology, 3rd edn, Edward Arnold, London

Corsellis J A N , Bruton C J, Freeman-Browne D 1973 The aftermath of boxing. Psychological Medicine 3: 207–303

Crapper D R, Krishnan S S, Dalton A J 1973 Brain aluminium distribution in Alzheimer's disease and experimental neurofibrillary degeneration. Science (New York) 180: 511–513

Crapper D R, Krishnan S S, Quittkat S 1976 Aluminium neurofibrillary degeneration and Alzheimer's disease. Brain 99

Crapper D R, Quittkat S, Krishnan S S, Dalton A T, De Boni V 1980 Intranuclear aluminium cortex in Alzheimer's disease, dialysis encephalopathy and experimental aluminium encephalopathy. Acta Neuropathologica 50: 19–24

Davis P J M, Wright E A 1977 A new method for measuring cranial cavity and its application to the assessment of cerebral atrophy at autopsy. Neuropathology and Applied Neurobiology 3: 341–358

Dekaban A S, Sadowsky D 1978 Changes in brain weight during the span of human life: relation of brain weight to body height and body weight. Annals of Neurology 4: 345–356

Dicks D, Myers R E, Kling A 1969 Uncus and amygdala lesions. Effects on social behaviour in the free ranging rhesus monkey. Science 165: 69–71

Duyckaerts C, Hauw J J, Piette F, Raunsard C, Poulain R, Bethaux P, Eseourolle R 1985 Cortical atrophy in senile dementia of Alzheimer type is mainly due to decrease in cortical length. Acta Neuropathologica (Berlin) 66: 72–74

Fuller S 1911 A study of the miliary plaques found in brains of the aged. American Journal of Insanity 68: 147–217

Glenner G G, Henry J H, Fujihara S 1981 Congophilic angiopathy in the pathogenesis of Alzheimer's disease. Annals of Pathology (Paris) 1: 120–129

Glenner G G, Page D L 1976 Amyloid amyloidosis and amyloidogenesis. In: Richter G W, Epstein M A (eds) International Review of Experimental Pathology 15, Academic Press, New York, p 1–92

Hall T C, Miller A K H, Corsellis J A N 1975 Variations in the human Purkinje cell population according to age and sex. Neuropathology and Applied Neurobiology 1: 267–292

Herzog A G, Kemper T H 1980 Amygdaloid changes in ageing and dementia. Archives of Neurology 37: 625–629

Hirano A 1965 Slow, latent and temporate virus infections. In: Gajdusek D C, Gibbs C J (eds) Monograph No 2. National Institute of Health, p 23–27

Hirano A, Dembither H M, Jurlald L T, Zimmerman H M 1968 The fine structure of some intraganglionic alterations. Journal of Neuropathology and Experimental Neurology 27: 167–182

Ihara Y, Abraham C, Selkoe D J 1982 Antibodies to paired helical filaments in Alzheimer's disease do not recognise normal human brain proteins. Nature 304: 327–329

Iqbal K, Wisniewski H M, Grundke — Iqbal I, Korthals J K, Terry R D 1975 Chemical pathology of neurofibrils. Neurofibrillary tangles of Alzheimer's presenile-senile dementia. Journal of Histochemistry and Cytochemistry 23: 563–569

Iqbal K, Wisniewski H M, Shelanski M L, Brostoff S, Liwnez B H, Terry R D 1974 Protein changes in senile dementia. Brain Research 77: 337–343

Kidd M 1965 Alzheimer's disease — an electronmicroscopical study. Brain 87: 307–320

Klatzo I, Wisniewski H, Streicher E 1965 experimental production of neurofibrillary degeneration. 1. Light microscopic observations. Journal of Neuropathology and Experimental Neurology 24: 187–199

Lassen L A, Feinberg I, Lane M H 1960 Bilateral studies of cerebral oxygen uptake in young and aged normal subjects and in patients with organic dementia. Journal of Clinical Investigation 39: 491–500

Mc Kinley M P, Bolton D C, Prusiner S B 1983 A protease-resistant protein is a structural component of the scrapie prion. Cell 35: 57–62

Mandybur T I 1975 The incidence of cerebral amyloid angiopathy in Alzheimer's disease. Neurology 25: 120–126

Mann D M A, Sinclair K G A 1978 The quantitative asessment of lipofuscin pigment, cytoplasmic RNA and nucleolar volume in senile dementia. Neuropathology and Applied Neurobiology 4: 129–135

Mann D M A, Neary D, Yates P O, Lincoln J, Snowden J S, Stanworth P 1981 Alterations in protein synthetic capability in Alzheimer's disease. Journal of Neurology, Neurosurgery and Psychiatry 44: 97–102

Mann D M A, Yates P O 1982 Ageing, nucleic acids and pigments. In: Smith W T, Cavanagh J B (eds) Recent advances in neuropathology 2. Churchill Livingstone, Edinburgh

Mann D M A, Yates P O, Marcyniuk B 1984 Alzheimer's presenile dementia, senile dementia of Alzheimer type and Down's syndrome in middle age form an age related continuum of pathological changes. Neuropathology and Applied Neurobiology 10: 185–207

Miller C A, Levine E M 1974 Effects of aluminium salts on cultured neuroblastoma cells. Journal of Neurochemistry 22: 751–758

Nauta W J H 1961 Fibre degeneration following lesions of the amygdaloid complex in the monkey. Journal of Anatomy 95: 515–531

O'Brien L, Shelley K, Towfighi J, McPherson A 1980 Crystalline ribosomes are present in brains from senile humans. Proceedings of the National Academy of Sciences USA II: 2260–2264

Oyanagi S 1974 An electron microscopic observation on senile dementia with special references to transformation of neurofilaments to twisted tubules and a structural connection of Pick bodies to Alzheimer's neurofibrillary changes. Advances in Neurological Science 18: 77–88

Pearson R C, Esiri M M, Hiorns R W, Wilcock G K, Powell T B 1985 Anatomical correlates of the distribution of the pathological changes in the neocenter in Alzheimer's disease. Proceedings of the National Academy of Sciences USA 82: 4531–4534

Perry E K, Tomlinson B E, Blessed G, Bergmann K, Gibson P H, Perry R H 1978 Correlation of cholinergic abnormalities with senile plaques and mental test scores in senile dementia. British Medical Journal 2: 1457–1459

Perry R H, Tomlinson B E, Candy J M, Blessed G, Foster J F, Bloxham C A, Perry E K 1983 Cortical cholinergic deficit in mentally impaired Parkinsonian patients. Lancet 2: 789–790

Powers J M, Spicer S S 1977 Histochemical similarity of senile plaque amyloid to apudamyloid. Virchows Archives: A Pathology, Anatomy and Histology 376: 107–115

Prusiner S B 1984 Some speculation about prions, amyloid and Alzheimer's disease. The New England Journal of Medicine 310: 661–663

Prusiner S B, McKinley M P, Bowman K A et al 1983 Scrapie prions aggregate to form amyloid-like birefringent rods. Cell 35: 349–358

Rodey G E, Good R A, Yunis E J 1971 Progressive loss in vitro of cellular immunity with ageing of mice susceptible to autoimmune disease. Clinical and Experimental Immunology 9: 305–311

Roth M, Tomlinson B E, Blessed G 1966 Correlation between scores for dementia and counts of senile plaques in cerebral grey matter of elderly subjects. Nature 209: 109–110

Scheibel M E, Scheibel A B 1975 Structural changes in the ageing brain. In: Brody H, Harmand D, Ordy J M (eds) Ageing 1: Clinical morphologic and neurochemical aspects in the ageing central nervous system. Raven Press, New York

Schlaepfer W W 1978 Observations on the disassembly of isolated mammal neurofilaments. Journal of Cell Biology 76: 50–60

Scheibel M E, Lindsay R D, Tomiyasu V, Scheibel A B 1975 Progressive dendritic changes in ageing human cortex. Experimental Neurology 47: 392–403

Schliwa M, van Blerkom J 1981 Structural interrelation of cytoskeletal components. Journal of Cell Biology 90: 222–235

Scholtz C L 1938 Studien zur Pathologie der Hirngefässe, II Die drusige Entartung der Hirnarterien und Capillaren (Eine Form seniler Gefässerkrankung). Zeitschrift für die gesamte Neurologie und Psychiatrie 162: 694–715

Scholtz C L, Brown A 1978 Lipofuscin and transsynaptic degeneration. Virchows Archives: A Pathology Anatomy and Histology 281: 35–40

Scholtz C L, Swettenham K, Brown A, Mann D M A 1981 A quantitative study of the striate cortex and lateral geniculate body in normal blind demented subjects. Neuropathology and Applied Neurobiology 7: 103–114

Sekhon S S, Maxwell D S 1974 Ultrastructural changes in neurones of spinal anterior horns of ageing mice with particular reference to the accumulation of lipofuscin pigment. Journal of Neurocytology 3: 59–72

Shelanski M L, Wisniewski H M 1969 Neurofibrillary degeneration. Archives of Neurology 20: 199–206

Shirahama T, Skinner M, Westermark P, Rubinow A, Cohen A, Brun A, Kemper T L 1982 Senile cerebral amyloid. American Journal of Pathology 107: 41–50

Terry R D 1980 Structural changes in senile dementia of the Alzheimer type. In: Amaducci L, Davison A N, Antuono P (eds) Ageing of the brain and dementia. Ageing vol 13. Raven Press, New York

Terry R D, Peck A, DeTeresa R, Schechter R, Hordupion D S 1981 Some morphometric aspects of the brain in senile dementia of the Alzheimer type. Annals of Neurology 10: 184–192

Terry R D, Wisniewski H 1970 The ultrastructure of the neurofibrillary tangle and the senile plaque in Alzheimer's disease and related conditions. In: Wolstenholme G E W, O'Connor M (eds) A Ciba Foundation Symposium. Churchill Livingstone, London

Tomlinson B E, Blessed G, Roth M 1968 Observations on the brains of non-demented old people. Journal of Neurological Science 7: 331–356

Tomlinson B E, Blessed G, Roth M 1970 Observations on the brains of demented old people. Journal of Neurological Sciences 11: 205–242

Tomlinson B E, Corsellis J A N 1984 Ageing and the dementias. In: Adams J H, Corsellis J A N, Duchen L W (eds) Greenfields neuropathology, 4th edn. Edward Arnold, London

Tomlinson B E, Henderson G 1976 Some quantitative cerebral findings in normal and demented old people. In: Terry R D, Geshaw S (eds) Neurobiology of Ageing, Vol 3. Raven Press, New York

Tomlinson B E, Irving D, Blessed G 1981 Cell loss in the locus caeruleus in senile dementia of Alzheimer type. Journal of Neurological Sciences 49: 419–428

Torack R M 1978 Current evaluation of pathological correlates of dementia. In: Torack R M (ed) The pathologic physiology of dementia. Springer, Berlin

Troper S, Bannister C M, Lincoln J, Mann D M A, Yates P O 1980 Nuclear inclusions in Alzheimer's disease. Neuropathology and Applied Neurobiology 6: 245–253

Virchow R 1860 Cellular pathology. Churchill, London

Weisenberg R C, Timasheff S M 1970 Aggregation of microtubules subunit protein. Effects of duralent cations colchicine and rublostine. Biochemistry 9: 4110–4116

Whitehouse P J, Hedreen J C, White C L, Price D L 1983 Basal forebrain neurons in the dementia of Parkinson's disease. Annals of Neurology 13: 243–248

Wilcock G K, Esiri M M 1982 Plaques, tangles and dementia. A quantitative study. Journal of Neurological Science 56: 343–356

Wilkins R L, Brody I A 1969 Alzheimer's Disease (Translation of: Uber eine eigenartige Erkrankung der Hirnrinde. 1907 Zentralblatt für die gesamte Neurologie und Psychiatrie 177–179). Archives of Neurology 21: 109–110

Wilks S 1864 Clinical notes on atrophy of the brain. Journal of Mental Science 10: 381–392

Willard M, Simon C 1981 Antibody decoration of neurofilaments. Journal of Cell Biology 89: 198–205

Wisniewski H M 1979 Neurofibrillary and synaptic pathology in senile dementia of the Alzheimer's type (SDAT). In: Glen A I M, Whalley L J (eds) Alzheimer's disease: early recognition of potentially reversible deficits. Churchill Livingstone, Edinburgh

Wisniewski H M, Bruce M E, Fraser H 1975 Infectious etiology of neuritic (senile) plaques in mice. Science 190: 1108–1110

Wisniewski H M, Iqbal K 1980 Ageing of the brain and dementia. Trends in Neuosciences 3: 226–228

Wisniewski H M, Narang H K, Terry R D 1976 Neurofibrillary tangles of paired helical filaments. Journal of Neurological Science 27: 173–181

Wisniewski H, Shelanski M L, Terry R D 1964 Effects of mitotic spindle inhibitors on neurotubules and neurofilaments in anterior horn cells. Journal of Cell Biology 39: 224–229

Wisniewski H, Terry R D 1968 An experimental approach to the morphogenesis of neurofibrillary degeneration and the argyrophilic plaque. In: Wolstenholme G E W, O'Connor M (eds) Alzheimer's disease and related conditions. Churchill Livingstone, London, p 223–241

Wisniewski H M, Terry R D 1973 Reexamination of the pathogenesis of senile plaque In: Timmerman H M (ed) Progress in neuropathology, Vol 2. Grune & Stratton, New York

Wright J R, Calkins E, Breen W T, Stolte G, Schultz R T 1969 Relationship of amyloid to ageing. Review of the literature and a systemic study of 83 patients derived from a general hospital population. Medicine 48: 39–60

Alzheimer's disease: neurobiochemistry

INTRODUCTION

Since 1975 there has been an unprecedented research input into Alzheimer's disease with a more detailed description of the neurochemical abnormalities, even if a pathophysiological explanation is still elusive.

Two important questions have been addressed in an attempt to achieve a biochemical understanding of Alzheimer's disease: firstly, the molecular nature of the proteins in senile plaques and neurofibrillary tangles, and secondly the biochemical features of those neurones which are affected by plaques and tangles or which have suffered premature cell death. The second question of the nature of the selective vulnerability of neurones is an intriguing one which can be applied generally to degenerative disease of the central nervous system.

BIOCHEMICAL NATURE OF PLAQUES AND TANGLES

Senile plaques are variable both in size and, to some extent, in their main components, and this may depend upon the stage of plaque formation. The main components are dystrophic neuronal processes, or neurites, which encircle the plaque and often contain paired helical filaments which are structurally similar to those found in the neurofibrillary tangle. A glial component consists largely of microglia and some astrocytic processes, and centrally there is an amyloid core (see Chapter 7). The precise nature of the amyloid substance has attracted much speculation, and with the recent development of a method for isolating plaque cores (Allsop et al, 1983) the amino-acid composition and sequence of a core protein has been established (Masters et al, 1985). The amino-acid composition is very similar to that of amyloid isolated from pial vessels in Alzheimer's cases (Glenner & Wong, 1984), and neither protein resembles amyloid found elsewhere in the body.

Interestingly, the amyloid core protein does share some characteristics with protein of the neurofibrillary tangle. The neurofibrillary tangle is the other hallmark of Alzheimer's disease and is found within perikarya throughout the cortex and particularly in pyramidal cells. Silver stains reveal at the light-microscope level thick fibrillary material which can be resolved on electron microscopy as paired helical filaments (Kidd, 1963; Terry, 1963). Paired helical filaments are remarkably insoluble in a variety of protein solvents and resistant to proteolytic enzymes, a feature shared with the amyloid core protein (Allsop et al, 1983; Ihara et al, 1983). The amino-acid composition of paired helical filament protein (Ihara et al, 1983) resembles that of both amyloid core protein and pial amyloid (Kidd et al, 1985). However, whether more than one protein is involved and the precise nature of paired helical protein are not yet resolved. Recent evidence suggests that it is not derived from neurofilament (Wischik et al, 1985).

SELECTIVE VULNERABILITY OF NEURONES IN ALZHEIMER'S DISEASE

Although cerebral atrophy in Alzheimer's disease may give the impression of widespread degeneration, the pathological changes appear to involve selective populations of neurones. Neurofibrillary tangles and senile plaques are found throughout the cerebral cortex, but are particularly dense within the temporal cortex and hippocampus, where similar changes are seen in normal old age. Within the cerebral cortex neurofibrillary tangles are found predominantly within pyramidal cells and are uncommon in subcortical structures, with the important exception of certain projection nuclei such as nucleus basalis, substantia nigra and dorsal raphe (see elsewhere in this volume and for review Tomlinson, 1980). Senile plaques are also uncommon outside the cerebral cortex, although they may be found in the claustrum, putamen and subcortical white matter (Rudelli et al, 1984). Within the cerebral cortex itself senile plaques are found in greatest numbers in layers 3 and 5 (Perry et al, 1984; Morrison et al, 1985).

Neuronal loss in Alzheimer's disease is selective, with involvement of cortical (Terry et al, 1982; Mountjoy et al, 1983), nucleus basalis (White-house et al, 1982; Nagai et al, 1983; Rogers et al, 1985) and locus caeruleus neurons (Tomlinson et al, 1981; Bondareff et al, 1982). Less dramatic losses can be seen in normal old age, although there are important differences; whether cell numbers in nucleus basalis are stable throughout life is uncertain (Whitehouse et al, 1983; McGeer et al, 1984). The underlying mechanism of this selective neuronal damage is a major challenge to understanding degenerative disease of the central nervous system. One approach is to seek biochemical characteristics of these neurones which may be common to each, and considerable attention has been directed towards neurotransmitter systems in degenerative disease. This approach is exemplified by Parkinson's disease, in which the neuronal loss can be defined in terms of the dopaminergic nigrostriatal system. However, although the involved neurones may be defined in terms of the neurotransmitter which they release, this may only be a marker and need not provide information on the pathophysiology of the selective degeneration. Indeed, the neurotransmitter receptors which a cell expresses may be as important as the neurotransmitter which is released.

Current studies of neurotransmitter systems in degenerative disease indicate that in general the neuronal loss cannot be defined in terms of a single neurotransmitter. The degeneration in Parkinson's disease is more diverse than the obvious dopamine deficit with additional involvement of noradrenergic, cholinergic and peptide systems (for review see Agid et al, 1986). Similarly, the neurotransmitter abnormalities in Alzheimer's disease are clearly more widespread than the observed cholinergic deficit (for review see Rossor, 1982; Hardy et al, 1985). However, the importance of assessing neurotransmitter systems in Alzheimer's disease lies in the fact that specific clinical features may relate to discrete neurochemical deficits, and the modulation of synaptic transmission may provide an opportunity for therapeutic intervention. The changes in neurotransmitter systems observed in Alzheimer's disease are detailed below, and the possible relationships to histopathological and clinical features discussed.

METHODOLOGY OF POST-MORTEM NEUROCHEMISTRY

Many chemical markers are surprisingly stable after death and provide an opportunity to analyse discrete areas of brain in Alzheimer's disease and to compare with a control group. The majority of data is derived from post-mortem studies, although some information is available from biopsy tissue which circumvents many of the pitfalls of post-mortem analyses.

Chemical markers vary in their post-mortem stability and need to be chosen with care. Acetylcholine, for example, is labile after death, but the biosynthetic enzyme choline acetyltransferase (ChAT), which is confined to cholinergic neurons, is remarkably stable. Most neuropeptides possess surprisingly high stability in post-mortem brain, provided the tissue is not disrupted; this contrasts with the rapid breakdown in plasma and might be due to protection within the neuron from peptidase activities. In addition to the problem of stability, a number of factors need to be considered in addition to the disease under scrutiny which can influence the neurochemical profile. These include age, sex, mode of death or the agonal state, and ante-mortem drug therapy. It is necessary to allow for these factors and to match carefully the two groups before attributing any neurochemical change to the disease itself (for reviews see Bird & Iversen, 1982; Rossor, 1986). Finally, interpretation of neurotransmitter and receptor concentrations may be ambiguous, since it can be difficult to distinguish between losses due to neuronal damage and those due to alterations in turnover. Combinations of quantitative radio immunoassay, immunohistochemistry and specific mRNA analysis may help to resolve these problems.

TRANSMITTER DEFICITS IN ALZHEIMER'S DISEASE

Acetylcholine

The discovery of a cholinergic deficit has fostered a dramatic output of neurochemical data on Alzheimer's disease (for reviews see Rossor, 1982; Coyle et al, 1983; Hardy et al, 1985). The biochemical observation that led to detailed examination of the cholinergic system was reduced activity within cerebral cortex of the enzyme choline acetyltransferase (ChAT) (Bowen et al, 1976; Davies & Maloney, 1976; Perry et al, 1977). This enzyme catalyses the synthesis of acetylcholine from acetyl CoA and choline, and since it is stable post-mortem and confined to acetylcholine neurones, it is a good marker for cholinergic neurones in autopsy studies. However, the enzyme is not rate-limiting for acetylcholine synthesis, and the functional significance of the low enzyme activity was uncertain until it was demonstrated that acetylcholine synthesis and release from tissue prisms prepared from biopsy tissue was reduced (Sims et al, 1983; Francis et al, 1985).

The greatest loss of ChAT activity, of up to 80%, is found in the temporal cortex and is not unexpected in view of the major histopathological changes occurring in that area. However, important advances in the neuroanatomy of the cholinergic system have been made from animal studies, and it is now clear that the majority of ChAT activity is found within the terminals of an ascending projection from the basal forebrain (Wenk et al, 1980; Johnston et al, 1981; Mesulam et al, 1984). The cell bodies of the cholinergic projection to cortex in the rat lie in the septal and ventral pallidal areas, and the homologous regions in the human are the medial septal nucleus, diagonal band of Broca and nucleus basalis of Meynert, the latter area lying within the substantia innominata. Large multipolar neurones are present in these nuclei which are similar to those found in animal studies and which also stain intensely for acetylcholinesterase, are ChAT immunoreactive and are believed to be the origin of the cortical projection (Rossor et al, 1982; Nagai et al, 1983; Mesulam et al, 1984; McGeer et al, 1984). These cells are reduced in number and in size in Alzheimer's disease (Whitehouse et al, 1982; McGeer et al, 1984; Pearson et al, 1983) and thus the reduced ChAT activity can be related to loss of those projection neurones and their terminals within the cortex. Choline uptake, which is also a specific marker of cholinergic terminals, is reduced in cortex, providing further evidence of damage to this projection system (Rylett et al, 1983).

In contrast to the loss of presynaptic markers of cholinergic neurones in cerebral cortex, the muscarinic cholinergic receptors, assayed using [3]HQNB as ligand, are normal (Davies & Verth, 1978; Bowen et al, 1979), although some loss of binding has been reported from temporal lobe (Rinne et al, 1985). Recently M_1 and M_2 subtypes of muscarinic receptors have been reported in Alzheimer's disease in which a selective loss of M_2 receptors was found (Mash et al, 1984). The M_2 receptor appear to be presynaptic and would thus provide further evidence of damage to ascending cholinergic receptor with preservation of the post-synaptic receptors. The relative preservation of post-synaptic receptors is an important observation, since it may provide a basis for enhancement of cholinergic transmission (see elsewhere in this volume).

Noradrenaline and dopamine

Early biochemical studies indicated that the neurochemical changes were not confined to the cholinergic system and that additional abnormalities occurred in the noradrenergic system with reduced concentrations of noradrenaline and metabolites in cerebral cortex (Adolfsson et al, 1979; Mann et al, 1982; Cross et al, 1983; Arai et al, 1984; Francis et al, 1985). Activity of dopamine-β-hydroxylase, the biosynthetic marker enzyme of noradrenergic neurones, is also reduced in cerebral cortex, as is noradrenaline uptake into terminals in biopsy tissue (Cross et al, 1980; Benton et al, 1982). The localization of noradrenaline in cerebral cortex is similar to cholinergic markers in that it is confined to terminals arising from brain stem without any cortical noradrenergic cells. The cell bodies lie within the locus caeruleus in the dorsal pons, and axons project caudally into cerebellum and spinal cord and rostrally to cerebral cortex. The reduced concentration of noradrenaline can be related to loss of cells from the locus caeruleus (Tomlinson et al, 1981; Bondareff, 1982; Mann et al, 1984) and more specifically to a loss of dopamine-β- hydroxylase immunoreactive cells (Iversen et al, 1983). In contrast to the loss of pre-synaptic noradrenergic markers both α and β adrenergic receptor binding sites are unchanged (Bowen et al, 1979; Cross et al, 1984).

Dopamine

In contrast to noradrenaline, dopamine concentrations within cerebral cortex are normal, although low concentrations of both dopamine and metabolite have been found in amygdala and striatum (Adolfsson et al, 1979; Arai et al, 1984). The apparent sparing of the mesocortical system with changes in striatal dopamine is of interest and may relate to the development of akinesia in a proportion of patients with Alzheimer's disease (Pearce, 1974).

5-hydroxytryptamine (5HT)

As with the cholinergic and noradrenergic projections, there is also a serotonin projection from the brain stem to cerebral cortex. There is now an increasing body of evidence for an abnormality in this system, with low concentrations of 5HT and its metabolite 5-hydroxyindoleacetic acid (5HIAA) in cerebral cortex (Adolfsson et al, 1979; Cross et al, 1983; Arai et al, 1984) and reduced uptake of 5HT in tissue prisms prepared from biopsy tissue (Benton et al, 1982).

The cells of origin of the serotonergic projection lie predominantly within the dorsal raphe nucleus in the caudal mesencephalon. Large numbers of neurofibrillary tangles are found in this nucleus and there also appears to be a reduction in the number of large polygonal neurones which may be serotonergic (Ishii, 1966; Curcio & Kemper, 1984). The biochemical deficit in cerebral cortex may relate to those histopathological changes in the dorsal raphe.

A number of different ligands have been used to define 5HT receptor binding sites in cerebral cortex which are reduced in Alzheimer's disease. The loss mainly involves the $5HT_2$ receptor which can be defined by using ^{3}H-ketanserin as ligand (Bowen et al, 1979; Cross et al, 1984; Reynolds et al, 1984). Reynolds et al (1984) reported a 42% loss of $5\text{-}HT_2$ receptors binding, which was considered to be due to reduced density rather than reduced affinity; this is notable in that it is the only classical receptor population analysed to date which is reduced in Alzheimer's disease. Alterations in receptor density may, like concentrations of neurotransmitters, reflect alterations in turnover, but it is equally probable that the loss of $5HT_2$ receptors reflects neuronal loss. The precise localization of these receptors is not yet clear, but recent evidence suggests that they exist on cholinergic terminals in cortex, and thus may be only a further marker of the damage to the ascending cholinergic projection (Quirion et al, 1985).

Amino-acids

The amino-acids aspartate, glutamate and γ-aminobutyrate (GABA) are all of interest in Alzheimer's disease as cortical transmitters, but they are difficult to measure reliably in autopsy tissue and, in particular, it is difficult to distinguish the transmitter pools of aspartate and glutamate from the metabolic pools. One approach is to measure the potassium-evoked release of aspartate and glutamate from tissue prisms, but this requires fresh biopsy tissue. Smith et al (1983) found no difference in release between Alzheimer cases and a series of controls.

GABA is a widely distributed inhibitory transmitter which may be used by as many as a third of all central synapses in the mammalian brain. It is found predominantly in local interneurones and thus, in the cortex, contrasts with the cholinergic and monoaminergic projection systems. As such it may provide information in Alzheimer's disease of the transmitter identity of the cells involved in the widespread cortical pathology. The activity of the marker enzyme for GABA neurons, glutamic acid decarboxyllase (GAD), is reduced in autopsy tissue from Alzheimer cases (Bowen et al, 1976; Davies, 1979). However, the activity of GAD can be profoundly influenced by the agonal state, and so this may be a non-specific abnormality, especially since the activity is normal in biopsy samples (Spillane et al, 1977). The concentration of GABA itself is less sensitive to the influence of the agonal state and is stable over the time-course of human post-mortem studies (Spokes et al, 1979). GABA concentrations are reduced, but only by 20–30% in the temporal cortex and this is confined to younger cases (Rossor et al, 1982, 1984). Due to the presence of GABA in non-neuronal tissue the precise relationship of neurotransmitter concentration to GABA neurones is uncertain. GABA receptor binding sites are unaltered (Bowen et al, 1979; Cross et al, 1984).

Neuropeptides

The recent discovery of neuropeptides has increased dramatically the list of neurotransmitter candidates in the mammalian brain. In general, peptides are found in much lower concentration than the classical neurotransmitters and many co-exist in cholinergic, monoamine and GABA neurons (for review see Iversen, 1982; Emson, 1983). They are remarkably stable in post-mortem tissue and provide further opportunity to define the biochemical characteristics of the neuronal loss of Alzheimer's disease.

A variety of peptides are found in the cerebral cortex, but many of these are present in very low concentrations, and only scattered immunoreactive fibres are seen immunohistochemically. Three peptides, however, somatostatin, cholecystokinin and vasoactive intestinal polypeptide (VIP), are found in relatively larger concentrations, and perikaryal staining can be demonstrated. To this list of cortical peptides can be added neuropeptide Y which co-exists with somatostatin in a proportion of cortical neurones (Vincent et al, 1982).

Both cholecystokinin and VIP-like immunoreactivities are normal in Alzheimer's disease (Rossor, 1980, 1981; Perry et al, 1981; Ferrier et al, 1983), but somatostatin-like immunoreactivity is reduced (Davies et al, 1980; Rossor et al, 1980; Ferrier et al, 1983). Interestingly, neuropeptide Y, which co-exists in at least a proportion of somatostatin neurones, is unchanged (Allen et al, 1984). The loss of somatostatin is found throughout the cerebral cortex, although it may be confined to the temporal cortex in patients dying over the age of 80 years (Rossor et al, 1984). The distribution of the somatostatin loss in Alzheimer's disease is very similar to the ChAT deficit, and this has raised the possibility that the peptide co-exists within cholinergic neurones, although animal lesion studies do not support this (McKinney et al, 1982). Recently it has been reported that the number of somatostatin receptors is reduced in cerebral cortex in addition to the concentration of somatostatin itself (Beal et al, 1985).

RELATIONSHIP OF NEUROCHEMICAL CHANGES TO HISTOPATHOLOGY

It is clear from the foregoing discussion that some of the neurochemical abnormalities can be related to specific pathological features (Table 8.1).

Table 8.1 Neurotransmitter correlates of histopathological features in Alzheimer's disease

Pathological feature	Neurotransmitter of neurones involved
Cell loss	
Nucleus basalis ofMeynert	Acetylcholine
Locus caeruleus	Noradrenaline
Nucleus dorsal raphe	5-HT
Cerebral cortex	Not yet established
	?somatostatin + others
Neurofibrillary tangles	Somatostatin + ?others
Senile plaques	Probable non-specific involvement of neurites. Immunostaining observed for ChAT, tyrosine hydroxylase, somatostatin, cholecystokinin and VIP.

Thus the reduced ChAT activity, acetylcholine synthesis and choline uptake into synaptosomes can be attributed to the cholinergic cell loss from the nucleus basalis. To what extent there is additional damage to cholinergic terminals with relative preservation of perikarya, or whether some of the nucleus basalis pathology can be attributed to shrinkage as a retrograde phenomenon subsequent to cortical damage, is not yet clear (Pearson et al, 1983.) Similarly the low concentrations of cortical noradrenaline, reduced dopamine-β-hydroxylase activity and noradrenaline uptake into tissue prisms can be attributed to the loss of neurones from the locus caeruleus. The 5HT damage may also relate to the high density of neurofibrillary tangles and loss of large polygonal cells from the dorsal raphe nucleus (Curcio & Herzog, 1984). The relationship of neurotransmitter changes to other histopathological features of Alzheimer's disease is, however, less clear.

In addition to the neuronal loss from the subcortical nuclei there is clear neuronal loss from the cerebral cortex in Alzheimer's disease in excess of that which is found with normal ageing. Numbers of large neurones are reduced, and this is more severe in younger patients (Terry et al, 1981; Mountjoy et al, 1983). The neurotransmitter identities of these cells are unknown. It is unlikely that they are cholinergic, since the number of intrinsic cortical cholinergic neurones is small compared with the ascending projection. It is tempting to relate directly the loss of somatostatin to cortical neuronal loss and, although this might explain some of the cell loss, there are certain inconsistencies. If the change in somatostatin is due to neuronal fall-out, then one would predict a commensurate loss of co-existing transmitters. There is recent evidence to suggest that cortical peptidergic neurones are also GABAergic (Hendry et al, 1984), and yet GABA markers are not consistently altered and the co-existent neuropeptide Y is also found in normal concentrations. Either the somatostatin deficit reflects alterations in turnover, or somatostatin neurones are lost, but this constitutes only a very small proportion of cortical cells.

Neurofibrillary tangles are clearly not confined to a single neurotransmitter system, since they are found in the cholinergic nucleus basalis, noradrenergic locus caeruleus and serotonergic raphe nucleus, as well as cerebral cortical neurons. Many tangle-containing neurones are also somatostatin-immunoreactive (Roberts et al, 1985), but it is likely that other neurones are involved as well. There is now good evidence for multiple neurotransmitter involvement in plaque formation. Studies of plaques in aged monkeys have revealed acetylcholinesterase staining (Struble et al, 1982) and more specifically ChAT immunoreactive fibres (Kitt et al, 1984), indicating involvement of cholinergic terminals, presumably from the ascending projection. This is not, however, a specific involvement, since immunoreactive tyrosine hydroxylase fibres, the biosynthetic marker enzyme for dopamine and noradrenaline neurones, are also present (Kitt et al, 1984). Recently somatostatin-immunoreactive neurites have been reported in plaques of Alzheimer cases (Morrison et al, 1985; Armstrong et al, 1985), and interestingly cholecystokinin and VIP-like immunoreactive fibres have also been observed (Roberts et al, 1985) despite normal concentrations on radio-immunoassay. It would appear that nerve terminals are involved irrespective of their neurotransmitter status, and Golgi studies also implicate a variety of local neurones contributing to the neurites of hippocampal plaques (Probst et al, 1983).

CLINICAL SIGNIFICANCE OF TRANSMITTER DEFICITS IN ALZHEIMER'S DISEASE

Do any of these neurotransmitter changes help either with diagnosis or with treatment of Alzheimer's disease? Currently the diagnosis of Alzheimer's disease is clinical with autopsy confirmation, although biopsy is occasionally performed. Changes in concentrations of neurotransmitters in CSF have been sought which might reflect the central abnormalities. Reduced acetylcholinesterase activity in CSF has been reported (Soininen et al, 1984) but not confirmed by others (Davies, 1979; Wood et al, 1982). Of greater potential interest is the reduction in CSF somatostatin which has been found by many groups (Oram et al, 1981; Wood et al, 1982; Soininen et al, 1984; Serby et al, 1984) in clinically diagnosed cases. Unfortunately this does not appear to be disease-specific, since it is found in a variety of other conditions including depression (Rubinow et al, 1983), an important differential diagnosis of cognitive impairment.

The potential for treatment lies in the significance of a given transmitter deficit and the ability to influence synaptic transmission. The ChAT activity in the cerebral cortex correlates with the severity of dementia at the time of death (Perry et al, 1978; Wilcock et al, 1982). This need not of course imply a direct causal link and may only reflect the severity of disease, although other neurotransmitter abnormalities do not show as close a correlation (Francis et al, 1985), and moreover manipulation of the cholinergic system in human and animal studies alters cognitive function (Drachman et al, 1978). However, final proof of the importance of the cholinergic deficit is improvement with enhancement of cholinergic transmission, and clinical trials have been disappointing (see elsewhere in this volume), although this may partly be due to the inadequacy of safe cholinergic agonists.

In conclusion a diversity of transmitter deficits are found in Alzheimer's disease, and the hypothesis that the disease is due specifically and solely to a cholinergic deficit can be rejected. However, of the many reported changes in Alzheimer's disease, the cholinergic deficit remains the most consistent and well-studied change, and the results of further studies to define the clinical correlates of this and the other transmitter deficits are awaited.

REFERENCES

Adolfsson R, Gottfries C G, Ross B E, Winblad B 1979 Changes in brain catecholamines in patients with dementia of Alzheimer type. British Journal of Psychiatry 135: 216–223
Agid Y, Taquet H, Cesselin F, Epelbaum J, Javoy-Agid F 1986 Neuropeptides and Parkinson's disease. In: Emson P, Rossor M, Tohyama M (eds) Peptides and neurological disease. Progress in Brain Research (in press)
Allen J M, Ferrier I N, Roberts G W, et al 1984 Elevation of neuropeptide Y (NPY) in substantia innominata in Alzheimer's type dementia. Journal of the Neurological Sciences 64: 325–331
Allsop D, Landon M, Kidd M 1983 The isolation and amino acid composition of senile plaque core protein. Brain Research 259: 348–352
Arai H, Kosaka K, Iizuka T 1984 Changes in biogenic amines and their metabolites in post mortem brains from patients with Alzheimer's type dementia. Journal of Neurochemistry 43: 388–393
Armstrong D M, LeRoy S, Shields D, Terry R D 1985 Somatostatin-like immunoreactivity within neuritic plaques. Brain Research 338: 71–79
Beal M F, Mazurek M F, Tran V T, Chattha G, Bird E D, Martin J B 1985 Reduced numbers of somatostatin receptors in the cerebral cortex in Alzheimer's disease. Science 229: 289–291
Benton J S, Bowen D M, Allen S J, et al 1982 Alzheimer's disease as a disorder of the isodendritic core. Lancet i: 456
Bird E D, Iversen L L 1982 Human brain post-mortem neurochemistry. In: Lajtha A (ed) Handbook of neurochemistry, Vol 2. Plenum Press, New York, pp 225–251
Bondareff W, Mountjoy C Q, Roth M 1982 Loss of neurons of origin of the adrenergic projection to cerebral cortex (nucleus locus caeruleus) in senile dementia. Neurology 32: 164–168
Bowen D M, Smith C B, White P, Davison A N 1976 Neurotransmitter-related enzymes and indices of hypoxia in senile dementia and other abiotrophies. Brain 99: 459–496
Bowen D M, Spillane J A, Curzon G, et al 1979 Accelerated aging or selective neuronal loss as an important cause of dementia. Lancet i: 11–14
Coyle J T, Price D L, DeLong M R 1983 Alzheimer's disease: a disorder of cortical cholinergic innervation. Science 219: 1184–1190
Cross A J, Crow T J, Perry E K, Perry R H, Blessed G, Tomlinson B E 1981 Reduced

dopamine-beta-hydroxylase activity in Alzheimer's disease. British Medical Journal 282: 93–94

Cross A J, Crow T J, Johnson J A, et al 1983 Monoamine metabolism in senile dementia of Alzheimer type. Journal of the Neurological Sciences 60: 383–392

Cross A J, Crow T J, Johnson J A, et al 1984 Studies on neurotransmitter receptor systems in neocortex and hippocampus in senile dementia of the Alzheimer type. Journal of the Neurological Sciences 64: 109–117

Curcio C A, Kemper T 1984 Nucleus raphe dorsalis in dementia of the Alzheimer type: neurofibrillary changes and neuronal packing density. Journal of Neuropathology and Experimental Neurology 43: 359–368

Davies P 1979 Neurotransmitter- related enzymes in senile dementia of the Alzheimer type. Brain Research 171: 319–327

Davies P, Maloney A F J 1976 Selective loss of central cholinergic neurons in Alzheimer's disease. Lancet ii:1403

Davies P, Verth A H 1978 Regional distribution of muscarinic acetylcholine receptors in normal and Alzheimer type dementia brains. Brain Research 138: 385–392

Davies P, Katzman R, Terry R D 1980 Reduced somatostatin-like immunoreactivity in cases of Alzheimer's disease and Alzheimer senile dementia. Nature 288: 279–280

Drachman D A 1977 Memory and cognitive function in man: does the cholinergic system have a specific role? Neurology 27: 783–790

Emson P C 1983 Chemical neuroanatomy. Raven Press, New York

Ferrier I N, Cross A J, Johnson J A, et al 1983 Neuropeptides in Alzheimer type dementia. Journal of the Neurological Sciences 62: 159–170

Francis P T, Palmer A M, Sims N R, et al 1985 Neurochemical studies of early-onset Alzheimer's disease. New England Journal of Medicine 313: 7–11

Glenner G G, Wong C W 1984 Alzheimer's disease. Initial report of the purification and characterisation of a novel cerebrovascular amyloid protein. Biochemical Biophysical Research Communications 120: 885–890

Hardy J, Adolfsson R, Alafuzoff I, et al 1985 Transmitter deficits in Alzheimer's disease. Neurochemistry International 7: 545–563

Hendry S H C, Jones E G, De Felipe J, Schmechel D, Brandon C, Emson P C 1984 Neuropeptide-containing neurons of the cerebral cortex are also GABAergic. Proceedings of the National Academy of Science 81: 6526–6530

Ihara Y, Abraham C, Selkoe D J 1983 Antibodies to paired helical filaments in Alzheimer's disease do not recognise normal brain proteins. Nature 304: 727–730

Ishii T 1966 Distribution of Alzheimer's neurofibrillary changes in the brain stem and hypothalamus of senile dementia. Acta Neuropathologica 6: 181–187

Iversen L L, Rossor M N, Reynolds G P, et al 1983 Loss of pigmented dopamine beta-hydroxylase positive cells from locus coeruleus in senile dementia of Alzheimer type. Neuroscience Letters 39: 95–100

Johnston M V, McKinney M, Coyle J T 1981 Neocortical cholinergic innervation: a description of extrinsic and intrinsic components in the rat. Experimental Brain Research 43: 159–172

Kidd M 1963 Paired helical filaments in electron microscopy of Alzheimer's disease. Nature 197: 192–193

Kidd M, Allsop D, Landon M 1985 Senile plaque amyloid, paired helical filaments and cerebrovascular amyloid in Alzheimer's disease are all deposits of the same protein. Lancet i:278

Kitt C A, Mobley W C, Struble R G, et al 1984 Contribution of catecholaminergic systems to neurites in plaques of aged primates. Annals of Neurology 16:118

Kitt C A, Price D L, Struble R G, et al 1984 Evidence for cholinergic neurites in senile plaques. Science 226: 1443–1445

Mann D M, Yates P O, Hawkes J 1982 The noradrenergic system in Alzheimer and multi-infarct dementias. Journal of Neurology, Neurosurgery and Psychiatry 45: 113–119

Mann D M A, Yates P I, Marcyniuk B 1984 A comparison of changes in the nucleus basalis and locus caeruleus in Alzheimer's disease. Journal of Neurology, Neurosurgery and Psychiatry 47: 201–203

Mash D C, Flynn D D, Potter L T 1984 Loss of M2-receptors in cerebral cortex in Alzheimer's disease and experimental cholinergic denervation. Science 228: 1115–1117

Masters C L, Simms G, Weinmann N A, Bayreuther K, Multhaup G, McDonald B L 1985

Amyloid plaque core protein in Alzheimer's disease and Down's syndrome. Proceedings of the National Academy of Science 82: 4245–4249

McGeer P L, McGeer E G, Suzuki J, Dolman C E, Nagai T 1984 Aging, Alzheimer's disease and the cholinergic system of the basal forebrain. Neurology 34: 741–745

McKinney M, Davies P, Coyle J T 1982 Somatostatin is not co-localised in cholinergic neurons innervating the rat cerebral cortex–hippocampal formation. Brain Research 243: 169–172

Mesulam M-M, Mufson E J, Levey A I, Wainer B H 1984 Atlas of cholinergic neurons in the forebrain and upper brainstem of the macaque based on monoclonal choline acetyltransferase immunohistochemistry and acetylcholinesterase histochemistry. Neuroscience 12: 669–686

Morrison J H, Rogers J, Scherr S, Benoit R, Bloom F E 1985 Somatostatin immunoreactivity in neuritic plaques of Alzheimer's patients. Nature 314: 90–92

Mountjoy C Q, Roth M, Evans N J R, Evans H M 1983 Cortical neuronal counts in normal elderly controls and demented patients. Neurobiology of Aging 4: 1–11

Nagai R, McGeer P L, Peng J H, McGeer E G, Dolman C E 1983 Choline acetyltransferase immunohistochemistry in brains of Alzheimer's disease patients and controls. Neuroscience Letters 36: 195–199

Oram J T, Edwardson J A, Millard P M 1981 Investigation of cerebrospinal fluid neuropeptides in idiopathic senile dementia. Gerontology 27: 216–223

Ottersen O P, Storm-Mathisen J 1984 Neurons containing or accumulating transmitter amino acids. In: Bjorklund A, Hokfelt T, Kuhar M J (eds) Handbook of chemical neuroanatomy, Vol 3. Elsevier, Amsterdam, ch V, p 141–246

Pearce J 1974 The extrapyramidal disorder of Alzheimer's disease. European Neurology 12: 94–103

Pearson R C A, Sofroniew M V, Cuello A C, et al 1983 Persistence of cholinergic neurons in the basal nucleus — a brain with senile dementia of the Alzheimer's type demonstrated by immunohistochemical staining for choline acetyltransferase. Brain Research 289: 375–379

Perry E K, Perry R H, Blessed G, Tomlinson B E 1977 Necropsy evidence of central cholinergic deficits in senile dementia. Lancet i:189

Perry E K, Tomlinson B E, Blessed G, Bergman K, Gibson P H, Perry R H 1978 Correlation of cholinergic abnormalities with senile plaques and mental test scores in senile dementia. British Medical Journal ii: 1457–1459

Perry R H, Dockray G J, Dimaline R, Perry E K, Blessed G, Tomlinson B E 1981 Neuropeptides in Alzheimer's disease, depression and schizophrenia. Journal of the Neurological Sciences 51: 465–472

Perry E K, Atack J R, Perry R H, et al 1984 Intralaminar neurochemical distributions in human midtemporal cortex: comparison between Alzheimer's disease and the normal. Journal of Neurochemistry 42: 1402–1410

Probst A, Basler V, Bron B, Ulrich J 1983 Neuritic plaques in senile dementia of Alzheimer type: a Golgi analysis in the hippocampal region. Brain Research 268: 249–254

Quirion R, Richard J, Dam T V 1985 Evidence for the existence of serotonin type-2 receptors on cholinergic terminals in rat cortex. Brain Research 333: 345–349

Reynolds G P, Arnold L, Rossor M N, Iversen L L, Mountjoy C Q, Roth M 1984 Reduced binding of [^{3}H] ketanserin to cortical 5-HT$_2$ receptors in senile dementia of the Alzheimer type. Neuroscience Letters 44: 47–51

Rinne J O, Laakso K, Lonnberg P, et al 1985 Brain muscarinic receptors in senile dementia. Brain Research 336: 19–25

Roberts G W, Crow T J, Polak J M 1985 Location of neuronal tangles in somatostatin neurones in Alzheimer's disease. Nature 314: 92–94

Rogers J D, Brogan D, Mirra S S 1985 The nucleus basalis of Meynert in neurological disease: a quantitative morphological study. Annals of Neurology 17: 163–170

Rossor M N 1982 Neurotransmitters in CNS disease: dementia. Lancet ii: 1200–1204

Rossor M N 1986 Post-mortem neurochemistry of human brain. Progress in Brain Research 65 (in press)

Rossor M N, Emson P C, Mountjoy C Q, Roth M, Iversen L L 1980 Reduced amounts of immunoreactive somatostatin in the temporal cortex in senile dementia of Alzheimer type. Neuroscience Letters 20: 373–377

Rossor M N, Fahrenkrug J, Emson P, Mountjoy C, Iversen L, Roth M 1980 Reduced cortical choline acetyltransferase activity in senile dementia of Alzheimer type is not accompanied by changes in vasoactive intestinal polypeptide. Brain Research 201: 249–253

Rossor M N, Rehfeld J F, Emson P C, Mountjoy C Q, Roth M, Iversen L L 1981 Normal cortical concentrations of cholecystokinin-like immunoreactivity with reduced choline acetyltransferase activity in senile dementia of the Alzheimer type. Life Sciences 29: 405–410

Rossor M N, Garrett N J, Johnson A L, Mountjoy C Q, Roth M, Iversen L L 1982 A post-mortem study of the cholinergic and GABA systems in senile dementia. Brain 105: 313–330

Rossor M N, Svendsen C, Hunt S P, Mountjoy C Q, Roth M, Iversen L L 1982 The substantia innominata in Alzheimer's disease: an histochemical and biochemical study of cholinergic marker enzymes. Neuroscience Letters 28: 217–222

Rossor M N, Iversen L L, Reynolds G P, Mountjoy C Q, Roth M 1984 Neurochemical characteristics of early and late onset types of Alzheimer's disease. British Medical Journal 288: 961–964

Rubinow D R, Gold P W, Post R M, et al 1983 CSF somatostatin in affective illness. Archives of General Psychiatry 40: 409–412

Rudelli R D, Ambler W M, Wisniewski H M 1984 Morphology and distribution of Alzheimer neuritic (senile) and amyloid plaques in striatum and diencephalon. Acta Neuropathologica 64: 273–281

Rylett R T, Ball M J, Colhoun E H 1983 Evidence for high affinity choline transport in synaptosomes prepared from hippocampus and neocortex of patients with Alzheimer's disease. Brain Research 289: 169–175

Serby M, Richardson S B, Twente S, Sickerski J, Corwin J, Rotrosen J 1984 CSF somatostatin in Alzheimer's disease. Neurobiology of Aging 5: 187–190

Sims N R, Bowen D M, Smith C C T, et al 1980 Glucose metabolism and acetylcholine synthesis in relation to neuronal activity in Alzheimer's disease. Lancet i: 333–337

Smith C C T, Bowen D M, Sims N R, Neary D, Davison A N 1983 Amino acid release from biopsy samples of temporal neocortex from patients with Alzheimer's disease. Brain Research 264: 138–141

Soininen H, Jolkkonen J T, Reinikainen K J, Halonen T O, Riekkinen P J 1984 Reduced cholinesterase activity and somatostatin like immunoreactivity in the cerebrospinal fluid of patients with dementia of the Alzheimer type. Journal of the Neurological Sciences 63: 167–172

Spillane J A, White P, Goodhardt M J, Flack R H A, Bowen D M, Davison A N 1977 Selective vulnerability of neurons in organic dementia. Nature 266: 558–559

Spokes E G S, Garrett N J, Iversen L L 1979 Differential effects of agonal status on measurements of GABA and glutamate decarboxylase in human post-mortem brain tissue from control and Huntington's chorea subjects. Journal of Neurochemistry 33: 773–778

Struble R G, Cork L C, Whitehouse P J, Price D L 1982 Cholinergic innervation in neuritic plaques. Science 216: 413–415

Terry R D 1963 The fine structure of neurofibrillary tangles in Alzheimer's disease. Journal of Neuropathology and Experimental Neurology 22: 629–642

Terry R D, Peck A, De Terese R, Schechter R, Horoupian D S 1981 Some morphometric aspects of the brain in senile dementia of the Alzheimer type. Annals of Neurology 10: 184–192

Tomlinson B E 1980 The structural and quantitative aspects of the dementias. In: Roberts P J (ed) Biochemistry of dementia. Wiley, Chichester, ch 2, p 15

Tomlinson B E, Irving D, Blessed G 1981 Cell loss in the locus caeruleus in senile dementia of Alzheimer type. Journal of Neurological Sciences 49: 419–428

Vincent S R, Johansson O, Hokfelt T, et al 1982 Neuropeptide coexistence in human cortical neurons. Nature 298: 65–67

Wenk H, Bigl V, Meyer U 1980 Cholinergic projections from magnocellular nuclei of the basal forebrain to cortical areas in rats. Brain Research Reviews 2: 295–316

Whitehouse P J, Price D L, Struble R G, Coyle J T, DeLong M A 1982 Alzheimer's disease and senile dementia — loss of neurons in the basal forebrain. Science 215: 1237–1239

Whitehouse P J, Parhad I M, Hedreen J C, et al 1983 Integrity of the nucleus basalis of Meynert in normal aging. Neurology 33:159

Wilcock G K, Esiri M M, Bowen D M, Smith C C T 1982 Alzheimer's disease: correlation of cortical choline acetyltransferase activity with the severity of dementia and histological abnormalities. Journal of the Neurological Sciences 57: 407–417

Wischik C M, Crowther R A, Stewart M, Roth M 1985 Subunit structure of paired helical filaments in Alzheimer's disease. Journal of Cell Biology 100: 1904–1912

Wood P L, Etienne P, Gauthier L S, Cajal S, Nair N P V 1982 Reduced lumbar CSF somatostatin in Alzheimer's disease. Life Sciences 31: 2073–2079

Alzheimer's disease: epidemiology

INTRODUCTION

Senile dementia of Alzheimer type (SDAT) now presents a burden and a challenge to public health. Although mediaeval and Greco-Roman writers described feebleness of the mind in late life, more systematic descriptions have come only recently, with recognition that impairment of mentation is due to structural changes in the brain. It was in 1835 that James Cowles Prichard described what he called 'incoherence' or 'senile dementia', a state characterized by 'forgetfulness of recent impressions, while the memory retains a comparatively firm hold of ideas laid up in the recesses from times long past.' Seventy years later, Alzheimer (1907) described to the Munich medical society the neuropathology of what we believe to be the same disorder. Major scientific resources are now deployed in finding aetiological clues or pharmacological treatments for this condition.

There are at least four reasons why senile dementia of Alzheimer type has become a major problem for public health (Henderson, 1986a, 1986b). Firstly, there is the remarkable demographic shift in the human population during the last hundred years. Both in developed and less-developed countries, the epidemiological transition has brought about a marked increase in the numbers of persons surviving to a late age. The transition is from high fertility with high mortality to low fertility with low mortality. As a consequence, a doubling in the proportion of the very old is taking place in the human population in the space of a single generation. In 1980, there were 260 million person aged 65 years and over in the world. By AD2020, there will be 650 million. The comparable figures for Europe are 63 and 90 million respectively. For the very old, those aged 80 years and over, the world population in 1980 was 35 million. But in AD 2020 it will be 102 million, while Europe will increase from 10 to 19 million in that period (WHO, 1982). This increase has no precedent in the species' history. Some of the implications have been examined in an important paper by Fries (1980).

Alas, though, this is not the only demographic change. Not only are large number surviving to late age, but those who are afflicted by chronic

154

diseases, including dementia, are living longer after the onset of their disability. It is this phenomenom which Gruenberg (1977) has wryly called 'the failures of success'. This latter change is due in part to progress in medical care, particularly in the reduction of previously fatal illnesses. Gruenberg et al (1976) expressed it pointedly: 'The old man's friend, pneumonia, is dead — a victim of medical progress'.

The second reason for the public health importance of SDAT is its age-specific incidence rate and its chronicity. The chance of developing dementia probably rises steeply during the fifth, sixth and seventh decades of life (Hagnell et al, 1983). Having developed a dementia, many people continue to live for several more years, deteriorating slowly. The absolute number of afflicted persons therefore rises with age. But it will also rise markedly between the present and the early decades of the 21st century because of the demographic shift which is relentlessly swelling the denominator of those at risk.

A third reason is that the majority of cases of SDAT are not in institutional care, but are living in the community with spouses or relatives. As many as four-fifths of all cases probably live in the community. The burden this brings with it to families is very considerable. Without the contribution of these families, the medical and social resources of even the wealthiest country would be overwhelmed.

A fourth reason is that SDAT is a disorder of unknown aetiology. While biomedical research continues to make much progress in understanding the bichemical and ultra-structural features of the disorder, the discipline of epidemiology can offer some contributions to complement these advances. Although some biomedical workers regrettably assert that epidemiological studies are unlikely to yield clues to aetiology, and that the latter will come instead from the laboratory, it seems a better strategy to try to integrate laboratory findings and epidemiological studies. Both approaches may generate knowledge which the other may use for further advancement, and both can generate hypotheses best tested by the other.

Epidemiology will continue to try to identify risk factors for SDAT. It will try to help to complete the clinical picture, based on cases identified in the general population, as well as those already known to hospitals and clinics. Indeed, in searching for risk factors in case-control studies, the systematic bias in treated samples, sometimes called Berkson's bias (Berkson, 1946), is an important distortion. Cases which reach hospital or specialist services are only a sub-sample of all persons with the disorder. For example, at the general-practice level, Williamson et al (1964) showed in a celebrated study that as many as four-fifths of cases of dementia in the community were unrecognized by their own doctors. This is a study which could well bear replication some twenty years later. Such basic epidemiology suggests that clinicians do not have a close familiarity with the whole spectrum of levels of severity. Clearly, this is particularly relevant in early and therefore presumably mild cases. There may be clinical features at that stage which later become buried and hence permanently inaccessible, due to the very disease which one is attempting to unravel.

It is therefore important to study total populations of the elderly, so that a picture of the development and evolution of the disease can be traced. Such population-based studies should include longitudinal observations on states of benign senescent forgetfulness, as originally described by Kral (1962, 1978). Epidemiology also contributes to information useful for the organization of services and the deployment of scarce resources. Here, special attention can be accorded to the costs involved, both in domiciliary and institutional care, as well as the personal burden placed on those relatives caring for cases at home.

A further contribution from epidemiology is in the development of diagnostic criteria and instruments. Even if biomedical workers are eventually successful in finding the causes of SDAT or an effective pharmacological treatment for it, there will still be a need for acceptable screening instruments and for knowledge about risk factors, with a view to primary prevention. It has been said that the ultimate service provided by epidemiology is prevention, and it is towards this that most epidemiological research on dementia is aimed.

Knowledge about the epidemiology of dementia falls under the following headings: information on prevalence and incidence; the possibility of variation in incidence rates between populations or over time; identification of risk factors; determining the natural history of SDAT and its delineation from normal ageing; and the development of efficient methods for screening, both in the community and in general-practice settings.

INFORMATION ON PREVALENCE

For the dementias of later life, there have been many prevalence surveys and these have been set out in some detail in a number of publications from this Research Unit (Henderson & Kay, 1984; Henderson, 1986a, 1986b). The great majority of studies have been conducted in Northern Europe, Scandinavia, Japan and North America. There is remarkable consistency between the rates reported for dementia of moderate and severe degree. Rates for mild dementia are highly variable. All the reports refer to populations aged 65 years and over, although the exact age-composition is variable. There seems to be no good information on the prevalence of Alzheimer's disease in its presenile form; Mortimer (1983) has noted that reliable estimates of the prevalence of dementia are not yet available for younger adults.

A recurrent technical difficulty in epidemiology is comparability between field surveys. This is certainly the case with surveys of dementia. Yet it is important to identify and, if possible, overcome these sources of variation if we continue to believe that aetiological clues might emerge, were real differences in rates securely established. The sources of variation include the following. Firstly, the population denominator studied may have varied appreciably in the proportion of very old persons in it. A high proportion of very elderly in a community will increase its prevalence rate. Secondly, surveys vary in whether they have included persons living in nursing homes or other institutional care. Some studies have deliberately covered both this group and the elderly in the community (Kay et al, 1965). Others have been deliberately restricted to community residents (Kay et al, 1986). Thirdly, the time-reference may vary, some surveys being of point prevalence, other of one month, six months or one-year prevalence. For a disorder with a very low incidence rate but high chronicity, this problem matters rather less. Fourthly, communities may vary in the likelihood of survival of cases of dementia. Thus, where medical services are very limited and many fatal diseases, including infections, are endemic, those who do develop a dementia in later life are likely to survive for a much shorter time. Fifthly, the clinical information, in both its history and mental-state examination, varies considerably between surveys. Sixthly, there is criterion variance (Cloninger et al, 1979; Grove et al, 1981).

Unless standardized diagnostic criteria are set up and actually used with high reliability, case recognition may vary appreciably. Clearly, this point is specially relevant for the diagnosis of mild dementia, where there is considerable variation in the observed rates. For dementia, the problem is that the criteria should ideally apply across different cultures with the same validity. Yet population groups may differ markedly in literacy, education, premorbid intelligence and the currency of information typically used by the elderly in daily living. For example, the Mini-Mental State Examination (Folstein et al, 1975) would be quite unsuitable as a screening instrument in an Asian or African population. Indeed, it may not be applicable in those groups within Western communities which have had little opportunity for education, although it is a highly satisfactory instrument elsewhere. Seventhly, only a few surveys have attempted to differentiate between SDAT and multi-infarct dementia (MID), during the process of case-ascertainment.

In the present chapter, our concern is specifically with Alzheimer's disease. In Table 9.1 are shown those surveys where such a differentiation

Table 9.1 Surveys reporting the prevalence (%) of senile dementia and multi-infarct dementia. Reproduced from Henderson (1986b) with the kind permission of the British Medical Bulletin.

	Senile dementia	Multi-infarct dementia	Undifferentiated
Kay et al (1964)	1.8 (±0.7)	2.8(±0.9)	1.1(±0.6)
Åkesson (1969)	0.7	0.2	—
Bollerup (1975)	1.3	1.9	1.8
Hasegawa (1975)	1.2	2.7	0.6
Karasawa (1980)	0.6	1.7	2.3
Mölsä et al (1982)	1.0	0.8	0.2
Hasegawa (1982)	1.2	2.0	1.6

has been attempted. Because of the considerable variation in methods enumerated above, detailed interpretation of these surveys is not justifiable. As Henderson & Huppert (1984) have argued, it is among milder cases of dementia that inter-observer variation will be greatest.

Liston & LaRue (1983a, 1983b) and St Clair & Whalley (1983) have emphasized the danger of overestimating the number of MID cases when that diagnosis is achieved by a method such as the Hachinski scale (Hachinski et al, 1975). There, a low score is taken to indicate AD, but it should be borne in mind that a high score can be achieved by persons with a mixture of both dementias.

Is SDAT a Western disease?

If the epidemiological data allowed it, in terms of reliability and validity of case-ascertainment, it would be extremely important for aetiological research to determine if there is any regional variation in the occurrence of SDAT. As pointed out above, this could be determined with certainty only by studying incidence rates. Differences in prevalence might be due to different survival times under different conditions. Nevertheless, it would be reasonable to start with prevalence rates, using them as an indirect estimate of incidence. Unfortunately, all the available prevalence studies come from Western countries, with the single exception of the Japanese report. Despite the rates shown in Table 9.1, it is generally accepted that SDAT is considerably more common than MID. A frequent citation to support this are the autopsy findings of Tomlinson et al (1970), based on a series of 50 cases of dementia reaching necropsy in a teaching hospital. Such a sample must have undergone strong selection effects, although it is not possible to say in which direction this might have biased the presence of SDAT or of MID cases. Tomlinson and his colleagues reported that Alzheimer-type changes were found in 50% of his series, MID in 17% and a mixed pathology in 18%. A greater prevalance of SDAT is also the impression of most clinicians in Western countries, although, as we have emphasized, it is not the pattern in the data reported by Kay et al, (1964) and by Bollerup (1975). The consensus seems to be that SDAT is substantially the more common disorder (Mortimer et al, 1981).

Consistently, though, Japanese epidemiologists find that MID is the more common dementia. They also confirm that it is much more commonly encountered in clinical practice. It is therefore more than reasonable to propose that SDAT may be more common in Western countries than in Japan. Furthermore, the Japanese observations suggest that not only is MID more common there, but that SDAT is rarer, so that the overall rates are rather similar to those in Western countries. This suggests that two processes might be at work: one promoting the occurrence of MID in Japan, and the other causing a lower occurrence of SDAT. If it were possible to confirm the latter, the situation would be analogous to that encountered by Marmot & Syme (1976) in their studies of coronary heart disease in Japanese men in Japan, Hawaii and California.

Information is urgently needed on the prevalence, and if possible the incidence, of AD in developing countries. Here, to this writer's knowledge, there is very limited information at present. This leads to the impression that dementia in the elderly is extremely rare in such settings. But the elderly there are essentially a survival élite. Furthermore, accurate knowledge of age is not always practicable. Osuntokun (personal communication, 27 November 1984) reports that in a survey of neurological disorders, conducted by his colleagues and himself in a community of 20 000 people in Nigeria, where 5% were aged 65 or over, no person with senile dementia was encountered. He goes further in saying that SDAT is unknown in Nigerians. It should be recalled, though, that Lambo (1966) described cases of senile dementia amongst the clientele of Aro Hospital, Abeokuta, and that rates rose markedly with age amongst the elderly patients, just as they do in developed countries.

If we want to find aetiological clues, establishing regional variation in rates would be a major contribution. There is a strong justification for the hypothesis that SDAT is more common in developed countries. One would have to acknowledge that this might be due to ethnic differences in vulnerability, either alone or interacting with environmental effects. Using an evolutionary perspective on the occurrence of disease in human populations, Boyden (1980) and Boyden et al (1981) have put forward the concept of an 'evodeviation'. In this, a disease is seen as the consequence of some exposure to which the human species is not adapted. Coronary heart disease is such an example. It should be borne in mind that the parts of the brain which are principally affected in AD, those concerned with memory, thinking and information processing, subserve those functions which have been acquired more recently in the evolution of higher primates. On the question of vulnerability and ethnicity, it is notable that there is so far no evidence for a difference in the occurrence of AD in whites and blacks in the United States, although the blacks are largely of West African stock.

The diagnosis of AD in field surveys

The foregoing shows how important it is to develop an adequate epidemiological technology for inter-regional comparisons. This is a priority for the Division of Mental Health in the World Health Organization, which is seeking to establish common diagnostic criteria and common case-finding instruments (WHO, 1986). Clinicians and epidemiologists alike are fully aware that the diagnosis of AD during life can be only by exclusion: it is essentially a neuropathological diagnosis. The problem of case ascertainment in field surveys is known to be considerable. We do not yet know how reliably the diagnosis can be made in such a setting, or the proportion of cases so diagnoses which could be subsequently confirmed to be AD by autopsy. These difficulties facing epidemioloists have been starkly described by Gajdusek and his colleagues: 'Until criteria are established for diagnosis, it seems almost pointless to attempt an epidemiologic analysis. . . At this stage, there does not even appear to be any reliable information on the accuracy of clinical diagnosis in a large enough series of patients with AD. Therefore, no estimate is available on the degree of case ascertainment that might be expected from population surveys.' (Masters et al, 1981). The study by Ron et al, (1979) is an important exception, showing that in 51 hospital patients diagnosed as having presenile dementia, that diagnosis had to be subsequently rejected in 31% at follow-up 5 to 15 years later. Masters et al are correct, though, in that no information has been obtained about reliability and validity of the diagnosis of SDAT in the field setting. The importance of this technical problem for epidemiological research cannot be overemphasized. It is an obstacle in case-control studies, because it will lead to dilution of the effect of risk factors. In case-control studies, there are likely to be special investigations available, such as CAT scans, which will improve diagnostic accuracy and therefore homogeneity amongst the cases. But no such investigations may be feasible in prevalence studies in the community.

One approach which would circumvent most problems in diagnosis in the course of field surveys is to work with brains rather than persons. De Wolfe Miller et al (1984) has reported an autopsy series on all available patients dying in a teaching hospital ($N=99$). These authors reported that the count of plaques and tangles increased monotonically from the age of 71 years, and there was no variation with gender or race. The age-specific presence of many plaques and tangles, suggesting the development of AD, was as follows: <55 years 0%; 55–64 years 2.6%; 65–74 years 4.5%; 75–84 years 19.6%; 85+ 45.5%. While such studies have the strength of a more certain diagnosis of AD, this advantage is offset by the biases introduced through the strong selection effects on persons who not only reach hospital, but die there and subsequently have a necropsy. We see as one solution the value of attempting to have post-mortem follow-up on all cases of dementia identified in prospective longitudinal field surveys. Even modest success in such an endeavour would be an improvement on the autopsy samples available so far.

INCIDENCE

Because of the difficulties involved, few studies of the incidence of Alzheimer's disease in general population samples have been undertaken. The reasons are obvious. Firstly, it is necessary to have a large enough sample as the denominator out of which new cases will arise. Secondly, each member of the cohort has to be re-examined after an adequate interval has elapsed, usually several years. Thirdly, when studying a sample of elderly persons, information must be collected on members of the cohort who have died, since they may have become cases of the disorder. Indeed, it is known that the mortality rate in AD is substantially increased (Kay, 1962; Varsamis et al, 1972; Henderson & Kay, 1984).

The studies of incidence we shall consider here are those by Åkesson (1969), Bergmann et al (1971), Jarvik et al (1980) and Hagnell et al (1981, 1983). In his celebrated study of the elderly in two Swedish islands, Åkesson combined a prevalence survey with a follow-up three years later. Based on a total population of 4198 aged 60 year and over, he found a three-years incidence of 0.52% for arteriosclerotic psychosis (MID) and 0.38% for senile psychosis (likely to be SDAT).

In Newcastle upon Tyne, in two samples of the elderly (n= 294 and 466) Bergmann et al (1971 undertook follow-up studies two to four years after the initial interview. These authors subtracted from the total denominator those cases who had a dementia at the first interview. They found an annual incidence rate of 0.7% for arteriosclerotic dementia and 0.8% for senile dementia.

Jarvik and her colleagues undertook a follow-up study on an unusual sample. They re-examined those persons available from the adult twins series originally examined by Kallmann. They succeeded in re-examining 22 of these individuals, six years after the initial cognitive assessment. Their finding was an incidence rate of 16% for dementia over the six years. They did not differentiate between SDAT and MID. These authors have proposed that persons who reach the age of 80 without developing a dementia may have passed the period of maximum risk. That is, there may be a plateau in the incidence rate. Mortimer et al (1981) have examined in some detail the evidence for this hypothesis. They conclude that 'the age-specific incidence of senile dementia has yet to be assessed in a true community study'.

By far the best data on incidence, fulfilling this aim, come from the remarkable work by Hagnell and his colleagues (Hagnell et al, 1981, 1983). Hagnell has worked with the total adult population of the southern Swedish town, given the name of Lundby. This population had originally been examined in 1947 by Essen-Möller (1956). Hagnell himself re-examined the population 10 years later (Hagnell, 1966) and then with his colleagues 25 years later. On this unique set of data, they have been able to calculate the incidence rate for dementia in a total population over a long period. Furthermore, they have distinguished between MID and SDAT on clinical grounds. The first report of their 25-years finding (Hagnell et al, 1981) showed that the incidence of dementia had decreased during that period. The question was whether this decrease was in SDAT or MID. A decreased incidence of stroke might have explained the overall drop. But further analysis of their data (Hagnell et al, 1983) showed that the decrease occurred in both types of dementia. They have reported an incidence rate for senile dementia (equivalent to a clinical diagnosis of AD) of 0.7% for men and 0.5% for women, aged 70 to 79 years. For the age group 80+, the incidence increased to 1.9% for men and 2.5% for women. Estimates which could throw light on the possibility of a plateau in the incidence curve are too unstable because of the numbers involved in both the numerator and denominator.

Mortimer (1983) points to the findings which are consistent over three autopsy studies that the characteristic neuropathological features of AD decrease in persons over the age of 90 years. He has gone on to suggest that this may be due to their being a survival élite, such people perhaps being specially resistant to the aetiological agents causing AD. But an alternative explanation would be that very elderly people who develop AD, including those in their 90s, may die earlier. When they come to autopsy, it would not be surprising that the histological features of the disease were less developed.

RISK FACTORS

Knowledge about risk factors offers two things: the possiblity of intervention for persons at high risk, and the unravelling of the aetiological puzzle through finding a coherence amongst an array of risk factors. Sluss et al, (1981) assert that there are no known risk factors for Alzheimer's disease other than age. Nevertheless, both they and Mortimer et al (1981) acknowledge that there is information on some suggested factors, although none has been adequately established. The reader should be aware that most of the work on risk factors has been conducted on AD with earlier onset, though not necessarily in its presenile form. There is much less information on risk factors established in cases with onset in very late life, where the disorder is more benign. The risk factors presently proposed are: age, a family history of AD, a family history of Down's syndrome or lymphomas, Down's syndrome itself, head injury, and thyroid disease. A recent finding of great interest is that cases of Alzheimer's disease have an excess of ulnar loops in their fingerprint patterns (Weinreb, 1985). Such a finding is also present in Down's syndrome. Clearly, the ulnar loops are present before birth, so that they may provide a biological marker of increased risk.

We have already seen how the expectation of AD increases rapidly with age, at least up to around 80 years. But there are many other disorders to which this also applies.

There seems little doubt that a family history of AD increases the risk. Sjögren et al (1952) were the first to conduct an inquiry into the clinical genetics of Alzheimer's disease. A further contribution was made by Larsson et al (1963). The material used by these authors was a series of probands, in about half of whom a diagnosis of AD had been neuropathologically established at autopsy. All available relatives were then examined to look for both AD and SDAT. Both groups of authors found a definite effect, in which there was an excess of cases amongst first-degree relatives of the probands.

Subsequently, Heston et al (1981) undertook a major genetic study, examining the relatives of 125 probands. Here, the diagnosis of AD had been established neuropathologically in all cases. Furthermore, in this work, the age of onset of the disorder ranged from 40 to 98 years. Heston and his colleagues used not only a hospital-based control group, but also the known incidence rates in the general population, when comparing morbidity rates in the probands' relatives. This applied to Down's syndrome and the lymphomas as well as AD itself. The finding was a substantial increased risk of AD and SDAT in first-degree relatives. They also noted that the risk was stronger where the age of onset of AD had been earlier in the index case. Where a proband's parent had been affected and where the age of onset in the proband was under the age of 70, the risk to siblings was nearly 50%. By contrast, where there was no other family history and the age of onset in the proband was later than 70 years, the risk was no greater than that for the general population. There was then the remarkable finding of an excess of Down's syndrome, lymphomas and a group of diseases characterized by impaired immune function, all of these occurring more frequently in relatives of the probands. It should be noted that for Down's syndrome and the lymphomas the increased risk was associated with earlier age of onset of AD in probands. More recently Heyman et al (1983) reported an excess of thyroid disease in cases of AD, compared to controls. They confirmed this in a second study (Heyman et al 1984).

The association between AD and Down's syndrome does not hold only between relatives. It also holds for individuals. That is, if they live long enough, persons with Down's syndrome have a very high, possibly absolute, incidence of AD (Ellis et al, 1974). Heston (1984) has provided a detailed examination of this association.

Much interest should be accorded to the finding by Heyman et al (1984) of an increased frequency of head injury in cases of AD, compared to their controls. This finding has now been replicated by Mortimer et al (1985). In the latter study, the average time elapsing between the head injury and the onset of the dementia was no less than 35 years. Bias in reporting remains a possible interpretation. The information about head injury is obtained from relatives. Relatives of cases of dementia might more thoroughly review their afflicted members' past, in an attempt to recall past events to which the dementia might be attributed. This is a phenomenon familiar to all who have conducted research on life events. There, what Bartlett (1932) called 'effort after meaning' can explain why people tend to report much misadventure and exposure to stress as an explanation of the presence of disease. The same phenomenon of selective recall pervades all research using the case-control design. Accordingly, it is now necessary to confirm this promising finding about head injury by conducting prospective studies of persons known to have suffered a head injury in the past. Such a design should be entirely feasible in many teaching hospital settings.

The finding of an excess of thyroid disease in the relatives of probands remains a puzzle. Heyman et al (1984) did not find that any particular thyroid disorder was involved.

Reasoning underlying risk factor research

Some effort is now required to find possible aetiologies which might underlie these proposed risk factors. Not only might this help understanding of the links in the causal chain, but it might generate hypotheses about further risk factors. The family clustering of cases could be brought about by means other than genetic effects. Although no pathologist has yet succeeded in identifying a transmissible agent, the possibility remains that family clustering could be due to this. Walley & Holloway (1985) have reported a non-random occurrence of AD within geographical areas of Edinburgh.

Another possibility which could provide a unifying basis for the risk factors of age, Down's syndrome and head injury, is damage caused by free oxygen radicals (Dormandy, 1983; Clark et al, 1985; Harman, 1985). Caution has to be observed in prematurely adopting a new and enthusiastically pursued area of knowledge as a satisfactory explanation for previous puzzles. The presence of free oxygen radicals is known to increase markedly in later life, to be caused by trauma and to be particularly toxic to the brain. Futhermore, the enzyme superoxide dismutase is dependent on a gene on the 21 chromosome. But the hypothesis does not fit well with the very long lapse time between the head injury and the onset of dementia. As proposed by Mortimer et al (1985) damage to the blood-brain barrier is possible more likely, leading to subsequent immunological events within the brain, which normally is an immunologically-privileged area.

G. A. Broe and ourselves have considered another starting point for causal hypotheses. Since the brain is embryologically ectoderm, one might expect an increased incidence of degenerative changes in other ectodermal tissues in cases of AD. Accordingly, one might predict an increased incidence of cataract and senile macular degeneration.

There is also a rationale for looking at demographic differences in rates. For example, if a social class gradient were found, this would be a most important starting point for further research. It could be due to different levels of exposure to some unidentified toxin or other environmental experience. The frequent co-existence of dementia and depression, which has given rise to an appreciable clinical literature, could conceivably be due to a common aetiological basis.

FUTURE DIRECTIONS

It will be amply clear that epidemiological work on Alzheimer's disease has already made substantial gains. There are a number of important technical difficulties which are currently being tackled with energy. The issues which now have to be faced have been set out by Henderson (1986a, 1986b). There are three:

1. Tasks which are peculiar to each new study. For example, identifying the elderly in a population, or obtaining an unbiased sample of treated cases, either in the community or in institutional care. Neither of these tasks is trivial.
2. Issues best solved by international collaboration between investigators. These include the construction of common instruments, such as the Geriatric Mental State Examination (Copeland et al, 1976, in press), as well as common diagnostic criteria, such as those recently proposed by McKhann et al (1984) for the disorder. These instruments and criteria should also make it possible to grade levels of severity, so that comparisons can be made between surveys. This would be of the greatest use in studies of natural history, which require measurement of change over time.
3. Most important of all, there is the task of bringing real creativity to the problem, generating bold new hypotheses, and vigilance for serendipitous findings.

Amongst these issues, more should be said about those which are demanding but essentially soluble.

The sample

From what has already been said, it will be apparent that much thought and effort is required for an adequate sample to be obtained. Anyone embarking on a study of dementia in the general population must firstly determine what the true denominator is and how it is to be sampled, so that an estimate may be made of the numerator — the latter being the cases. Only in this way will a realistic prevalence or incidence figure be achieved. In many countries, including Australia, there is no publicly available age-specific list with the names of all persons in the population, let alone the elderly. The electoral rolls do not usually give the date of birth. As a consequence, a survey cannot begin until one has firstly done a census to determine who and where the elderly persons are. This can be extremely expensive. Care must also be taken in deciding on the geographical boundaries for this study. Some areas may have an over-or under-representation of the elderly, particularly the very elderly, due to intramigration effects. There is then the problem of including those individuals who are already in institutional care. Should all those living in nursing homes or hospitals in the area be included? Could this then be an overestimate? If some are to be excluded from the survey, on what basis should this be determined?

In some countries with advanced systems of health care and social security, general practitioner lists may be an adequate sampling frame. In this writer's experience, where a fee-for-service form of private practice exists, many general practitioners may not be able to provide an exhaustive list of their elderly patients. This is because some old persons, possibly those of special relevance, may not have consulted the doctor for many years. With increasing recognition of the needs for privacy and confidentiality, access to lists of names and addresses, let alone with birth dates to determine age, is becoming much more difficult. Indeed, this is already posing a serious problem in psychiatric epidemiology more generally, as Robins (1977) has reported.

Diagnostic criteria

Establishing diagnostic criteria should logically precede the development of case-finding instruments. The latter must serve the former. Scientifically adequate and internationally accepted diagnostic criteria for dementia are now needed, but more than that we need criteria for the clinical diagnosis of AD during life. These should include adequate gradings of severity. At the time of writing, the most ubiquitous criteria are those of DSM-III (American Psychiatric Association, 1980). Kay et al (1985) have described the difficulties encountered, as well as the variation in rates, when they estimated the prevalence of dementia and depression in a community sample in Hobart, Tasmania, using different diagnostic criteria applied to the same body of clinical information. Jorm & Henderson (1985) have pointed to the deficiencies in the DSM-III criteria for dementia. Essentially, there are two.

Firstly, they require the investigator to view the disorder as categorical rather than dimensional. But it is obvious that dementia is graded in severity, and that its nominal point of onset is man-made and arbitrary. We therefore need a cut-off, in the way that hypochromic anaemia is established. This has so far not been achieved, other than with reference to social performance, which could vary between social classes, certainly for mild dementia, and also considerably between geographic or cultural groups.

Secondly, the DSM-III criteria are very broad. For example, criterion B requires the presence of 'memory impairment', without further specification being provided. The consequence is the danger of diagnostic unreliability when clinicians or survey workers use these criteria in different ways. Jorm and Henderson have proposed some strategies for overcoming these difficulties.

Attention to diagnostic criteria for international use is timely, because the World Health Organization is preparing for the Tenth Revision of the International Classification of Diseases (ICD-10). This Revision will have sizeable differences from its predecessors. It will include revised glossary definitions, but also new elements in the form of clinical diagnostic guidelines and research-oriented diagnostic criteria. ICD-10 will also provide specific criteria for diagnosis of Alzheimer's disease, within the dementias. Considerable headway has already been achieved in this with the publication of proposed criteria for precisely this purpose by McKhann et al (1984).

In our own view, some provision should be made for the possibility that there is more than one type of SDAT. As a minimum, there may be two types: one with earlier onset, a more rapid deterioration and an emphasis on parietal features, while the second is of later onset, has a more benign course and may have more frontal signs. Jorm (1985) has provided a detailed examination of the issues to be faced in establishing such a typology of Alzheimer's disease.

For the diagnosis of mild dementia, there are particular difficulties in establishing diagnostic criteria (Henderson & Huppert, 1984). The problem is severe enough in Western populations. It is much greater in populations where education is limited, particularly in the elderly, or where there is much illiteracy. There, many of the cognitive tasks used in neuropsychological tests would make little sense. The principle task in any population is to demonstrate a significant drop in cognitive performance. This applies to the domains of intelligence , memory and specific areas of higher cortical function. Next, clouding of consciousness must be excluded before a diagnosis of dementia can be made. In Western and non-Western populations alike, this may prove very difficult because of the high prevalence of disease, subnutrition or prescribed medication. It is well established that large numbers of our elderly are consuming medication with anticholinergic properties which may therefore impair memory and cognition.

The criteria McKhann et al (1984) for Alzheimer's disease are by far the most thorough available to date. Furthermore, they appear to most workers to be suitable for use in survey settings. They allow the diagnosis of 'probable Alzheimer's disease' in the absence of neuropathological evidence, although special investigations are required, in addition to clinical information. Procedures such as a CAT scan can prove a major obstacle to case-ascertainment in surveys.

Instruments

There is at present no established instrument in widespread use for the ascertainment of Alzheimer's disease in field surveys. This means that epidemiological research on this diagnosis has not yet reached the stage achieved for most psychiatric disorders, with instruments such as the Diagnostic Interview Schedule (DIS) (Robins et al, 1981), or the Present State Examination (PSE) (Wing et al, 1974). Indeed, in the course of the Epidemiologic Catchment Area (ECA) studies in the United States, the DIS has the Mini-Mental State Examination grafted onto its end as its sole cognitive component. It is therefore not possible to make a diagnosis of dementia on the DIS. The same holds for the PSE. A diagnosis of dementia, but not Alzheimer's disease, can be made with the Geriatric Mental State Examination (GMS) (Copeland et al, 1976), as used in the

US–UK Cross National Diagnostic Study. It is also achieved by the Comprehensive Assessment and Referral Evaluation (CARE) developed in the US–UK Study in London and New York (Gurland et al, 1977, 1984). Using a shortened version of the GMS, called the GMS-6, Kay and his colleagues found that diagnostic criteria for dementia were better met by the Mini-Mental State Examination than by items in the GMS-6 itself (Kay et al, 1985).

There is now a new and promising instrument, the CAMDEX, currently under development in the Department of Psychiatry, Cambridge. Rosen et al (1984) have developed a rating scale for the diagnosis of Alzheimer's disease, but its utility in a field setting has not been determined. In the construction of any instrument which will allow the diagnosis of Alzheimer's disease, there are three necessary components: a history of the onset of the disorder and the current level of functioning, usually to be obtained from an informant such as a spouse or a close relative; a neuropsychiatric examination of the individual, including the assessment of any features of depression or of clouding of consciousness; and a neuropsychological examination. Wherever possible, a diagnosis of Alzheimer's disease should not be made on the basis of a single clinical examination.

Screening

By screening, we mean the identification of probable cases of Alzheimer's disease through the application of a relatively brief test to large numbers of the elderly, either in the community, in primary care or in some special group such as retirement homes. Such screening is usually the first part of a two-phase design (Deming, 1977; Duncan-Jones & Henderson, 1978) in which all of the probable cases are subsequently given a more thorough examination, but a proportion of probable normals are also re-examined, so that case-rates can be estimated for the whole sample. Some authors have already noted that screening for dementia may bring a number of practical difficulties. Eastwood & Corbin (1981) and Cooper & Bickel (1984) have pointed out the formidable load on diagnostic services which such a procedure would cause. There are nevertheless some practical and scientific reasons for justifying screening. Both the old person's doctor and family are at some advantage in managing the person if they know that cognitive impairment is present. It will influence the pattern of the doctor's prescribing and the family's attitude to any difficult behaviour which arises. There are also important scientific reasons for screening, because it provides the only practicable way for estimating prevalence or incidence in larger samples.

The screening instruments presently available are for dementia, not specifically Alzheimer's disease. The best-known are the Mini-Mental State Examination (Folstein et al, 1975; Anthony et al, 1982) and the package developed by Pfeffer et al (1981). In the Hobart prevalence study by Kay et al, (1985) the Mini-Mental State Examination performed very satisfactorily. On the basis of an examination taking no more than 5 minutes, conducted by a trained lay interviewer, it gave 100% sensitivity and 86% specificity against these authors' use of DSM-III criteria. This was for dementia of moderate and severe degree. But if mild dementia was included, the respective values changed to 59% and 93%. The package used by Pfeffer et al (1981) gave 93% sensitivity and 80% specificity for mild dementia. That instrument took some 15 minutes to administer, one of its components being the Mini-Mental State. From that finding, it seems likely that the small amount of extra time is well spent for the detection of milder cases.

The demands made of a screening instrument for dementia are considerable. As emphasized above, the main task is to demonstrate the deterioration in cognitive performance, presumed to have been at a previously higher level. Furthermore, this has to be achieved without having examined the individual at an earlier time. All information is therefore retrospectively obtained and is likely to have some unreliability. Jorm (1986) has introduced an innovative approach. He has advocated a test which will compare controlled and automatic processing of information. It is known that everyone performs better at tasks involving automatic processing. In dementia, it is believed that the impairment is much greater for controlled or effortful information; and that impairment of automatic processing comes only much later. A discrepancy between performance on the two parts of the tests suggests the presence of a probable dementia. Further development of this test with appropriate community norms is now being undertaken.

At present, there is no brief screening instrument for Alzheimer's disease itself, but only for dementia in general. Our own view is that a specific screening test for Alzheimer's disease is not practicable, because the clinical diagnosis of this disorder is extremely demanding and could not be contained in a brief instrument.

CONCLUSION

There is already much useful information on Alzheimer's disease from epidemiological studies. In the future, special priority should be accorded to longitudinal studies and to case-control designs; both of these hold the greatest promise for advancing knowledge on aetiology and prevention. Because of its public health importance, and because it remains a disorder of unknown aetiology, energetic attempts are being made for epidemiological research to complement laboratory-based studies of Alzheimer's disease. Any advance towards an understanding of its aetiology is a contribution to science and to human well-being.

ACKNOWLEDGEMENT

The writer expresses appreciation to Professor D. W. K. Kay, Professor G. A. Broe and Dr A. F. Jorm for their participation in discussions about the epidemiology of dementia. Ms Debra Rickwood generously assisted with the bibliography.

This chapter is based on material previously published (Henderson, 1986b) with the kind permission of the British Medical Bulletin.

REFERENCES

Åkesson H O 1969 A population study of senile and arteriosclerotic psychoses. Human Heredity 19: 546–566

Alzheimer A 1907 (On a peculiar disease of the cerebral cortex) Uber eine eigenartige Erkrankung der Hirnrinde. Allgemeine Zeitschrift für Psychiatrie und Psychisch-Gerichtlich Medicin 64: 146–148 Translation: Wilkins R H, Brody I A 1969 Alzheimer's Disease. Archives of Neurology 21: 109–110

American Psychiatric Association 1980 Diagnostic and statistical manual of mental disorders, 3rd edn DSM III. Division of Public Affairs, American Psychiatric Association, Washington DC

Anthony J C, Niaz U, LeResche L A, Von Korff M R, Folstein M F 1982 Limits of the 'Mini-Mental State' as a screening test for dementia and delirium among hospital patients. Psychological Medicine 12(2): 397–408

Bartlett F C 1932 Remembering: a Study of experimental and social psychology. Cambridge University Press, London

Bergmann K, Kay D W K, Foster E M, McKechnie A A, Roth M 1971 A follow-up study of randomly selected community residents to assess the effects of chronic brain syndrome and cerebrovascular disease. In: New prospects in the study of mental disorders in old age. Proceedings of the V World Congress of Psychiatry, Mexico, 25 November–4 December. Excerpta Medica, Amsterdam

Berkson J 1946 Limitations of the application of fourfold table analysis to hospital data. Biometrics Bulletin 2: 47–53

Bollerup T R 1975 Prevalence of mental illness among 70-year-olds domiciled in nine Copenhagen suburbs. Acta Psychiatrica Scandinavica 51: 327–339

Boyden S 1980 The need for an holistic approach to human health and well-being. In: Stanley N F, Joske R A (eds) Changing disease patterns and human behaviour. Academic Press, London

Boyden S, Millar S, Newcombe K, O'Neill B 1981 Environment lifestyle and health: problems and principles. In: The ecology of a city and its people: the case of Hong Kong, Australian National University Press, Canberra, p 325–354

Clark I A, Cowden W B, Hunt N H 1985 Free radical-induced pathology. Medical Research Review 5(3): 1–36

Cloninger C R, Miller J P, Wette R, Martin R L, Guze S B 1979 The evaluation of diagnostic concordance in follow-up studies: I A general model of causal analysis and a methodological critique. Journal of Psychiatric Research 15: 85–106

Cooper B, Bickel H 1984 Population screening and the early detection of dementing disorders in old age: a review. Psychological Medicine 14: 81–95

Copeland J R M, Kelleher M J, Kellett J M, Gourlay A J, Gurland B J, Fleiss J L, Sharpe L 1976 A semi-structured clinical interview for the assessment of diagnosis and mental state in the elderly: The Geriatic Mental State Schedule. I. Development and reliability. Psychological Medicine 6: 439–449

Copeland J R M, Henderson A S, Dewey M E 1985 Manual for the Geriatric Mental State. in press

Deming W E 1977 An essay on screening or on two-phase sampling applied to surveys of a community. International Statistical Review 45: 29–37

De Wolfe Miller F, Hicks S P, D'Amato C J, Landis J R 1984 A descriptive study of neuritic plaques and neurofibrillary tangles in an autopsy population. American Journal of Epidemiology 120(3): 331–341

Dormandy T L 1983 An approach to free radicals. Lancet ii: 1010–1014

Duncan-Jones P, Henderson S 1978 The use of a two-phase design in a population survey. Social Psychiatry 13: 231–237

Eastwood R, Corbin S 1981 Investigation of suspect dementia. Lancet i:1261

Ellis W G, McCulloch J R, Corley C L 1974 Presenile dementia in Down's syndrome: ultrastructural identity with Alzheimer's disease. Neurology 24: 101–106

Essen-Möller E 1956 Individual traits and morbidity in a Swedish rural population. Acta Psychiatrica Scandinavica, Suppl 100

Folstein M F, Folstein S E, McHugh P R 1975 'Mini-mental state'. A practical method for grading the cognitive state of patients for the clinician. Journal of Psychiatric Research 12: 189–198

Fries J F 1980 Aging, natural death and the compression of morbidity. New England Journal of Medicine 303: 130–135

Grove W M, Andreasen N C, McDonald-Scott P, Keller M B, Shapiro R W 1981 Reliability studies of psychiatric diagnosis: theory and practice. Archives of General Psychiatry 38: 408–413

Gruenberg E M 1977 The failures of success. Milbank Memorial Fund Quarterly 55: 3–24

Gruenberg E M, Hagnell O, Öjesjö L, Mittelman M 1976 The rising prevalence of chronic brain syndrome in the elderly. Paper presented at the Symposium on Society Stress and Disease: Aging and Old Age, Stockholm, 14–19 June

Gurland B, Kuriansky J, Sharpe L, Simon R, Stiller P, Birkett P 1977 The Comprehensive Assessment and Referral Evaluation CARE Rationale, development and reliability. International Journal of Aging and Human Development 8(1): 9–42

Gurland B, Golden R R, Teresi J A, Challop J 1984 The short-care: an efficient instrument for the assessment of depression, dementia and disability. Journal of Gerontology 19(2): 166–169

Hachinski V C, Iliff L D, Phil M, Zilhka E, Du Boulay G H, McAllister V L, Marshall J, Ross Russell R W, Symon L 1975 Cerebral blood flow in dementia. Archives of Neurology 32: 632–637

Hagnell O 1966 A prospective study of the incidence of mental disorder. Svenska Bokforlaget (Scandinavian University Books), Stockholm

Hagnell O, Lanke J, Rorsman B, Ojesjö L 1981 Does the incidence of age psychosis decrease? A prospective longitudinal study of a complete population investigated during the 25-year period 1947–1972: the Lundby Study. Neuropsychobiology 7(4): 201–211

Hagnell O, Lanke J, Rorsman B, Ohman R, Ojesjo L 1983 Current trends in the incidence of senile and multi-infarct dementia. Archives of Psychiatry and Neurological Sciences 233: 423–438

Harman D 1985 Role of free radicals in aging and disease. In: Johnson H A (ed) Relations between normal aging and disease. Raven Press, New York

Hasegawa K 1975 An epidemiological study on age-related dementia. Japanese Journal of Geriatrics 12: 258–264

Hasegawa K 1982 Kanagawa-ken. The report of the health status of the aged in Kanagawa Prefecture. Section of Health of Kanagawa-ken

Henderson A S 1986a Developments in the epidemiology of senile dementia. In: Tansella M (ed) L'approccio epidemiologica in psichiatria. Patron, Bologna

Henderson A S 1986b The epidemiology of Alzheimer's disease. British Medical Bulletin January 42(1): 3–10

Henderson A S, Huppert F A 1984 The problem of mild dementia. Psychological Medicine 14: 5–11

Henderson A S, Kay D W K 1984 The epidemiology of mental disorders in the aged. In: Kay D W K, Burrows G (eds) Handbook of studies in psychiatry and old age. Elsevier, Amsterdam

Heston L L, Mastri A R, Anderson V E, White J 1981 Dementia of the Alzheimer type. Clinical genetics natural history and associated conditions. Archives of General Psychiatry 30: 1085–1090

172 DEMENTIA

Heston L L 1984 Down's Syndrome and Alzheimer's disease: defining an association. Psychiatric Developments 4: 287–294

Heyman A, Wilkinson W E, Hurwitz B J, Schmechel D, Sigmon A H, Weinberg T, Helms M J, Swift M 1983 Alzheimer's disease: genetic aspects and associated clinical disorders. Annals of Neurology 14: 507–515

Heyman A, Wilkinson W E, Stafford J A, Helms M J, Sigmon A H, Weinberg T 1984 Alzheimer's disease: a study of epidemiological aspects. Annals of Neurology 15(4): 335–341

Jarvik L F, Ruth V, Matsuyama S S 1980 Organic brain syndrome and aging: a six-year follow-up of surviving twins. Archives of General Psychiatry 37: 280–286

Jorm A F 1985 Subtypes of Alzheimer's dementia: a conceptual analysis and critical review. Psychological Medicine 15: 543–553

Jorm A F 1986 Controlled and automatic information processing in senile dementia: a review. Psychological Medicine 16(1): 77–88

Jorm A F, Henderson A S 1985 Possible improvements to the diagnostic criteria for dementia in DSM-III. British Journal of Psychiatry 147: 394–399

Karasawa A 1980 The report on the health status of the aged in Tokyo. Tokyo Metropolitan Government, Tokyo

Kay D W K 1962 Outcome and cause of death in mental disorders of old age: a long-term follow-up of functional and organic psychoses. Acta Psychiatrica Scandinavica 38: 249–276

Kay D W K, Beamish P, Roth M 1964 Old age mental disorders in Newcastle upon Tyne. Part I. A study of prevalence. British Journal of Psychiatry 110: 146–158

Kay D W K, Henderson A S, Scott R, Wilson J, Rickwood D, Grayson D A 1985 Dementia and depression among the elderly living in the Hobart community: the effect of the diagnostic criteria on the prevalence rates. Psychological Medicine 15: 771–788

Kral V A 1962 Senescent forgetfulness, benign and malignant. Canadian Medical Association Journal 86: 257–260

Kral V A 1978 Benign senescent forgetfulness. In: Katzman R, Terry R D, Bicks K L (eds) Alzheimer's disease: senile dementia and related disorders. Raven Press, New York

Lambo T A 1966 Psychiatric disorders in the aged: epidemiology and preventive measures. West African Medical Journal 15: 121–124

Larsson T, Sjögren T, Jacobson G 1963 Senile dementia: a clinical, sociomedical and genetic study. Acta Psychiatrica Scandinavica Suppl 167: 1–259

Liston E H, LaRue A 1983a Clinical differentiation of primary degenerative and multi-infarct dementia: a critical review of the evidence, Part I: Clinical studies. Biological Psychiatry 18: 1451–1465

Liston E H, LaRue A 1983b Clinical differentiation of primary degenerative and multi-infarct dementia: a critical review of the evidence Part II: Pathological studies. Biological Psychiatry 18: 1467–1484

Marmot M G, Syme L 1976 Acculturation and coronary heart disease in Japanese-Americans. American Journal of Epidemiology 104: 225–247

Masters C L, Gajdussek D C, Gibbs C J 1981 Problems of case ascertainment and diagnosis in the epidemiology of dementia occurring in geographic isolates and worldwide. In: Mortimer J A, Schuman L M (eds) Epidemiology of dementia. Oxford University Press, New York

McKhann G, Drachman D, Folstein M, Katzman R, Price D, Stadlan E M 1984 Clinical diagnosis of Alzheimer's disease: report of the NINCDS-ADRDA Work Group under the auspices of Department of Health and Human Services Task Force on Alzheimer's Disease. Neurology 34: 939–944

Mölsä P K, Marttila R J, Rinne U K 1982 Epidemiology of dementia in a Finnish population. Acta Neurologica Scandinavica 65: 541–552

Mortimer J A 1983 Alzheimer's disease and senile dementia: prevalence and incidence. In: Reisberg B (ed) Alzheimer's disease. Free Press, New York,p: 141–148

Mortimer J A, Schuman L M, French L R 1981 Epidemiology of dementing illness. In: Mortimer J A, Schuman L M (eds) The epidemiology of dementia, Oxford University Press, New York, p: 3–23

Mortimer J A, French L R, Hutton J T, Schuman L M 1985 Head injury as a risk factor for Alzheimer's disease. Neurology 35(2): 264–267

Pfeffer R I, Kurosaki T T, Harrah C H, Chance J M, Bates D, Detels R, Filos S, Butzke C 1981 A survey diagnostic tool for senile dementia. American Journal of Epidemiology 114(4): 515–527

Robins L N 1977 Problems in follow-up studies. American Journal of Psychiatry 134: 904–907

Robins L N, Helzer J E, Croughan J, Ratcliff K S 1981 National Institute of Mental Health Diagnostic Interview Schedule. Its history characteristics and validity. Achives of General Psychiatry 38: 381–388

Ron M A, Toone B K, Garralda M E, Lishman W A 1979 Diagnostic accuracy in presenile dementia. British Journal of Psychiatry 134: 161–168

Rosen W G, Mohs R C, Davis K L 1984 A new rating scale for Alzheimer's disease. American Journal of Psychiatry 141(11): 1356–1364

Sjögren T, Sjögren H, Lindgren A G H 1952 Morbus Alzheimer and morbus Pick: a genetic clinical and patho-anatomical study. Acta Psychiatrica et Neurologica Scandinavica Suppl 82

Sluss T K, Gruenberg E M, Kramer M 1981 The use of longitudinal studies in the investigation of risk factors for senile dementia — Alzheimer type. In: Mortimer J A, Schuman L M (ed) The epidemiology of dementia. Oxford University Press, New York

St Clair D, Whalley L J 1983 Hypertension, multi-infarct dementia and Alzheimer's disease. British Journal of Psychiatry 143: 274–276

Tomlinson B, Blessed G, Roth M 1970 Observations on the brains of demented old people. Journal of Neurological Sciences 11: 205–242

Varsamis J, Zuchowski T, Maini K K 1972 Survival rates and causes of death in geriatric psychiatric patients. Canadian Psychiatric Association Journal 171: 17–22

Weinreb H J 1985 Fingerprint patterns in Alzheimer's disease. Archives of Neurology 4250–54

Whalley L J, Holloway S 1985 Non-random geographic distribution of Alzheimer's presenile dementia in Edinburgh, 1953–76. Lancet i:578

World Health Organization 1982 World Health Statistics Quarterly 35(3&4): WHO, Geneva

World Health Organization 1986 Senile dementia: research and action. Technical Report Series in press

Williamson J, Stockoe I H, Gray S, Fisher M, Smith A, McGhee A, Stephenson E 1964 Old people at home: their unreported needs. Lancet I: 1117–1120

Wing J K, Cooper J E, Sartorius N 1974 Measurement classification of psychiatric symptoms. Cambridge University Press, Cambridge

Alzheimer's disease: the clinical picture

INTRODUCTION

This chapter is addressed to an exposition of the clinical picture of Alzheimer's disease. Thus its content provides base material for other aspects of the disease considered elsewhere in this volume and its context requires mention of issues that are considered in greater depth in other chapters. It is to be hoped, therefore, that the reader will accept patiently some degree of overlap with those other chapters.

The original description by Alzheimer (1907) emphasized that both the clinical picture and the pathological findings were distinct from other disorders recognized at that time. He described a 51-year-old woman whose first symptom was morbid jealousy, which was soon followed by a rapidly progressive amnesia. She became unable to find her way round her own home and at times believed that someone wished to kill her. In the asylum, she presented a picture of marked helplessness, being completely disorientated in time and place. Her reaction to her doctor varied: sometimes she treated him as a visitor to her own home, at other times she believed that he was trying to make an assault upon her life or upon her chastity. Due to her poor understanding she screamed if anyone tried to examine her. At times, she appeared to be subject to auditory hallucinations and called out to her husband and daughter. Some insight was preserved, in so far as she sometimes remarked that she was unable to understand anything. Cognitive testing showed that her comprehension was defective and there was some impairment of naming. Her speech was repetitive, with some verbal paraphasias. Her reading was affected in that she drifted from line to line and her vocal inflection did not accord with the sense of the text. Her writing displayed omissions and perseverations, and she rapidly lost the thread of this task. She seemed unable to comprehend the function of objects presented to her, although she could still use her hands normally; her gait was also preserved. She deteriorated progressively and died four and a half years after the onset of her illness, to fall under the knife which she had needlessly feared whilst alive. In both the title and the text of his paper, Alzheimer specified the cerebral cortex as the seat of the pathology.

Since the original description there have been differences of opinion concerning the relationship between the pre-senile form of the disease ('Alzheimer's disease') and the disease in old age ('senile dementia of the Alzheimer type'). Comparison of presenile and senile forms of the disease in clinically diagnosed patients, using clinical features, neuropsychology and e.e.g. data, had not shown any major differences between the two groups (Pearce & Pearce, 1979; Sulkava & Amberla, 1982; Sulkava, 1982). It seems more reasonable to regard age as a pathoplastic factor rather than an artificial watershed between two domains. The term 'Alzheimer's disease' will thus be applied to both senile and presenile forms of the illness.

SOURCES OF INFORMATION

In any chronic disabling condition, it is necessary to point out that information about the disorder comes from different sources with different viewpoints. Only after considering the basis of our data can we hope to integrate a satisfactory picture.

Patients

The patients' ability to reflect on their handicaps depends very much on the stage of the illness. Patients will rarely be able to volunteer a spontaneous account of their difficulties, but this should not blind the doctor to the possibility that answers to specific questions can be appropriate and accurate. Adequate description is rendered impossible by severe overall affliction or significant aphasia. Memory deficits may interfere with the presentation of current symptoms, although earlier features may still be accurately portrayed. Severe dysarthria may make the patients' comments very difficult to understand. On the other hand, visuospatial disorder or mild memory disturbance is compatible with satisfactory description of symptoms.

Informants

It is of course essential to interview an informant, who will often be a relative. There is no need to emphasize the necessity of gleaning independent information, but it is necessary to be reminded that the relatives' accounts are not 'objective'. The two main factors which interfere with the relatives' accounts are, firstly, the difficulty in assessing the behaviour of the patient and, secondly, the emotional reactions of the relatives themselves.

   The patient with Alzheimer's disease may have multiple neuropsychological handicaps, physical symptoms and secondary psychiatric symptoms. It is often difficult for the trained professional to evaluate this complex tapestry of handicaps and the relative contribution of different impairments to the overall picture. It is thus hardly surprising that an untutored lay relative may experience difficulty in summarizing the patients' difficulties. As memory disturbances are prominent, they often serve as the peg for all symptoms, so that anomia is interpreted as amnesia for words and dressing 'apraxia' as forgetting how to get dressed. Problems with manual operations or gait may be construed as weakness. Although much is known about the way psychological disorders present with physical symptoms, neuropsychiatry offers a rich and often uncharted field where symptoms of organic brain disease are interpreted in psychodynamic terms. A dense amnesia may thus be interpreted as a desire to forget or a retreat into the past.

When taking a history, it is important to assess the effects of the relatives' emotional reactions on the account which they are giving. Many relatives cope with severe burdens when looking after affected patients. In such cases, the consultation is often the occasion for a display of loyalty. Symptoms may be minimized and the amount of nursing care required may not be made plain. Some relatives seem to cope well as long as they can avoid ruminating on current disabilities or the prospect of future deterioration. Great importance may be attached to something which medically appears to be of minor significance, such as dental hygiene or bowel habit.

Mental State Examination

At least some aspects of Mental State Examination can be carried out on all patients. Observation may show evidence of self-neglect or difficulty in feeding. It is important to establish whether the patient's clothing and grooming are the result of his or her own endeavours, or reflect the care of nurses or relatives. When speech is relatively unimpaired by dysphasia or dysarthria, euthymic patients usually preserve the social aspects of speech and engage in light conversation which would pass for normal in a café or cocktail party, but is inappropriate during a medical consultation. Following the observations of Jung (1910) on delayed reaction times or flustered responses to emotionally significant verbal stimuli, one can note that our patients usually respond normally to questions concerning their emotional wellbeing, but become apprehensive, evasive or slow to answer after questions related to their cognitive function; the opposite pattern obtains in depressive states. Patients who appear relatively normal while their attention is engaged may become distressed and agitated if left to their own devices, which appears to be a response to their realization that they do not know where they are or how they came to be there. Patients suffering from delusions usually display the emotions appropriate to their abnormal beliefs.

Patients can usually comment on their current emotional state, but it is necessary to ask informants about other mood-related features, such as sleep disturbance, poor appetite, weight loss, social withdrawal and apathy. Unfortunately, changes in these functions may prove to be due to brain damage rather than clearly attributable to a mood disorder and treatable as such (Post, 1975). Patients may be able to comment on thought-blocking secondary to anxiety, particularly if it is elicited in the interview; most other aspects of the cognitive process are too recherché for comment. Thought content may be dominated by misinterpretations of events secondary to dementia, e.g. failure to find objects is interpreted as theft. Sensory stimuli may also be misinterpreted. Rapport is usually good in the undeluded patient. Insight may not be obviously present, but if the patient's attention is drawn to his or her failings, some deficiency is usually acknowledged.

Investigations

The role of special investigations is dealt with elsewhere in this volume. The rationale in clinical practice is to discover treatable disorders which can produce the clinical features of dementia: in other words, their importance is due to their ability to *refute* a diagnosis of progressive brain decay rather than providing evidence in support of such a diagnosis. In writing about the clinical features of dementia, it is important to place this in the context of the over-zealous application of this diagnostic label. Investigations of patients with a clinical diagnosis of dementia failed to support this diagnosis in virtually one-quarter of cases, both in a presenile series (Marsden & Harrison, 1972) and in a series of mixed ages (Smith et al, 1976). Follow-up studies of presenile patients with a diagnosis after investigation of dementia suggest that mis-labelling may be even more common, as the catamnesis bore out the diagnosis in only 43–69% of cases (Nott & Fleminger, 1975; Ron et al, 1979).

Psychological testing may be of value, but it is important to be aware of its limitations. One major problem is in the application of a cross-sectional analysis to a longitudinal process. It is also important to know how experienced the psychologist is in the assessment of such problems. In some countries (such as the United States and Finland) a separate speciality of neuropsychology has evolved, but such a development has not occurred in the UK. Despite this, some clinical and experimental psychologists have attained considerable expertise in assessing patients with known or suspected brain damage. A second problem with traditional psychological examination is the artificial nature of the test situation. The strangeness of the test procedure to the patient may be experienced as frightening and interfere with an accurate assessment. It is sometimes difficult, therefore, to establish the relationship between information obtained by psychological assessment and that obtained by more naturalistic techniques (De Renzi et al, 1968).

When discussing tests with the psychologist, it is worth discriminating between tests originally devised to assess intelligence in normal people, such as the Wechsler Adult Intelligence Scale (Wechsler, 1955) and Raven's Progressive Matrices (Raven, 1958), compared with those tests designed to assess specific cognitive deficits, for example prosopagnosia (Benton et al,

1983). It is also important to assess whether a focal cognitive impairment may have produced widespread impairment. For example, defective comprehension in Wernicke's aphasia may produce impairment on many tests which are supposed to tap non-linguistic functions (a diagnostic error recorded by Marie, 1926). Similarly, slowness may produce a spurious verbal-performance discrepancy on the Wechsler Adult Intelligence Scale, as all the performance subscales are timed and all but one of the verbal scales are untimed. It is equally important to consider the role of emotional factors, and there is now a considerable literature on the cognitive deficits associated with some emotional disorders, e.g. 'pseudodementia' (Post, 1975; Wells, 1982) and 'dementia syndrome of depression' (Folstein & McHugh, 1978). Although necessary, these observations are not new, for over a century ago Griesinger warned against confounding melacholia with dementia (Griesinger, 1865). Clinical experience suggests that this phenomenon is commoner with increasing age, a contention implicitly supported by some reviews (Post, 1975, 1982) and consistent with the views of Bleuler (1951) on the pathoplastic influence of age on the occurrence of amnesia.

Despite the disadvantages inherent in disorganizing the patient's usual lifestyle, one of the most powerful investigations available is admission for observation as a day patient or inpatient. When the diagnosis is unclear, this procedure generates valuable extra information about the patient's disabilities. In an institutional setting, nurses and remedial therapy staff have the opportunity to establish the exact nature of the patient's disabilities and also to comment on retained abilities and inconsistencies in the picture. Changes during the day can be noted: for example, a patient was referred with incontinence of urine and sometimes faeces, but this incontinence only occurred in the morning and was part of a clear diurnal mood variation. Fluctuations in memory may occur pari passu with fluctuations in conscious level found in confusional states, and may be associated with variation in the general level of sensory stimulation. Nursing staff are especially well placed to note patients' ability to orientate themselves in the ward and learn its routine; they are equally well placed to observe changes in symptoms related to the presence of medical staff or relatives.

MAJOR FEATURES

The major features of Alzheimer's disease are usually defined as amnesia, agnosia/apraxia, aphasia and neurophysical changes. These topics will be reviewed in turn before discussing other associated features and the course of the disorder.

Amnesia

Memory disorder is one of the most striking features of Alzheimer's disease. It occurs in 92–100% of pathologically confirmed cases (Sjögren et al, 1952;

Sim & Sussman, 1962; Lauter, 1968). It is a common presenting feature and often appears to be the best guide to deterioration in the patient. In the early stages of the disease, it is usually apparent as a mild forgetfulness which could be passed for normal. Relatives may state that the forgetfulness is abnormal for the patient but still better than their own memory, with the implication that the current performance is within the range of adult norms although impaired for that particular individual. Provided the memory disorder is pure, one finds on testing that the immediate recall or registration (e.g. digit span forwards) is satisfactory and memory for events in the distant past is also intact; the deficit is in the short-term memory (e.g. recalling information after a few minutes' delay) which represents a deficit of new learning.

In the first stage of memory deficit, it is very difficult to be confident about a diagnosis of Alzheimer's disease because the deficit appears relatively mild and, during testing, patients may appear quite anxious, sufficiently anxious to account for the performance failure. It is necessary, therefore, to follow patients up over a period of time in order to assess deterioration. In patients with Alzheimer's disease, the deficit in new learning will steadily increase. At this stage, one finds that day-to-day activities in familiar surroundings are usually unimpaired, but when patients are faced with new situations, or have to positively recall something different, mistakes are made and often the patients become flustered when presented with novel problems. They may at this stage be able to comment on their anxiety when faced with the unexpected, or may simply become distressed without being aware of the reason.

As the memory deterioration continues, patients require more and more prompting. The relatives frequently become exasperated at this stage, because they can tell the patient to do something and the patient will repeat the instruction accurately but then fail to carry the action out. If patients are doing something where all the visual cues are in front of them, they may be able to complete the activity, but if they look up and away from the task they might quite simply wander off, having forgotten all about it. The memory deficit at this stage is already so severe that it is difficult to keep patients occupied with any activity. Stressful events result in endlessly repeated requests for reassurance from the patient. Each request appears totally new for the patient, who shows no awareness of any previous reply. Testing at this stage will usually show a consistent dense amnesia, of the kind seen in patients with Korsakoff's psychosis (Constantinidis et al, 1978).

With further progression of the illness, the patient begins to live in the past. The names of children may be forgotten and the children themselves not recognized. The patient begins to behave as a much younger person and talks about his or her long-dead parents. Misrecognition of relatives usually places them as siblings or parents, and patients may deny that they are married, causing considerable embarrassment to their harassed spouse. In the end stages of illness, assessment of memory is virtually impossible, but the patient does not appear to show any signs of recognition for familiar faces.

Agnosia/apraxia

The second characteristic feature of Alzheimer's disease lies in the domain of agnosia/apraxia. Patients may show some degree of prosopagnosia (agnosia for faces). It can be difficult to assess this deficit in the presence of amnesia, in that failure to recognize a face may be due to memory impairment rather than inability to discriminate the physiognomy. However, it is possible to demonstrate difficulties in some patients by tests which do not rely on memory, such as matching two photographs of the same person. Non-recognition of the patients' own face is part of the so-called 'mirror sign'. The essence of this feature is that patients are seen talking to their own reflection in the mirror. It depends on the patients being unable to recognize their own face in the mirror and being unable to apperceive that the person in front of them is a reflection in a mirror rather than another human being. An experimental study of the behaviour of patients in front of a mirror was carried out by Ajuriaguerra et al (1963). Patients showed a range of abnormal behaviour. The mildly affected patients could recognize themselves but could not point out parts of their body on the mirror image; the most severely affected patients with 'Alzheimerized' dementia could not accept that the image was their own reflection even when told that this was the case, and often conversed with the image as though it were a normal person. The mirror sign was noted in 17% of Sjögren's small series of patients (Sjögren et al, 1952).

There are problems in the definition of apraxia. The definition of most neurological symptoms (such as sensory extinction, apraxia, or agnosia) suggests that all other relevant functions are intact. Hécaen (1981) defines apraxia as 'an impairment of the ability to carry out purposeful movements by an individual who has normal primary motor skills (strength, reflexes, co-ordination) and normal comprehension of the act to be carried out (no agnosia, no general intellectual impairment)'. Nevertheless, the purity of the definition of apraxia is not always maintained. Some so-called apraxic disturbances appear to be secondary to linguistic impairments (De Renzi et al, 1968). Despite his own definition, Hécaen (1981) includes in his study motor disorders which he regards as secondary to disorders of visuospatial perception and to disorders of body awareness — 'somatospatial apraxias'. Such secondary apraxias often characterize patients with Alzheimer's disease.

Patients may have considerable difficulty in locating objects in space. When asked to point to a pen on the table in front of them, they may search their environment minutely but unsystematically and look in quite bizarre places such as under their chair before their eyes actually light on the object. Once having located it, they experience considerable difficulty in letting go of it. Consequently, their attention may be directed inappropriately during a consultation. They may appear to be distracted by objects in their environment, but this distraction is quite different from the distractibility seen in the 'frontal lobe syndrome', where the patient is distracted by new sensations presented in any modality and relinquishes excessively easily any object or sensation which was previously being attended to. The disorder of location is also seen in the relationship between different objects in the environment. When asked to write on a piece of paper, they may choose to start in an odd place on the page. If there is any writing already on the page, they appear to be attracted to this stimulus as though by magnetism. If asked to carry out a copy of a simple drawing, they appear to have great difficulty in keeping their copy separate in space from the original and often start attaching their own copy to the original or even drawing over it. This feature was described in 1935 by Mayer-Gross as the 'closing-in phenomenon' and is also part of Balint's syndrome (De Renzi, 1982).

Patients also have difficulty in understanding the relationship between themselves and other objects. This disorder tends to be manifest as difficulty in dressing (dressing 'apraxia'). The act of getting dressed involves a very complicated sequence of spatial relationships between one's body and one's clothes. Patients with impairment in this area find tremendous difficulty in the correct orientation of themselves vis-à-vis articles of clothing. One patient reported that she had so much difficulty putting on her bra correctly that she used to keep it on for days at a time instead of taking it off each night, to avoid the distress of trying to put it on again the following day. Patients may try to put clothes on inside out or put their left arm through the right armhole of a shirt. Patients who wear spectacles may be seen fumbling with them for some length of time and even putting them on upside down. Given this disorder, feeding seems to be surprisingly well preserved, although problems do occur in this context. This type of disorder is also seen in the patients' writing and in their calculations. The closing-in phenomenon may also be relevant to the fact that patients often seem to attach themselves to their relatives and may follow a spouse around the house. The patients' ability to walk about can be affected, as they find it difficult to judge the height of objects that they perceive, such as steps. A flat floor with a change in colour or floor-covering may be misapprehended as a step or barrier.

Given all the patients' impairments, it is difficult to establish the presence of a pure apraxia in the sense defined by Hécaen above. Patients often perform badly on tests for apraxia, for whatever reason. It has been suggested that patients often have some gait apraxia which is clinically distinct from the Parkinsonian features which they may develop later. Such a gait disorder was described in 72% of the material presented by Sjögren et al (1952). Apraxia/agnosia was recorded in 34% of the large series of

Lauter (1968) and in 72% of the smaller series of Sjögren et al (1952). Pearce & Miller (1973) noted spatial disorientation in 75% of their patients, and Sulkava (1983) found disorders of orientation and higher visual functions in 78–89% of his patients.

Aphasia

The third major disturbance in Alzheimer's disease is aphasia. Initially this is manifest as a mild anomia, which the patient may be the first to complain of. In testing for anomia, it is important to establish that the patient's perception of the stimulus is correct, because failure of location and recognition has been established as a major source of error in naming by dements (Rochford, 1971).

As the language disorder progresses, some defects of comprehension may be evident. Initially this tends to be limited to more complicated sentence structures. The patients' speech tends to be generally fluent, although less rich than usual due to anomia. Routine social utterances appear to be relatively well preserved — described as 'empty speech'. The patients may make literal paraphasic errors in which letters in a word are substituted for incorrect letters. The patients' language function may appear relatively normal to the supporters and only on formal testing is it clear to what extent aphasia is present. Repetition may also be defective. As the disorder develops, language may become increasingly incomprehensible and the patient may produce less and less speech, finally becoming mute. The patient thus displays a progression from anomia through a fluent aphasia of the Wernicke kind to global aphasia (Albert et al, 1981), In the series of Lauter (1968) some form of language disorder was noted in 82%; Sjögren et al (1952) found language disorder in all their patients. Receptive aphasia was noted in 67% and 71% of Sulkava's presenile and senile series (Sulkava, 1983) and in 82% of the series of Pearce & Miller (1973). Dyslexia and dysgraphia have been noted slightly less frequently (53% and 55% by Pearce & Miller, 1973).

Neurophysical disorders

In the early stages of the disease, the patient is often physically well preserved and it is only towards the end of the course of the illness that physical symptoms appear. As Alzheimer noted in his original description, it may not be easy to carry out a full physical examination, particularly those aspects which require the active cooperation of the patient. Some of the problems encountered in examining mentally disordered patients have been discussed by Kampmeier (1977).

The earliest features appear to be those of Parkinsonism, in particular bradykinesia and rigidity of cog-wheel type; tremor is usually absent and never marked (Pearce, 1974). Parkinsonism was noted in 62% of the patients of Pearce (1974); Sulkava (1983) found that all his patients were akinetic and approximately two-thirds of them were rigid. Gait apraxia has been mentioned, but with progression of the disease it is more usual to see the gait disorders associated with Parkinsonism. These features provide a further handicap for the cognitively compromised patient.

Apart from aphasic difficulties, the patients will often show some non-aphasic speech disorder. Dysarthria was reported in 67% of patients by Sjögren et al (1952). Speech may be disorganized by the occurrence of perseveration, repetition of words (pallilalia), and repetition of parts of words (logoclonia) (Constantinidis et al, 1978).

Epilepsy is comparatively frequent: Sjögren et al (1952) reported an incidence of 22%, whereas Lauter (1968) reported an incidence of 9%. Pearce & Miller (1973) found that it occurred in 16% of the patients at some point but was not a major feature, often occurring as an isolated seizure or as a late complication. Most of their patients had generalized seizures, but partial seizures did occur.

On inspection of the physique, patients usually appear normal, although muscle-wasting has been noted as an end-stage phenomenon. Local amyotrophy of the hands has been noted in 9% of patients by Pearce (1974), always in association with Parkinsonism. On examination of muscle tone, some increase is usually noted, and this appears to be a combination of extrapyramidal rigidity with some pyramidal spasticity. Paratonia or gegen-halten (an inconstant resistance to passive movement proportional to the speed of the movement) has been described in association with rigidity (Sulkava, 1983).

Examination of the tendon reflexes may show some exaggeration, a finding in approximately 40% of patients (Sulkava, 1983). Primitive reflexes may also appear. The Babinski sign was positive in a small number of the patients studied by Sulkava (1983). The snout reflex was positive in the majority of patients studied by Sulkava (1983) and by Basavaraju et al (1981). The same authors noted the presence of grasp reflexes in a minority of patients. The palmomental reflex has been recorded in approximately half the patients studied by Pearce (1974) and Basavaraju et al (1981); unfortunately, the latter study also found it to be present in a third of healthy elderly controls. Basavaraju et al (1981) found the face–hand test to be helpful in discriminating between patients with Alzheimer's disease and normal controls, although there was still some overlap. This test relies on sensory extinction of a distal stimulus (the hand) by a proximal stimulus (the face), and may be positive if the stimuli are ipsilateral or contralateral: clearly, it necessitates a certain degree of cooperation on the part of the patient.

Involuntary movements are not usually regarded as an integral part of Alzheimer's disease, but they have certainly been reported. Some patients display small-amplitude, irregular and asymmetrical clonic contractions, which resemble those seen in 'jittery' babies. Action myoclonus is also sometimes present. Some form of myoclonus was reported in 2% of cases by Lauter (1968). Orofacial dyskinesia can occur and was reported in a quarter to a fifth of cases by Sulkava (1983). A few patients exhibit odd postures and writhing movements of the upper limbs, which appear to be associated with severe visuospatial disorganization. This is probably best considered to be a form of pseudo-athetosis.

Other major features

The emphasis on the previous points related to their possible help in diagnosis. The story would be misleading unless attention was also drawn to more general, non-specific features. The impairment of intellectual capacity clearly has important implications for the patients' behaviour, and it is often noted that the personality may become coarsened, whether by the loss of scintillation or by the exaggeration of the ego's unlovely aspects. Such organic personality changes have been referred to as 'androphrenias' by Sjöbring (1973), who notes that these defect states may show considerable intrapersonal variability. Reduced spontaneity has been recorded in the majority of patients (Pearce & Miller, 1973; Sjögren et al, 1952) and is often regarded as an early sign. This may give way to subsequent agitation and wandering. Goldstein (1952) has drawn our attention to the way in which patients may try to cope with their disabilities, for example by social withdrawal and avoidance of new situations. Patients may attempt to organize the environment in order to maintain the sameness of their situation. This so-called 'organic orderliness' is a significant early feature, and it seems likely that in a perverted form it is a factor in patients' restlessness in the later stages of illness.

Perplexity is an important but unsung feature of organic states (Lezak, 1978), and is a very unpleasant experience. The combination of prolonged disability and uncertain grasp fosters emotional disequilibrium, and all the features of a neurasthenic state may appear — debility, irritability, misery, anxiety, emotional lability and anhedonia. More specific psychological reactions will be discussed below; their presence or absence does not diminish the importance of recognizing the more pervasive problem of demoralization (Frank, 1979).

In the early stages of the illness, patients usually display some form of insight into their impairment, even if it is only a catastrophic reaction when faced with a memory test. Extensive deterioration is clearly not compatible with any significant grasp of their disability, but even in mild stages insight may be distorted by amnesia, perplexity, or retained psychological defence mechanisms. As in children, the tension in the carer can be communicated and exacerbate interpersonal difficulties. Social behaviour can usually be understood in terms of the patients' specific impairments, previous personality, life experiences and current circumstances. A pure picture of a 'frontal lobe syndrome' of moria (a vacuous euphoria), disinhibition and callousness is not usually seen, although moria has been reported in the series of Sjögren et al (1952). Such a clinical picture is most significant in the absence of other neurobehavioural deficits. The defects in our subjects' apperceptions necessarily entail some constraint on the ability to empathize with others, form long-term goals (and the plans to achieve them), and maintain control over their impulses. Anticipation is defective, even in comparison with patients suffering from Korsakoff's psychosis, and may be reduced to the level of a 4-year-old child (Ajuriaguerra et al, 1969). Social interaction is thus deflated. Despite these handicaps, there does appear to be a relative preservation of social behaviour in the earlier stages of the illness (Sim & Sussman, 1962; Albert, 1981).

From the cognitive point of view as from the social, normal performance depends on the integrated functioning of the whole brain. Factors such as attention and concentration are affected by most organic disorders, as is the ability to plan behaviour and successfully monitor the execution of that plan. Abstraction appears to depend both on linguistic function (De Renzi et al, 1966) and on the holistic or gestalt functions of the non-dominant hemisphere (Walsh, 1978), thus justifying Goldstein's emphasis on the concrete attitude as a manifestation of brain damage. Many diffuse and focal lesions can produce disorders such as perseveration (Allison, 1966) and catatonia (Gelenberg, 1976). In the end stages of dementia, it becomes extremely difficult to make realistic assessments of the patient and to differentiate between different syndromes (Drachman et al, 1981; Sim, 1979). It is also important to acknowledge that pathoplastic features may be important in organically induced states, just as they are in functional states. Premorbid personality has been considered to play an important role in the genesis of mental disturbance in the context of arteriosclerotic dementia (Rothschild, 1944), the occurrence of jargon aphasia after brain damage (Weinstein & Lyerly, 1976), as well as in the evolution of psychotic symptoms associated with senile dementia (Post, 1944).

COMPLICATIONS

A variety of complications are associated with Alzheimer's disease and may lead to presentation or dominate the clinical picture.

Mood disorder

Many textbooks emphasize that the early stages of Alzheimer's disease are characterized by depression, which is usually described as an understandable response to the insight into failing cognition. This is certainly the impression one gets from clinical practice, although research has not borne out a causative association (Roth, 1955; Bergmann, 1978; Post, 1978). In the series of Larsson et al (1963), affective disorder in pure form was seen in 10% of patients and in combination with paranoia in a smaller number; Sim & Sussman (1962) found depression in 55% of their 22 patients. It is of course true that both affective disorder and dementia are common in the elderly, and chance coincidence would be expected to occur reasonably frequently.

Aside from those patients who have depressive symptoms, it is common to see patients who have a fluctuating level of anxiety which varies with the extent to which their symptoms are brought to their attention. The patient may become excessively fearful when going to see the doctor, due to the anxiety provoked by failing routine memory tests, and detailed testing may result in catastrophic reaction. It is interesting to observe that the anxiety associated with such conditions is remembered, even though the reason for its occurrence has been forgotten and the answers to the appropriate questions have also been forgotten. Affect-laden memories appear far more resistant and robust than memory of neutral material, no doubt due to the limbic system's intimate involvement with both emotion and memory. It has even been suggested that 'without emotion there is no cognition' (Tucker, 1981). The presence of anxiety seems to be an important factor in those occasions when the patient wanders off and becomes lost.

Dependency

The awareness of some form of impairment in oneself encourages the adoption of the sick role. If the presence of ministering relatives allows it, the patient may display abnormal illness behaviour by becoming excessively dependent on others and professing disability even in the face of activities which are still potentially possible. The advantage of such dependency is three-fold. By refusing to tackle any task, the patient spares him or herself the pain of failing. Similarly, the fear associated with the reduced grasp of the environment is circumvented by limiting the environment to the carer and the carer's provisions. Finally, there is the human need for contact, support and succour, which may be assauged by this ploy (Henderson, 1974).

Paranoid symptoms

In association with memory disorder, patients often display some degree of paranoid misinterpretation. In patients with focal brain damage, paranoid reactions are particularly associated with aphasias characterized by defective comprehension and poor insight (Benson & Geschwind, 1975), an observation which is also relevant to our patients. Paranoid symptoms were apparent in 19% of cases described by Lauter (1968) and were also common in the series of Larsson et al (1963), occurring in 11% of male patients and 23% of female patients in pure form, with a small number of additional cases with mixed affective and paranoid features. Inability to remember where something was placed is often reinterpreted as evidence that possessions have been stolen. With this kind of misinterpretation, the accused often seem to be people known to the patient, such as relatives and neighbours, as opposed to the more remote organizations and forces preferred by paranoid schizophrenics. Lauter (1968) describes the paranoid ideas as less fantastic than in schizophrenia, 'pale' and unsystematized. Because of the emotional power of the paranoid misinterpretation, accusations seem to be remembered better than neutral information.

Confusional states

The failing brain appears, understandably, more sensitive to generalized insults such as toxins, metabolic disorders and infections (Strub, 1982). Thus we find that acute confusional states are relatively common in the course of the disease. The occurrence of such cases no doubt explains the bad prognosis of acute confusional states in the elderly (Roth, 1955), because so many of them are in fact acute on chronic disorders rather than purely acute ones. Appropriate medical intervention in these cases cannot thus return the patient to normal, though it can return patients to their functioning prior to the super-added insult. In the series described by Pearce & Pearce (1979), a confusional state was noted at presentation in 13% of their presenile patients and 48% of their senile patients.

Other physical problems

The increased incidence of falls and of epilepsy renders patients liable to head injury. Apart from the brain damage which may be incurred by the trauma itself, there is also an increased incidence of subdural haematoma. Assessment of chronic progressive failure incurred by a subdural haematoma in addition to the nature of the disease itself is exceedingly difficult, and many cases go undetected. It is not clear to what extent treatment would have improved the symptoms, as some of these blood clots may simply be filling the space vacated by atrophied brain tissue. Other injuries may also occur, including fractures due to falls.

Constipation is often a severe problem and, unless examined for, is overlooked. It is important to consider this as a possible cause of agitation and it may require repeated enemas to alleviate the problem.

In the end stages of the disease, the patient may be incontinent (describe in 85% of end-stage patients in the series of Pearce & Miller, 1973) and patients are usually also immobile due to a combination of rigidity and spasticity. Infections became a serious problem at this stage, with urinary tract infections, chest infections and pressure sores presenting a considerable challenge to the nursing care of the patient.

ONSET AND COURSE

The medical understanding of Alzheimer's disease includes an insidious onset with a progressive course. When describing the onset of the illness, relatives often seem to date it unusually precisely. In this instance they are usually referring to the occasion on which they themselves first became aware of the problem, or sometimes are using a memorable occasion as a sort of milestone (Sim, 1979). More detailed questioning usually reveals symptoms prior to the informant's conception of the 'onset', and the informant has some difficulty in specifying temporal details of these, as one would expect with a gradually evolving process.

The youngest case of Alzheimer's disease known to me is that presented by Malamud & Lowenberg (1929), a man who died at the age of 23. The exact age of onset is unclear from the account presented, but he was normal until the age of 7 and showed a final progressive decline in his last year of life. The age of onset presented by other authors is clearly dependent on the context in which they are working (e.g. neurology or psychiatry), and on their exclusion of presenile or senile cases from their series. The youngest case reported by Lauter (1968) is of a 26-year-old, but the illness is exceedingly rare under the age of 45.

It is important to note that the occurrence of complications, from whatever cause, can impose stepwise shifts on the course of the illness. If we allow for this effect, the course of the illness never shows improvement, and overall there is progressive deterioration. The rate of progression displays some variability both within and between patients. Within the individual patient there may be phases of the illness when the symptoms appear to be static. There are at least four possible reasons for this: firstly, the disease process in the brain may be truly static; secondly, the disease process may be progressive but depend on a threshold effect to become clinically apparent (as in the sudden onset of a Korsakoff's psychosis due to a chronic nutritional deficiency); thirdly, relatives may mistake or deny evidence of progression; fourthly, our assessments may be too insensitive, or have too poor a signal-to-noise ratio, for us to detect a true deterioration. These factors may, of course, co-exist.

The recorded duration of illness varies from less than a year (Larsson et al, 1963) to twenty years (Lauter, 1968). The duration of illness is strongly related to the age group of the patient. Younger age groups have a longer duration of illness, on average lasting six to seven years (Lauter, 1968; Sjögren et al, 1952). Authors who have studied a broad age range of patients have been able to make comparisons between their younger and older patients. Sulkava (1983) reported an average illness duration of 6.1 years in his presenile group and 3.9 years in the senile group, a difference statistically significant at the 1% level. Pearce & Pearce (1979) have found similar differences, their 51–60 year-old-age group having a mean duration of 6.7 years and their group aged 81 and over having a mean duration of 3.6 years. Within the geriatric age range, Constantinidis (1978) had a younger group with mean age of 68 and mean survival of 6.8 years, and an older group with mean age 80 whose mean survival was 1.7 years. Similar findings are presented by Roth (1955) in a slightly different fashion. Of his patients with 'senile psychosis' aged 60–69, 40% were dead at 6 months and 50% at 2 years, whereas in his patients aged 80 and over, 81% were dead at 6 months and 90% at 2 years. The mortality of patients has been compared with the mortality of the same aged population by Larsson et al (1963). The highest excess mortality was in fact observed in the younger patients (aged 74 or less), and with increasing age the excess mortality dwindled. The authors calculated that the onset of dementia shortened the life of their subjects by approximately 4 years on average. Wang (1978) has carried out similar calculations. He produces a similar figure for senile patients, with a reduction of approximately 5 years in life expectancy; the figure for the presenile patients is much greater, being approximately 15 years.

In describing the course of Alzheimer's disease, it has been commonplace to divide it into three stages. This approach is adopted by Sjögren et al (1952), Lauter (1968) and Pearce & Miller (1973). The initial stage is characterized cognitively by the presence of amnesia, and behaviourally by a reduction of spontaneity. During this phase, there may already be some spatial disorientation and possibly some word-finding difficulty, but not a frank aphasia. In this phase, the course may seem to be relatively indolent and benign, and there is some debate as to whether the syndrome of benign senescent forgetfulness is entirely distinct or represents an especially slow form of mild amnesia due to Alzheimer's disease (Kral, 1978).

The second stage is characterized by the evolution of more widespread cognitive impairment. In addition to the already existing amnesia, some 80–85% of patients will show aphasic difficulties, predominantly of the fluent variety. Visuospatial disorganization with secondary apraxia is seen in approximately three-quarters of the patients, and a similar proportion are affected by the physical changes of Parkinsonism, spasticity and general difficulty with locomotion. The frequency of perseveration is estimated to range from 66% (Pearce & Miller, 1973) to 89% (Sjögren et al, 1952).

The third stage represents one of severe cognitive and physical impairment. Incontinence is frequent, and the patient may develop contractures. Primitive reflexes are most likely to be elicited in this final stage. Motor stereotypies have been commented upon by both Lauter (1968) and Sjögren et al (1952). It is in this stage that some components of the Klüver-Bucy syndrome have been recorded (Pearce & Miller, 1973). However, it is clear from a study of this syndrome that the complete clinical picture is incompatible with the severe disability present in the final stages of Alzheimer's disease (Poeck, 1969).

The single commonest cause of death in Alzheimer's disease (other than the condition itself) is pneumonia, which was found in 43% of autopsied patients by Libow (1978) and in 59% of patients by Sulkava (1983). Of the latter series, 27% had pulmonary embolism or deep vein thrombosis, and 14% had no obvious immediate cause of death. The patients of Libow (1978) had a mean weight of 50 kilograms, which is illustrative of the wasting found in this disease. It is interesting to note from the series of Larsson et al (1963) that one patient had succeeded in committing suicide, and the yearly incidence of attempted suicide was 0.8% for males and 0.3% for females.

The clinical features and course depend considerably on the age of the patient. It has already been pointed out that the older patients are likely to have a shorter illness. This is perhaps best regarded as due to factors which are related to the age of the patient rather than the presence of Alzheimer's disease, because the *excess* mortality is actually less in the older patients than in the younger patients. It thus seems most likely that old patients die earlier on in the course of the illness when they are displaying perhaps only a memory deficit or a few mild symptoms, rather than the full-blown picture of the disorder.

These earlier deaths are presumably more often due to coincident diseases and less often due to factors intimately related to Alzheimer's disease. Constantinidis (1978) has demonstrated that younger patients show a more severe cognitive impairment and more widespread and severe histopathological changes at necropsy in association with a longer duration of illness. In his most severe group, all patients had amnesia and 91% had aphasia and/or agnosia/apraxia, whereas his least severe group had amnesia in 84% and other disorders in only 16%. He also noted that the time interval between the onset of the amnesia and the onset of additional features was the same in all groups (between 3 and 4 years). Other authors have also reported that, in the geriatric age group, the combination of amnesia, aphasia and perceptuospatial disorders is associated with a high mortality (McDonald, 1969; Hare, 1978; Naguib & Levy, 1982). Similar observations were made on a mixed-age series by Kaszniak et al (1978), who found that, of 14 measures of cognitive function, 8 were statistically significantly associated with increased mortality at one year. The measures included assessments of memory, perceptuospatial organization and language, but the strongest associations were with linguistic measures. This accords with the observation of Ajuriaguerra et al (1960) that constructional 'apraxia' precedes aphasia in the evolution of senile dementia. The occurrence of the so-called Alzheimerized dementia in the geriatric age group thus appears to be simply due to the fact that the patient has lived long enough to display those changes rather than their being due to differences in the disease process itself.

PRESENTATION

From the foregoing remarks, it is clear that the presentation of the disorder will depend firstly on the type of lifestyle the patient is living, and secondly on the features of the illness. With a more active life the disease will come to notice more readily than in subjects who have a routine pattern of activity or possibly are already supported by carers for another reason. Failing memory is the commonest initial presenting complaint (made by the informant rather than the patient), and occurred in 87% of cases reported by Sulkava (1983) and in all the pathologically confirmed cases of Sim & Sussman (1962). Amnesia will be detected sooner in someone who is working full-time in an exacting post rather than in more sheltered settings. The present cultural expectation appears to be that all old people will show some forgetfulness, and going a bit 'senile' is not sufficient grounds for a medical consultation in old people (Levy & Post, 1982). This expectation appears to be even more marked in some developing countries (Awad-El-Kariem, 1983). Some patients will present with spatial disorientation, often because they are becoming lost in familiar surroundings. Presentation with aphasia is relatively unusual, possibly because it evolves later in the disorder. Often the presentation may be based on a complication, such as paranoia, which occurred in 60% of Sulkava's series. Patients may even present with a coincident illness and be found to suffer from significant cognitive impairment on routine examination or become conspicuous by their abnormal behaviour on admission to hospital.

PRACTICAL PROBLEMS

Problems concerned with the provision of services, support from relatives and ethical difficulties are dealt with elsewhere in this volume, but a brief mention of some relevant difficulties will be made here. In considering testamentary capacity, patients with uncomplicated amnesia with or without spatial disorientation may be able to make a valid will, provided that they are reminded sufficiently of their belongings and the claims due upon their estate. Apart from the mildest anomia, any linguistic impairment is likely to include defective comprehension and thus make significant inroads on the appropriateness of making a will. The occurrence of confusional states or paranoid misinterpretations will obviously render the patient unfit for this purpose. It should be noted that, at a time when the patient can consider the problems involved, his or her signature may be unrecognizable due to spatial disorientation.

An increasingly common problem is the question of fitness to drive. Motor vehicles are dangerous and responsible for much disability and death in our country. Here, we would suggest a cautious attitude. The presence of significant amnesia may well lead to distraction on the part of the driver and, if the driver is being reminded, may lead to sudden, unexpected manoeuvres to correct the mistake. The presence of spatial disorientation means not only that patients are liable to lose their way when navigating the vehicle, but their ability to judge speed and direction is also impaired. These handicaps are obviously incompatible with safe driving, as well as creating hazards for pedestrians. Ethical problems are encountered when patients are reluctant to give up their licences but appear to their medical advisors to be significantly impaired. Each case obviously requires assessment on its own merits, balancing one's duty of confidentiality against one's duty to society (British Medical Association, 1981).

The third common problem which occurs is the question of leaving patients on their own. In the house, patients may follow the relatives around, never leaving them alone, and if left alone the patients may become extremely anxious, so that it takes considerable time for them to calm down when company is restored. Also, if left alone, the patient may 'escape' and wander off, becoming lost and causing anxiety to the carers. There are also practical implications in that provision of an attendance allowance may depend on whether or not it is considered safe for the patient to be left alone. On the other hand, some relatives' jobs may depend upon their ability to attend for some hours, during which time no one is available to attend to the patient. Once more, coping with this problem depends very much upon the individual case. Some patients manage if they are locked in when they are on their own, while others require different solutions.

WHAT DO RELATIVES COMPLAIN OF?

In practical terms, presentation and follow-up are usually instigated by relatives (or other supporters), and much care is also provided by them. Their complaints and the burden which they are prepared to bear are important determinants of service utilization. Many features of Alzheimer's disease are exceedingly wearing, if not frankly exasperating, and these problems must be recognized for effective diagnosis and support.

In the initial stages of the illness the main complaints are usually of affective disorder, which may be the first time that the patient has ever shown any emotional instability. Amnesia leads to endlessly repeated questions and demands for reassurance from the patient. The variability in amnesia due to superior retention of affect-laden material and decreased recall when anxious often gives the impression that some 'forgetting' is motivated; indeed, this sometimes appears to be a significant element in patients' behaviour.

Difficulties in telling the time from a clock or in dressing are usually tolerated fairly well, although the latter may not be understood and regarded as deliberate awkwardness when patients use the wrong armhole of a coat or cannot fasten buckles. Much more important is the fact that patients may continually follow the relatives round the house, and if patients are left on their own they may appear to be disorientated and wander out of the house and become lost. Failure to recognize the face of the carer is exceedingly distressing and undermines the supporter considerably. Defective comprehension is likely to lead to misunderstandings, especially when the patient appears to retain relatively fluent speech and can come out with everyday platitudes without any difficulty. With more severe disturbance, the patients' tendency to live in the past and to deny the birth of children or the fact of marriage causes further distress and bewilderment in relatives.

Paranoid misinterpretations due to amnesia are very destructive, especially as they seem to be directed at the people who provide the most care. The patients' daily rhythm is often disrupted, and patients may retire early and awaken even earlier, thus causing relatives worry and fatigue due to lost sleep. Spatial disorientation means that patients cannot toilet themselves in more advanced stages of the disease and may even fail to recognize what a toilet is, resulting in urination and defecation in inappropriate places. The occurrence of falls and decreased mobility adds further demands to the carers, and epileptic attacks of the partial type may pass undiagnosed but cause additional confusion and agitation.

All these frustrating disabilities can be explained to relatives in simple terms, although the concept of spatial disorientation is difficult to convey and comprehend. It is good medicine to offer appropriate explanations, but not necessarily to insist on their acceptance. Relatives may feel happier refusing to grasp the concept of progressive deterioration, and the choice should be left to them. Some relatives may be so exhausted or emotionally involved that they cannot assimilate appropriate explanations at an initial visit and they may benefit from repeated explanations or written advice. Special attention should be paid to fears that the relatives themselves might inherit the disease or indeed be suffering from it themselves. Some of the issues raised by the patients' illness can only be resolved after the patient has died and the relatives are going through the process of mourning. In many senses the clinical features of Alzheimer's disease represent a family disturbance, and the medical involvement includes some aspects of family therapy.

ALZHEIMER'S DISEASE IN RELATION TO CURRENT CONCEPTS OF DEMENTIA

In retrospect, the later 19th and earlier 20th century appears to have been a time of great activity in neuropsychiatry, in which detailed clinical observations were correlated with pathological findings: for example, Kahlbaum's clinical analysis of catatonia was complemented by post-mortem examinations he himself carried out (Kahlbaum, 1973). Alzheimer's original observation (1907) is very much apart of that tradition, in that he emphasized firstly the distinct clinical picture, secondly the distinct pathological findings, thirdly the fact of this specific clinicopathological congruence, and finally the importance of pursuing this approach in the definition of psychological illnesses.

We now know that the pathological changes described by Alzheimer are not unique to the disorder he described, at least in the senium; similarly, each of the symptoms which we have described may not be unique to this process, and the end stages of dementing illnesses often appear indistinguishable. These appears to be a trend for dementia to be regarded as a unitary phenomenon with global impairment of intellect and personality. Such an approach turns us away from the careful appraisal of symptoms and from making clinicopathological correlations. It is to be hoped that this exposition has shown that Alzheimer's disease does have cross-sectional and longitudinal clinical characteristics which may be of diagnostic and heuristic value, and that the overall picture is not an amorphous one.

ACKNOWLEDGEMENT

Many of these observations were made possible by a grant from the National Fund for Crippling Diseases, allowing me to gain further experience in dementia under the expert tutelage of Dr David Neary. I am also indebted to Dr David Jolley for his generous guidance and encouragement, and to Dr Ruth Dodwell for her patient support.

REFERENCES

Ajuriaguerra J de, Muller M, Tissot R 1960 A propos de quelques problèmes posés par l'apaxie dans les démences. Revue Neurologique 102: 640–642

Ajuriaguerra J de, Strejilevitch M, Tissot R 1963 A propos de quelques conduites devant le miroir de sujets atteints de syndromes démentiels du grand âge. Neuropsychologia 1: 59–73

Ajuriaguerra J de, Cordeiro J D, Steeb U, Fot K, Tissot R, Richard J 1969 A propos de la désintégration des capacités d'anticipation des déments dégénératifs du grand âge. Neuropsychologia 7: 301–311

Albert M L, Goodglass H, Helm N A, Rubens A B, Alexander M P 1981 Clinical aspects of dysphasia. Springer, Vienna

Albert M S 1981 Geriatric neuropsychology. Journal of Consulting and Clinical Psychology 49: 835–850

Allison R S 1966 Perseveration as a sign of diffuse and focal brain damage I & II. British Medical Journal ii: 1027–1032, 1095–1101

Alzheimer A 1907 Über eine eigenartige Erkrankung der Hirnrinde. Allgemeine Zeitschrift für Psychiatrie 64: 146–148

Awad-El-Kariem S M 1983 Attitudes of Sudanese populations to mental illness. In: Brown S (ed) Psychiatry in developing countries. Gaskell, London, p 1–3

Basavaraju N G, Silverstone F A, Libow L S, Paraskevas K 1981 Primitive reflexes and perceptual sensory tests in the elderly — their usefulness in dementia. Journal of Chronic Diseases 34: 367–377

Benson D F, Geschwind N 1975 Psychiatric conditions associated with focal lesions of the central nervous system. In: Reiser M F (ed) American handbook of psychiatry, vol 4. Organic disorders and psychosomatic medicine. Basic Books, New York, ch 9, p 208–243

Benton A L, Hamsher K de S, Varney N R, Spreen O 1983 Contributions to neuropsychological assessment: a clinical manual. Oxford University Press, New York

Bergmann K 1978 Neurosis and personality disorder in old age. In: Isaacs A D, Post F (eds) Studies in geriatric psychiatry. Wiley, Chichester, ch 3, p 41–75

Bleuler M 1951 Psychiatry of cerebral diseases. British Medical Journal ii: 1233–1238

British Medical Association 1981 The handbook of medical ethics. British Medical Association, London, p 12–13

Constantinidis J 1978 Is Alzheimer's disease a major form of senile dementia? Clinical, anatomical, and genetic data. In: Katzman R, Terry R D, Bick K L (eds) Alzheimer's disease: senile dementia and related disorders. Raven Press, New York, p 15–25

Constantinidis J, Richard J, Ajuriaguerra J de 1978 Dementias with senile plaques and neurofibrillary changes. In: Isaacs A D, Post F (eds) Studies in geriatric psychiatry. Wiley, Chichester, ch 6, p 119–152

De Renzi E 1982 Disorders of space exploration and cognition. Wiley, Chichester, pp 57–137

De Renzi E, Faglioni P, Savoiardo M, Vignolo L A 1966 The influence of aphasia and of the hemispheric side of the cerebral lesion on abstract thinking. Cortex 2: 399–420

De Renzi E, Pieczuro A, Vignolo L A 1968 Ideational apraxia: a quantitative study. Neuropsychologia 6: 41–52

Drachman D A, Fleming P, Glossor G, Long R 1981 Multidimensional assessment of dementia: a means of revealing distinctive clinical patterns. Transactions of the American Neurological Association 106: 17–21

Folstein M F, McHugh P R 1978 Dementia syndrome of depression. In: Katzman R, Terry R D, Bick K L (eds) Alzheimer's disease: senile dementia and related disorders. Raven Press, New York, p 87–93

Frank J D 1979 What is psychotherapy? In: Bloch S (ed) An introduction to the psychotherapies. Oxford University Press, Oxford, ch 1, p 1–22

Gelenberg A J 1976 The catatonic syndrome. Lancet i: 1339–1341

Goldstein K 1952 The effect of brain damage on the personality. Psychiatry 15: 245–260

Griesinger W 1865 The prognosis in mental disease. Journal of Mental Science 11: 317–327

Hare M 1978 Clinical check list for diagnosis of dementia. British Medical Journal ii: 266–267

Hécaen J 1981 Apraxias. In: Filskov S B, Boll T J (eds) Handbook of clinical neuropsychology. Wiley, New York, ch 8, p 257–286

Henderson S 1974 Care-eliciting behaviour in man. Journal of Nervous and Mental Disease 159: 172–181

Jung C G 1910 The association method. American Journal of Psychology 21: 219–269

Kahlbaum K L 1973 Catatonia. (Die Katatonie oder das Spannungsirresein, trans Levij V, Pridan T) Johns Hopkins University Press, Baltimore, Maryland, p 59

Kampmeier R H 1977 Diagnosis and treatment of physical disease in the mentally ill. Annals of Internal Medicine 86: 637–645

Kaszniak A W, Fox J, Gandell D L, Garron D C, Huckman M S, Ramsey R G 1978 Predictors of mortality in presenile and senile dementia. Annals of Neurology 3: 246–252

Kral V A 1978 Benign senescent forgetfulness. In: Katzman R, Terry R D, Bick K L (eds) Alzheimer's disease: senile dementia and related disorders. Raven Press, New York, p 47–51

Larsson T, Sjögren T, Jacobson G 1963 Senile dementia: a clinical, sociomedical and genetic study. Acta Psychiatrica Scandinavica 39: suppl 167

Lauter H 1968 Zur Klinik und Psychopathologie der Alzheimerschen Krankheit. Psychiatria Clinica 1: 85–108

Levy R, Post F 1982 The dementias of old age. In: Levy R, Post F (eds) The psychiatry of late life. Blackwell, Oxford, ch 5, p 163–175

Lezak M D 1978 Subtle sequelae of brain damage: perplexity, distractibility and fatigue. American Journal of Physical Medicine 57: 9–15

Libow L S 1978 Epidemiology — excess mortality and proximate causes of death. In: Katzman R, Terry R D, Bick K L (eds) Alzheimer's disease: senile dementia and related disorders. Raven Press, New York, p 315–319

Malamud W, Lowenberg K 1929 Alzheimer's disease: a contribution to its aetiology and classification. Archives of Neurology and Psychiatry 21: 805–827

Marie P 1926 A propos d'un cas d'aphasie de Wernicke considéré par erreur comme un cas de démence sénile. In: Travaux et mémoires, vol 1. Masson, Paris, p 161–164

Marsden C D, Harrison M J G 1972 Outcome of investigation of patients with presenile dementia. British Medical Journal ii: 249–252

Mayer-Gross W 1935 Some observations on apraxia. Proceedings of the Royal Society of Medicine 28: 1203–1212

McDonald C 1969 Clinical heterogeneity in senile dementia. British Journal of Psychiatry 115: 267–271

Naguib M, Levy R 1982 Prediction of outcome in senile dementia — a computed tomography study. British Journal of Psychiatry 140: 263–267

Nott P N, Fleminger J J 1975 Presenile dementia: the difficulties of early diagnosis. Acta Psychiatrica Scandinavica 51: 210–217

Pearce J 1974 The extrapyramidal disorder of Alzheimer's disease. Europe Neurology 12: 94–103

Pearce J, Miller E 1973 Clinical aspects of dementia. Baillière Tindall, London

Pearce J M S, Pearce I 1979 The nosology of Alzheimer's disease. In: Glen A I M, Whalley L J (eds) Alzheimer's disease: early recognition of potentially reversible deficits. Churchill Livingstone, Edinburgh, ch 20, p 93–96

Poeck K 1969 Pathophysiology of emotional disorders associated with brain damage. In: Vinken P J, Bruyn G W in collaboration with Critchley M, Frederiks J A M (eds) Handbook of clinical neurology, vol 3. Disorders of higher nervous activity. Elsevier, Amsterdam, ch 20, p 343–367

Post F 1944 Some problems arising from a study of mental patients over the age of sixty years. Journal of Mental Science 90: 554–565

Post F 1975 Dementia, depression, and pseudodementia. In: Benson D F, Blumer D (eds) Psychiatric aspects of neurologic disease. Grune & Stratton, New York, ch 6, p 99–120

Post F 1978 The functional psychoses. In: Isaacs A D, Post F (eds) Studies in geriatric psychiatry. Wiley, Chichester, ch 4, p 77–94

Post F 1982 Affective disorders in old age. In: Paykel E S (ed) Handbook of affective disorders. Churchill Livingstone, Edinburgh, ch 29, p 393–402

Raven J C 1958 Standard progressive matrices sets A, B, C, D and E. Lewis, London

Rochford G 1971 A study of naming errors in dysphasic and in demented patients. Neuropsychologia 9: 437–443

Ron M A, Toone B K, Garralda M E, Lishman W A 1979 Diagnostic accuracy in presenile dementia. British Journal of Psychiatry 134: 161–168

Roth M 1955 The natural history of mental disorder in old age. Journal of Mental Science 101: 281–310

Rothschild D 1944 The role of the premorbid personality in arteriosclerotic psychoses. American Journal of Psychiatry 100: 501–505

Sim M 1979 Early diagnosis of Alzheimer's disease. In: Glen A I M, Whalley L J (eds) Alzheimer's disease: early recognition of potentially reversible deficits. Churchill Livingstone, Edinburgh, ch 17, p 78–85

Sim M, Sussman I 1962 Alzheimer's disease: its natural history and differential diagnosis. Journal of Nervous and Mental Disease 135: 489–499

Sjöbring H 1973 Personality structure and development: a model and its application. Acta Psychiatrica Scandinavica suppl 244: 159–195

Sjögren T, Sjögren H, Lindgren Å G H 1952 Morbus Alzheimer and morbus Pick: a genetic, clinical and patho-anatomical study. Acta Psychiatrica et Neurologica Scandinavica suppl 82

Smith J S, Kiloh L G, Ratnavale G S, Grant D A 1976 The investigation of dementia: the results in 100 consecutive admissions. Medical Journal of Australia 2: 403–405

Strub R L 1982 Acute confusional state. In: Benson D F, Blumer D (eds) Psychiatric aspects of neurologic disease, volume II. Grune & Stratton, New York, ch 1, p 1–23

Sulkava R 1982 Alzheimer's disease and senile dementia of Alzheimer type: a comparative study. Acta Neurologica Scandinavica 65: 636–650

Sulkava R 1983 Alzheimer's disease: neurological, neuropsychological, neuropathological and genetic studies. Department of Neurology, University of Helsinki, Helsinki

Sulkava R, Amberla K 1982 Alzheimer's disease and senile dementia of Alzheimer type: a neuropsychological study. Acta Neurologica Scandinavica 65: 651–660

Tucker D M 1981 Lateral brain function, emotion and conceptualisation. Psychological Bulletin 89: 19–46

Walsh K W 1978 Neuropsychology: a clinical approach. Churchill Livingstone, Edinburgh

Wang H S 1978 Prognosis of dementia and related disorders in the aged. In: Katzman R, Terry R D, Bick K L (eds) Alzheimer's disease: senile dementia and related disorders. Raven Press, New York, p 309–313

Wechsler D 1955 Manual for the Wechsler adult intelligence scale. Psychological Corporation, New York

Weinstein E A, Lyerly O G 1976 Personality factors in jargon aphasia. Cortex 12: 122–133

Wells E C 1982 Pseudodementia and the recognition of organicity. In: Benson D F, Blumer D (eds) Psychiatric aspects of neurologic disease, volume II. Grune & Stratton, New York, ch 8, p 167–178

Alzheimer's disease: the prognosis

INTRODUCTION

In an age of unprecedented social and demographic change the prognosis of senile dementia of the Alzheimer type (SDAT), formerly referred to simply as senile dementia, has assumed greater importance than ever before. Studies such as those carried out by the Newcastle group (Kay et al 1964, 1970) provide reliable estimates of the prevalence of SDAT and highlight the significance of advanced age in this respect. Kramer (1980) has linked the findings of a Scandinavian study of prevalence with world-wide demographic changes and concluded that we are facing a frightening increase in the prevalence of SDAT in the last quarter of this century in both the more affluent societies and the less developed parts of the world. The so-called 'quiet epidemic'(1978) has profound implications for the future of medical services not only in the fields of geriatric medicine and geriatric psychiatry.

To the contemporary clinician it comes as something of a surprise to learn that our present predicament was anticipated by shrewd observers some 40 years ago. Writing of his experience in Edinburgh in the years 1937–1943, Post (1944) noted the disproportionate number of over-60s in the hospital population and from a study of the hospital records traced the trend back to the turn of the century. Among the many important observations made in this study were comments on the contemporary prognosis of various forms of mental illness in the older age group. His comment that cases of depression were a greater problem than the dementias in terms of extended bed occupancy is a measure of the change that has come over the scene in the intervening years.

Prompted, one suspects, by Post's work, Lewis (1946) produced a remarkable study citing evidence that the upward trend of the elderly in mental hospitals may go back at least to the 1860s. The work anticipates issues of present concern, such as how far mental hospital admission reflects prevalence of illness and the suitability of what we would now refer to as local authority homes for the elderly suffering from mental illness. Most important of all, Lewis pieced together the available evidence and accurately predicted the implications for psychiatric services of the relative and absolute increase in the elderly within society.

Several points of fundamental importance to the study of the prognosis of Alzheimer's disease have been clarified since the 1940s and thus improved our understanding of the issues. The belief that all forms of dementia were based on vascular change has been disproved by Roth & Morrissey (1952) and Roth (1955) who at the same time established a new and more satisfactory nosology of dementia. Subsequently the view that dementia was an accelerated form of ageing has been challenged in reports such as those by Bergmann (1977) and by pathological studies carried out by Bowen et al (1979). Finally, in reviewing the evidence Constantinidis (1978) offered strong support for the view that Alzheimer's disease and senile dementia were one and the same condition occurring in different age groups. Collectively these changes had a profound impact on our understanding of dementia and as a result have opened up to study many aspects of Alzheimer's disease, not least the prognosis.

Methodological problems, however, remain. The global term 'chronic brain syndrome' (CBS) is frequently employed in reports without attempting separation into senile dementia of the Alzheimer type (SDAT) and arteriosclerotic dementia (ASD) or its alternative title 'multi-infarct dementia'. Even the assumption that the ratio between cases of SDAT and ASD is constant in otherwise comparable societies is called into question by the findings of Vitaliano et al (1981) in their New York/Tokyo study. Gurland et al (1983) have raised similar doubts concerning prevalence.

The impact on prognosis of availability of services for the demented has not been clearly established. Smith (1983, 1984) has shown that residential care is available to a substantially higher proportion of the elderly in Denmark and the Netherlands than is the case in the United Kingdom. In theory, at least, the demented of these countries should enjoy better care and therefore a better prognosis, but this has not as yet been clearly demonstrated. To add to such difficulties Mann et al (1984) have recently shown marked differences in the style of caring for demented patients in London and New York. In the latter city greater input of medical and trained nursing resources is reported, as well as much higher use of drugs such as phenothiazines. Here again we await evidence that these differences are reflected in the prognosis.

It is against this background of progress in some areas, coupled with recently recognized problems in others, that the prognosis of Alzheimer's disease is reviewed under four headings largely avoiding that delicate issue — the quality of the patient's life.

SURVIVAL AS AN INDEX OF PROGNOSIS

Clearly the interval between the onset of a condition and death is an attractive measure of prognosis. To a degree the duration of time spent in hospital with a chronic condition leading up to death is even more attractive, since it can be measured with precision. It is, however, influenced by a number of factors such as availability of beds and social attitudes to admission. As a result comparisons must be treated with caution.

Kay's (1962) retrospective study of admissions to the Stockholm Psychiatric Hospital in the period 1931–1937 is perhaps the earliest reliable source of information on survival. The author based his conclusions on a restructuring of the original case record data in terms of the recently established nosology. Having discarded a substantial number of cases on the grounds that the onset of illness preceded the sixtieth birthday, he was left with 41 cases of SDAT and an equal number of ASD out of a total of 232 cases (35% organic).

By taking advantage of the highly efficient Swedish systems of data collection, Kay was able to follow up cases of dementia until death. He found that the mean survival time for the males suffering from dementia was 2.6 years and for females 2.3 years. In this instance he does not discriminate between SDAT and ASD. Fifty per cent of the dementia patients were dead within one year, 72% within three years and 82% within five years. By contrast, only 33% of functional cases died within five years.

Kay worked out the ratio of observed to expected survival time of patients using the elderly population of Stockholm as the reference standard. Overall, males suffering from dementia had a ratio of 0.34 and females 0.25, but sub-groups varied considerably, ratios of 0.5 being recorded for males under 70 with ASD and females over 70 with SDAT. Overall, women with ASD did badly, with a ratio of 0.16.

Camargo & Preston (1945) published an extended study of all admissions to the State Hospitals in Maryland over the age of 65 for the years 1938 to 1940. In all there were 683 patients of whom 85% were awarded a diagnosis of SDAT or ASD. The study notes a high early mortality following admission, 17% in the first month rising to 37% at the end of six months. This pattern of high mortality continued: almost half were dead at the end of the first year and two-thirds were dead at the end of three years. While detailed analysis by age groups is provided, rather less information is available on diagnosis. Nevertheless the authors reported that 66% of the ASD subjects died within three years and 70.7% of the SDAT subjects died within the same timespan. A sub-group of approximately one-third of the cohort were followed for five to six years, and it was found that 77.8% had died, with 11.7% still in hospital. Diagnostic details unfortunately were not provided on the extended follow-up cases.

The report notes a correlation between mortality and age, 53% of the 65–69 age group having died by the end of three years, the figure rising progressively to 82.4% for those over 80 at the time of admission. Since details of the 15% of patients not suffering from dementia were not provided separately, minor inaccuracies may exist in these figures.

In summary the 87 studies covering the period 1931–1943 have a number of points in common. Each is characterized by a high mortality in cases of dementia; secondly, cases of ASD generally had a better prognosis than SDAT, an exception being Kay's finding that in women over 70 SDAT had a better prognosis; thirdly, mortality rises steeply with age, and finally all report a high mortality in cases of dementia in the period immediately following admission.

Roth's (1955) Graylingwell study was of fundamental importance for two reasons. By placing the nosology of mental illness in old age on a sound basis it opened up the field for later workers. Central to Roth's argument was the issue of differing prognosis in the various categories of illness, and by providing data on survival rates at 6 and 24 months after admission to hospital he established reference standards which have been of great value in subsequent investigations.

The first to apply Roth's methodology were Shah et al (1969) when they studied all admissions over 60 to Saxondale Hospital, Nottingham in the years 1955–1960 and compared their results at 6 and 24 months after admission with Roth's Graylingwell figures. They found that survival in cases of dementia had improved and that the evidence for this was greater in cases of arteriosclerotic dementia than senile dementia. However, the upward trend was not statistically significant.

Further work along similar lines followed some years later. Blessèd (1982) studied all admissions over 65 to psychiatric care in Newcastle in the year 1976, and Christie (1982) looked at all admissions over 69 to Crichton Royal between 1974 and 1976. In the latter study patients between 65 and 69 were excluded, as were Graylingwell cases between 60 and 69 in order to achieve comparability. Both the Newcastle and Crichton studies revealed a significant increase in survival of cases of dementia at 6 and 24 months. They differed, however, in the contribution to the change made by the respective SDAT and ASD sub-groups, a finding which may be due to the difference in the lower age limits. Assuming the pattern described by Kay (1962) applies, it is likely that in the Newcastle study the inclusion of men between 65 and 69 weighted results in favour of increased survival of the ASD group

Table 11.1 Mortality rates for cases of dementia admitted to hospital in 1940s, 1960s, 1970s (as percentage)

| | At 6 months | | | At 24 months | | |
	SD	ASD	Combined	SD	ASD	Combined
Graylingwell 1948–9 (lower age limit 60)	59	33	55	82	73	80
Saxendale 1955–60 (lower age limit 60)	42	35	39	71	59	65
Newcastle 1976 (lower age limit 65)	31	36	32	68	68	68
Crichton Royal 1974–6 (lower age limit 70)	15	56	25	50	69	55

as a whole. By contrast the exclusion of women with SDAT under 70 in the Crichton study may have influenced the results in favour of the latter diagnostic group. Table 11.1 sums up the experience over time of the four British studies based on similar methodology.

Viewed retrospectively, the evidence suggests the there has been a steady if unspectacular increase in survival of cases of dementia admitted to British hospitals since World War 2 and that cases of SDAT have contributed substantially to this change.

Five-year follow-up was undertaken in two recent British reports. Whitehead & Hunt (1982) followed up 48 cases of CBS over 60, and Christie & Train (1983) followed up 152 similar cases over 65. Figure 11.1 illustrates their findings and compares them with the earlier work of Kay (1962) and Camargo & Preston (1945).

The results may be treated in pairs, the first from the 1930s and the second from the 1970s. Each pair contains one study based on a lower age limit of 60 and the other 65. The striking difference is that the mortality in the first year of the 1970s studies is substantially lower and that these differences, while diminishing, are still appreciable up to the three-year mark. Results converge at around 80% mortality at five years.

Canadian studies are divided on the issue of change in the prognosis in dementia. Duckworth et al (1979) employed Roth's approach to 100 randomly selected patients admitted to three hospitals in Toronto. Their organic group was small, totalling only 35 cases, of whom 23 suffered from SDAT and 5 from ASD. When compared with Roth's original Graylingwell group, survival rates showed statistically significant improvement at both 6 and 24 months. Kraus & McGeer (1982) compared a group of demented patients in the Kingston area with Goldfarb's (1969) New York group. Once again a statistically significant increase in survival of the Canadian cohort was reported. Inevitably questions of comparability arise. Cases are drawn from a variety of hospitals with possibly different admission and care policies, and at a higher level the legitimacy of comparing practice in Canada with either the United States or England may be called in question.

Thompson & Eastwood (1981) solved the problem of comparability by studying admissions with dementia to the same institution in Toronto over a 10-year period. They concluded that there was no statistically significant difference in survival over the period, although they did note an upward trend. It is possible that, as in the case of the previously quoted study by Shah et al (1969), the study was limited by the short timescale employed.

Studies quoted so far have been hospital-based, and with the exception of the last mentioned may have compared fundamentally dissimilar populations. Neither of these criticisms, however, can apply to the Lundby study from Sweden which has followed up meticulously a discreet population of some 2500 people of all ages over a 25-year period. In a recent progress report Hagnell (1982) has recorded a substantial rise in the prevalence of chronic brain syndromes when he compared the initial ten years

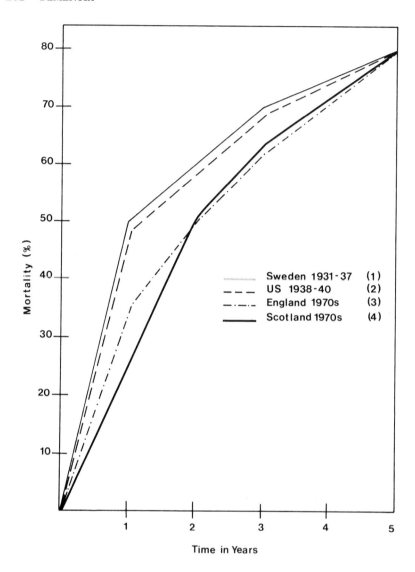

Fig. 11.1 Summary of survival patterns from various centres over time.
Sources
(1) Kay (1962)
(2) Camargo & Preston (1945)
(3) Whitehead & Hunt (1982) (supplementary to personal communication)
(4) Christie & Train (1983)

of his study with the subsequent fifteen. As yet the results for the diagnostic sub-groups, SDAT and ASD, have not been published. It is unlikely, however, that the relationship between these two sub-groups has undergone any radical change within the same community over a comparatively short period of time. The overall pattern of change, therefore, is likely to reflect the experience of the SDAT sub-group.

The author points out that the rising prevalence of chronic brain syndromes is not the product of rising incidence; indeed there is some evidence that this may actually be falling, except in the case of women under 80. Important though these results are, they must be interpreted with some caution, since the total number of cases involved is just over 40.

AGE AT ONSET AS A FACTOR IN PROGNOSIS

A recurring theme in several of the studies quoted is the shorter survival of patients with increasing age. However, there may be reason to doubt the existence of a simple linear relationship. Bondareff (1983) refers to two clinical sub-types of Alzheimer's disease identified as AD1 and AD2. The former is described as beginning in old age, is characterized by an insidious clinical course, fewer motor signs, less parietal lobe involvement and less evidence of the classical pathological features of the condition. AD2, on the other hand, is characterized by onset in middle age, a rampant clinical course and more marked features, both clinical and pathological.

More recently Rossor et al (1984) reported the neurochemical changes found in a series of 49 patients with Alzheimer's disease. They identified more widespread and severe cholinergic deficits in those dying in their 60s and 70s than those dying over 80. In addition, the younger patients showed other changes not evident in the older age group. The authors suggest that Alzheimer's disease in people under 80 may differ in important respects from older patients. As yet there is no substantial evidence that the less severe neurochemical changes in those dying after 80 is reflected in the prognosis. The evidence of both Bondareff and Rossor highlights the need for a large-scale longitudinal study to investigate the relationship between the prognosis on the one hand and age, clinical features and laboratory findings on the other.

TREATMENT AND PROGNOSIS

As in all chronic conditions lacking specific therapy, treatment is a complex and sometimes delicate issue. The evidence suggests that modern hospital treatment prolongs the patient's life without daring to evaluate the quality of those additional months or years.

Exactly how this improved survival has come about is not clear. Larsson et at (1963) suggested that improved survival was a by-product of developing medical services, with particular reference to the part played by antibiotics in controlling infection. Hagnell (1982) attributed the rising prevalence of dementia to similar factors.

Goldfarb (1967) studied cases of dementia in a variety of settings in New York. He emphasized their physical condition or viability as the most important factor determining survival. It is interesting also to note that he took the view that care in more elaborate settings did little or nothing to modify the prognosis of the severely impaired patient. Jarvik et al (1980), in an extended study of surviving twins, came to the conclusion that the above-average mortality of patients suffering from chronic brain syndrome was the product of the severity of the primary condition and was independent of coexisting physical illness.

Peck et al (1978) pursued the relationship between physical status and prognosis in a group of dementing patients, mostly women, admitted to the Jewish Home and Hospital for the Aged in New York. He concluded that the physical condition of the patient rather than the degree of dementia was the important factor in determining survival. Vitaliano et al (1981) in a subsequent report disputed that physical status was the dominant factor in determining survival. The authors put forward the interesting suggestion that survival time was reduced as the result of pathological processes underlying dementia, and in this respect cited the possibility of impairment of the immunological response as a major contribution.

CAUSE OF DEATH

Central to any discussion of prognosis in Alzheimer's disease is the question of the certified cause of death. Katzman (1976) has pointed out the paradox that, while between 60 000 and 90 000 people in the United States die with dementing illnesses annually, the condition is rarely, if ever, listed as the cause of death, a remarkable finding since, if so recorded, dementia would rank fifth among the major causes of death in that country. Gruenberg (1977) in his evocative title *Failures of success* makes the point that chronic conditions (among which he cites senile dementia) rarely, in themselves, prove fatal. Indeed, the whole essence of his argument is that by dealing with secondary problems such as infections we justify his title.

Identifying the cause of death has for long been one of the least satisfactory aspects of dementia. Kay (1962) noted that in the 1930s in Sweden non-specific causes of death predominated among the dementing population, which was in marked contrast with the general population of Stockholm of similar age.

The whole issue of the mechanism of death and the problem of awarding a specific cause adequate to explain the arrest of vital functions may be eased by a recent study by Kohn (1982), who reported on the autopsy findings of 200 patients over the age of 85 who died in hospital in Cleveland between 1967 and 1980. The study, which was not directed specifically towards the problems of cause of death in Alzheimer's disease, showed that overall some 30% of cases could not be given a cause of death, which would have been broadly acceptable in a younger age-group. The author concluded that against the background of progressive physiological decline with ageing, minor insults to the tissues exerted a disproportionate effect on those singularly vulnerable individuals and thus precipitated death in the absence of autopsy evidence of traditional causes. Kohn's suggestion may well apply with particular force to the demented if to the effects of age are added the systemic changes in dementia, as Goldfarb (1967) suggests. Together they may furnish a more satisfactory explanation of death than the doubtful causes often recorded.

PROGNOSIS COMPARED

Comparisons between SDAT and other forms of mental illness in the elderly fall naturally into two headings — the comparatively simple and measurable one of survival and the more debatable quality of life. The position regarding the former and to some degree the latter is admirably dealt with by Blessed & Wilson (1982) when, at 6 and 24 months, they compare the results for cases of senile dementia with affective illness, paraphrenia, acute confusion and arteriosclerotic dementia under the three basic headings of discharged, inpatient or dead. At neither point in time do the results reflect favourably on the senile dementia group, and in the case of the functional illnesses the results show a high degree of statistical significance at both points in time. When comparison is made with arterio-sclerotic dementia, there is little to choose in terms of outcome, although results marginally favour the ASD cases.

Such hospital-based findings, however, may prejudice the picture against the victims of SDAT. Reisberg et al (1982) outline a seven-stage pattern of deterioration of primary degenerative dementia based on a large number of cases. Their description of stages 1–4 and possibly stage 5 is compatible with reasonable quality of life and suggests very strongly that hospital experience does greatly distort the overall picture. The Newcastle studies of the early 1960s and the work of Williamson et al (1964) in Edinburgh indicate that the vast majority of patients live out their lives without hospital and perhaps even without family doctor involvement.

Since depression has been more extensively studied, more is known in comparative terms about the quality of life. Other studies bear out the findings of Blessed & Wilson with regard to hospital results. Post (1972) expressed the general disappointment with the results of treatment in the antidepressant era, and more recently Murphy (1983) showed that there is a high residual morbidity among the elderly treated for depression: indeed in a subsequent study Murphy & Grundy (1984) reported a disturbing upward trend in the demand for beds for older patients with depression and likened it to the trend already recorded in dementia. Nonetheless, the good results reported in approximately one-third of the elderly treated for depression place it way ahead of SDAT in prognosis.

The most invidious comparison is against paraphrenia, where the much improved results reported by Post (1966) are again in evidence in the more recent Newcastle and Crichton Royal studies.

CONCLUSIONS

We have learnt a lot about the prognosis of Alzheimer's disease, but this has served to show how little we actually know about the problem. Study of the subject is beset by difficulties, but a few points can be made with confidence. Patients are living longer. The change in the hospitalized group centres on the marked improvement in survival in the first year after admission. At five years this effect has been eliminated. Older patients survive for shorter periods, but this fact may conceal the important point that SDAT has relatively less impact on the life expectancy of the older subject.

Rossor's report of less severe damage in the very elderly with SDAT encourages speculation that for them effective treatment may come sooner than for their younger fellows. Success here would carry enormous benefits, not only to patients and their families, but also to the providers of care by reducing demand without radically altering life expectancy. If this came to pass, Gruenberg's (1977) cogent argument about the 'failures of success' would be reversed.

REFERENCES

Bergmann K 1977 Prognosis in chronic brain failure. Age and Ageing 6: suppl 61–66
Blessed G, Wilson I D 1982 The contemporary natural history of mental disorder in old age. British Journal of Psychiatry 141: 59–67
Bondareff W 1983 Age and Alzheimer's disease. Lancet 1: 1447
Bowen D M et al 1979 Accelerated ageing or selective neuronal loss as an important cause of dementia? Lancet 1: pp 11–14
Camargo O, Preston G H 1945 What happens to patients who are hospitalised for the first time when over sixty five years of age? American Journal of Psychiatry 102: PP 168–173
Christie A B 1982 Changing patterns in mental illness in the elderly. British Journal of Psychiatry 140: 154–159
Christie A B, Train J D 1983 S H A P E dementia and clinical experience. Health Bulletin 41: 283–291
Constantinidis J 1978 Is Alzheimer's disease a major form of senile dementia? Clinical, anatomical and genetic data. In: Katzman R, Terry R D, Bick K L Alzheimer's disease: senile dementia and related disorders (Aging Vol 7). Raven Press, New York
Dementia — the quiet epidemic, leader, British Medical Journal 1978 1: 1–2
Duckworth G S, Kedward H B, Bailey W F 1979 Prognosis in mental illness in old age. Canadian Journal of Psychiatry 24: 674–82
Goldfarb A I 1969 Predicting mortality in the institutionalized aged. Archives of General Psychiatry 21: 172–176
Gurland B et al 1983 The mind and mood of ageing. Croom Helm, London
Gruenberg E M 1977 The failures of success. Millbank Memorial Fund Quarterly, Health Society 55: 3–24

Hagnell O, Lanke J, Rorsman B 1981 Increasing prevalence and decreasing incidence of age psychosis. A longitudinal epidemiological investigation of a Swedish population. The Lundby Study Nordic Geronto-psychiatric Symposium. Nordisk Gerontologisk Tidsskrift, Norsam-Nyt, P 34–41

Jarvik L F, Ruth V, Mutsyama S S 1980 Organic brain syndrome and ageing. Archives of General Psychiatry 37: 280–286

Katzman R 1976 The prevalence and malignancy of Alzheimer's disease. Archives of Neurology 33: 217–218

Kay D W K 1962 Outcome and cause of death in mental disorders of old age. A long term follow-up of functional and organic psychoses. Acta Psychiatrica Scandinavica 38: 249–76

Kay D W K, Beamish K, Roth M 1964 Old age mental disorders in Newcastle upon Tyne, Part I. A study of prevalence. British Journal of Psychiatry 110: 146–158

Kay D W K, Bergmann K, Foster E M, McKechnie A A, Roth M 1970 Mental illness and hospital usage in the elderly. A random sample followed up. Comprehensive Psychiatry 11: 1, 26–35

Kohn R R 1982 Cause of death in very old people. Journal of the American Medical Association 247: 2793–2797

Kramer M 1980 The rising pandemic of mental disorders and associated chronic disease and disabilities. Epidemiological research as basis for the organisation of extramoral psychiatry. Acta Psychiatrica Scandinavica Suppl 285: 328–396

Kraus A S, McGeer C P 1982 The effect of dementia on mortality in the elderly institutionalized population. Canadian Journal on Aging 1: 40–47

Larsson T, Sjogren T, Jacobsen G 1963 Senile dementia. Acta Psychiatrica Scandinavica Suppl 167: 1–259

Lewis A J 1946 Ageing and senility: a major problem of psychiatry. Journal of Mental Science 92: 150–170

Mann A H, Jenkins R, Cross P S, Gurland B J 1984 A comparison of the prescriptions received by the elderly in long term care in New York and London. Psychological Medicine 14: 891–897

Murphy E 1983 the prognosis of depression in old age. British Journal of Psychiatry 142: 111–119

Murphy E, Grundy E 1984 A comparative study of bed usage by younger and older patients with depression. Psychological Medicine 14: 445–450

Peck A, Wolloch L, Rodstein M 1978 Mortality of the aged with chronic brain syndrome. In: Katzman R, Terry R D, Bick K L (eds) Alzheimer's disease: senile dementia and related disorders. Raven Press, New York

Post F 1944 Some problems arising from a study of mental patients over the age of 60 years. Journal of Mental Science 90: 554–565

Post F 1966 Persistent persecutory states of the elderly. Pergamon Press, London

Post F 1972 The management and nature of depressive illnesses in late life. A follow through study. British Journal of Psychiatry 121: 393–404

Reisberg B, Ferris S H, De Leon M J, Crook T 1982 The global deterioration scale for assessment of primary degenerative dementia. American Journal of Psychiatry 139:9: 1136

Rossor M N, Iversen L L, Reynolds G P, Mountjoy C Q, Roth M 1984 Neurochemical characteristics of early and late onset types of Alzheimer's disease. British Medical Journal 288: 961–964

Roth M 1955 The natural history of mental disorder in old age. Journal of Mental Science 101: 281–301

Roth M, Morrissey F D 1952 Problems in the diagnosis and classification of mental disorders in old age. Journal of Mental Science 98: 66–80

Shah K V, Banks G D, Merskey H 1969 Survival in atherosclerotic and senile dementia. British Journal of Psychiatry 115: 1283–6

Smith T 1983 Denmark — The elderly living in style. British Medical Journal 287: 1053–1055

Smith T 1983 Care of the elderly in the Netherlands. British Medical Journal i: 127–129

Thompson E G, Eastwood M R 1981 Survivorship and senile dementia. Age and Ageing 10: 29–32

Vitaliano P P, Peck A, Johnson D A, Prinz P N, Eisdorfer C 1981 Dementia and other competing risks for mortality in the institutionalized aged. Journal of the American Geriatrics Society 29(11): 513–519

Whitehead A, Hunt A 1982 Elderly psychiatric patients: a five year prospective study. Psychological Medicine 12: 149–157

Williamson J, Stokoe I H, Gray S, Fisher M, Smith A, McGhee A, Stephenson E 1964 The unreported needs of the elderly. Lancet 1: 1117–23

Multi-infarct dementia

INTRODUCTION

The blanket term 'cerebral atherosclerosis' has rightly fallen into disrepute as an adequate explanation for mental deterioration in the elderly. The extent of senile changes in the demented brain bears no constant relationship to the extent of atherosclerosis. Even in subjects in whom a vascular aetiology can be evoked, the process usually results from multiple small and large infarcts and not from a global reduction in flow secondary to occlusive arterial disease (Hachinski et al, 1974). Although the general emphasis in dementia has shifted from the blood vessels to the primary neurological degenerations, the importance of recognizing multi-infarct dementia lies in the fact that, in this group, the dementing process may be halted or prevented by effective treatment.

DEFINITION OF DEMENTIA

Single cortical infarcts may interfere with individual aspects of higher function but the aphasic patient, for example, is not usually considered demented. The American Psychiatric Association Diagnostic and Statistical Manual (1980) uses the term 'primary degenerative dementia' to cover organic mental deterioration without obvious aetiology and the definition thereby excludes patients in whom intellectual deterioration occurs in the context of an identifiable cause. In practice, most patients with Alzheimer's disease will fall into this category but so too will various 'secondary' dementias unless they are thoroughly evaluated. It may be more appropriate to consider dementia as a symptom complex and not as a disease per se. Cummings et al (1980) offered a useful operational definition. 'Dementia can be defined as an acquired persistent impairment of intellectual function with compromise in at least three of the following spheres of mental activity: language, memory, visuospatial skills, emotion or personality, and cognition (abstraction, calculation, judgment etc.).'. It therefore remains a clinical description without any supposition as to underlying aetiology. The definition is sensitive to the fact that few, if any, of the dementias are truly global: most present with certain aspects of higher function more affected than others. Excluded from the definition, however, is the type of focal deficit, such as amnesia or aphasia, which may reflect an isolated focal hemispheric lesion. The clinician is thus encouraged to give a detailed neurological description and, although the general category of dementia may be appropriate, differences in temporal, neurological and psychological profiles allow further subdivision.

DEMENTIA AND VASCULAR DISEASE

Dementia, when it occurs in the context of vascular disease, usually does so as a result of multiple small and large vessel occlusions giving rise to infarctions in focal areas (Fisher, 1968). Accordingly, the term multi-infarct dementia (MID) has been coined by Hachinski et al (1974). The lesions are commonly bilateral; single unilateral infarctions normally produce relatively well defined focal symptoms. Occasionally, however, a single lesion may give rise to a syndrome which fulfils many of the criteria of dementia; thus disorientation, dysphasia and memory disturbance have been reported after unilateral thalamic infarction (Castaigne et al, 1981; Graff-Radford et al, 1984) and a syndrome simulating Alzheimer's disease has been described in lesions of the angular gyrus (Benson et al, 1982). This syndrome refers to a symptom complex resulting from a lesion in the posterior portion of the middle cerebral artery territory and may comprise fluent dyshpasia, dyslexia, dysgraphia, acalculia, right/left disorientation, finger agnosia and constructional dyspraxia. Focal motor and sensory symptoms may be absent and the lesion may be too small to be visualized by computerized tomography (CT) of the brain. There may be a complaint of memory disturbance, typically restricted to word-finding difficulties. Insight usually remains. The history of acute onset differentiates this stroke syndrome from Alzheimer's disease, but what is important is that a discrete cerebral lesion can give rise to a syndrome which mimics a generalized dementia.

The neuropathological data provided by Tomlinson et al (1970) demonstrated that large cerebral infarcts (greater than 100 ml) are invariably associated with dementia, whereas when the volume of infarction is smaller, the location becomes more critical. Their criteria for dementia were extremely stringent, and so patients with the less florid intellectual impairment characteristic of multiple small infarcts may have missed inclusion.

The concept of multi-infarct dementia has proved useful in clinical practice and consistent with most of the studies using CT, cerebral blood flow and more recently positron emission tomography. The lesions may be cortical or subcortical, large or small and in any combination. Cummings & Benson (1984) have emphasized the differences in neuropychological profile which distinguish a primarily cortical from a subcortical dementia. Cortical dementias are characterized by dysphasia, amnesia, dyspraxia, agnosia and other focal deficits of higher function, whereas the subcortical dementias present with dysarthria, forgetfulness, slowness at abstract thinking and, usually, abnormalities of gait. A 'typical' cortical picture is seen in early Alzheimer's disease, whereas the neuropsychological profile of the lacunar state is more subcortical in type. The term multi-infarct dementia (MID) is used to encompass the lacunar state as well as the more usual situation in which intellectual decline occurs in the context of both deep and cortical infarcts. Most cases present with a combination of cortical and subcortical signs, a feature emphasized in the ischaemic score (Hachinski et al, 1975).

LACUNAR STATE

Lacunar infarcts are small deep-seated regions of ischaemic damage which leave behind cavities 2–15 mm in size. Typically they occur in patients with prolonged hypertension and result either from atherosclerosis or from a particular focal degeneration of small vessels termed lipohyalinolysis. Sites commonly involved are the thalamus, internal capsule, striatum and pons. Lacunar infarcts produce small strokes in elderly hypertensive subjects, many conforming to Fisher's original four types (pure motor, pure sensory, ataxic hemiparesis and dysarthria clumsy hand) (Fisher, 1967). As lacunes accrue, mental deterioration can occur, and the lacunar state is character-ized by a subcortical dementia (dysarthria, forgetfulness, intellectual slow-ness) as well as bilateral corticospinal and corticobulbar signs. Fisher (1968) felt that the impact of lacunes was much more on motor and sensory systems than on higher cortical function and he emphasized this by describing a patient who, though mentally alert, turned out to have 44 lacunes at necropsy.

Mental deterioration, when it occurs, generally lags behind the physical changes and it is unusual to see an Alzheimer-like clinical syndrome where intellectual deficit develops insidiously in the absence of focal motor signs. The condition of bilateral paramedian thalamic lacunar infarction (Castaigne et al, 1966; Guberman & Stuss, 1983), proves somewhat of an exception in that two small lacunes, placed strategically within the thalami, can produce a syndrome of subcortical dementia without motor signs, although this is extremely rare.

BINSWANGER'S DISEASE

Although much less frequent than the discrete small and large infarcts already described, Binswanger's subcortical arteriosclerotic encephalopathy is almost certainly a distinct syndrome in which subcortical dementia and prominent bilateral pyramidal tract signs are the predominant clinical features (Caplan & Shoene, 1978). The pathological hallmark of this condition is demyelinization secondary to advanced arteriosclerotic changes in the long penetrating vessels supplying the white matter (Burger et al,

1976; De Rueck et al, 1980). Lacunar infarcts involving the basal ganglia and thalamus usually coexist, and the clinical evolution resembles the lacunar state with repeated 'small strokes' leading to an accumulating deficit. Subjects usually have severe and persistent hypertension. The CT scan characteristically reveals enlarged ventricles and discrete infarcts involving the deep white matter (Rosenburg et al, 1979).

CEREBRAL AMYLOID ANGIOPATHY

Cerebral amyloid angiopathy, or congophilic angiopathy, is a well-recognized pathological condition characterized by amyloid deposition in small cortical and meningeal vessels (Mandybur et al, 1978). It has been described in elderly non-demented patients and is frequently, though not invariably, associated with Alzheimer-type changes. Patients usually present with intra-cerebral haemorrhage, which may be recurrent, and about a quarter will be demented (Gilbert & Vinters, 1983; Gilles et al, 1984). Not all patients with Alzheimer's disease have cerebral amyloid angiopathy, and in those that do, the distribution of severe Alzheimer cellular changes does not correlate with areas of prominent cerebral amyloid angiopathy (Vinters & Gilbert, 1983). Although the final diagnosis of cerebral amyloid angiopathy remains histological, it should be considered in any elderly normotensive patient presenting with a spontaneous intracerebral haemorrhage in an atypical site. Multiple small cortical infarcts are also a histological feature of this condition (Okazaki et al, 1979). If the patient is dementing, then the intellectual decline is probably due to Alzheimer's disease, but multiple discrete haemorrhages or infarcts can accelerate the process.

PREVALENCE OF MULTI-INFARCT DEMENTIA

Cummings & Benson (1983) have tabulated the findings of several large studies on the prevalence of the different types of dementia. They stress that since most are hospital-based, sample bias favours dramatically progressive disorders like MID and overestimates their prevalence. Seven surveys from the basis of their tabulation account for a total of 708 evaluations. Overall, MID was the final diagnosis in 13% of cases (ranging from as few as 8% in one series to as many as 34% in another.) Indeed, MID was second only to Alzheimer's disease as the major cause of dementia. Differences in prevalence are probably related to distinctive referral patterns and variations in diagnostic methods. In addition, the initial clinical diagnosis is not always accurate; indeed, in one prolonged follow-up study, Ron et al (1979) found that the initial diagnosis was erroneous in about 20% of cases of organic dementia when viewed in the context of subsequent clinical events (Ron et al, 1979). There may be a systematic tendency to overdiagnose MID, because stroke and dementia often coexist in the elderly, and patients with primary degenerative dementia may be misdiagnosed as MID because of this chance coincidence (Brust, 1983).

Series based on neuropathological classification may be even more biased, although the final diagnosis will be more precise. Tomlinson et al (1970) studied 50 demented brains using quantitative morphology to delineate Alzheimer's disease and attributed the dementia to a vascular aetiology in nine cases and a mixed vascular and Alzheimer's disease changes in a further nine cases. Incidentally, they confirmed Arab's (1954) original observation that there is no correlation between the distribution and density of arteriosclerotic plaques in the vessels and the distribution and density of senile Alzheimer-type plaques in the brain. In general, autopsy data suggest that, in the demented elderly, about 50% suffer from senile dementia of the Alzheimer type (SDAT), 20% have MID and about 20% have a combination of both conditions (Tomlinson et al, 1970; Jellinger, 1976). However, for the reasons already discussed, the figure of 20% diagnosed as MID almost certainly exaggerates the significance of this condition as a cause of intellectual impairment in the elderly. A further point that emerges from both the clinical and pathological data is that, whereas SDAT may be commoner in women, MID and mixed disorders prevail among men (Tomlinson et al, 1970.)

DIAGNOSIS

In most patients with MID, diagnosis is relatively simple because of the history of recurrent strokes and the presence of unequivocal focal neurological signs. Difficulties arise, however, when progressive intellectual failure is punctuated by one or more strokes of only mild severity. Hachinski et al (1975) developed an ischaemic score (Table 12.1) by attributing a numerical value to some of the clinical features of vascular dementia described by Slater and Roth in Mayer Gross et al (1969). The purpose of the score is to differentiate those patients in whom dementia is caused by multiple infarction from those with primary degenerative dementia.

Table 12.1   Ischaemic score. From Hachinski et al (1975). Reproduced by permission

Abrupt onset	2
Stepwise deterioration	1
Fluctuating course	2
Nocturnal confusion	1
Relative preservation of personality	1
Depression	1
Somatic complaints	1
Emotional incontinence	1
History of hypertension	1
History of strokes	2
Evidence of associated atherosclerosis	1
Focal neurological symptoms	2
Focal neurological signs	2

Abrupt onset refers to the onset of intellectual decline, and it is important not to confuse abrupt onset with sudden recognition. Patients may cope quite adequately despite considerable intellectual decline, provided they keep within familiar and stable surroundings. Intercurrent illness, necessitating hospital admission, or the death of a spouse, can then precipitate a crisis, falsely suggesting an acute onset. *Stepwise deterioration* refers to a decline in intellectual function characterized by relatively long plateaux of stable cognition interrupted by episodes of rapid deterioration. Each step represents the steep intellectual decline that follows a cerebral infarct too small or atypical to cause an obvious stroke. A *fluctuating course* implies a more 'sawtooth' temporal profile with improvement from one cerebral infarct followed by deterioration caused by the next.

Nocturnal confusion appears on the score, since relative daytime lucidity with intermittent episodes of nocturnal wandering are considered more characteristic of vascular dementia than SDAT (Roth, 1981). It is important to mention relative daytime lucidity because nocturnal exacerbations are a feature common to all types of dementia. Insight and emotional responsiveness tend to be preserved for longer in patients with MID than SDAT, and hence the inclusion of *relative preservation* of personality on the score. Perhaps as a consequence, *depressive symptomatology* is more frequently encountered in MID than SDAT. *Somatic complaints* refer to vague and usually inexplicable symptoms such as dizziness, unsteadiness or headache of which patients with MID often complain. Sometimes these undoubtedly reflect an underlying affective disorder; on other occasions an organic basis is suspected but not proven. Whatever their aetiology, this should be scored whenever non-specific symptoms without obvious physical counterparts are prominent.

Emotional incontinence refers to the rapid, inappropriate and inconsequential mood changes often displayed by patients with bilateral corticobulbar lesions. It can be prominent in the lacunar state and, by contrast, a most unusual sign in SDAT.

A history of *hypertension* and/or its confirmation on examination favour a diagnosis of MID, since hypertension is a major risk factor for all types of stroke, especially for recurrent lacunar infarction, a condition rarely seen in the absence of hypertension. The incidence of stroke is higher in patients with a history of associated *atherosclerosis* (ischaemic heart disease, claudication), and even when the history is negative, the finding of a carotid bruit or absent foot pulses would lend support to a vascular aetiology. A *history of strokes* certainly suggests MID but in itself is insufficient to make the diagnosis, since patients with Alzheimer's disease may also suffer from stroke.

Focal neurological symptoms include visual disturbances, brain stem abnormalities (such as dysarthria, dysphagia and ataxia) and episodes of sensory disturbance or weakness in the limbs. Symptoms may be transient, suggesting a TIA, or they may suddenly develop and persist as in completed stroke. Dysphasia, dyscalculia, dyspraxia, agnosia and other symptoms which may be due to focal cortical lesions are excluded simply because they have little discriminant value, since they are common to both SDAT and MID. These considerations also apply to the question of what constitutes a *focal neurological sign*, and again the score achieves greater discriminant function if we exclude signs attributable to cortical lesions. The exception is a homonymous hemianopia, which may be due to an occipital cortical lesion, since this is rarely, if ever, seen in Alzheimer's disease. Accordingly any visual-field defect of central origin is included as a focal sign.

Primitive reflexes are common to both groups and are therefore excluded unless they are clearly asymmetrical. Signs of brain-stem dysfunction (cranial nerve palsy, pseudobulbar palsy) are scored as focal signs. In the limbs, any evidence of a pyramidal tract disturbance is taken as a focal sign, even if it is restricted to an extensor plantar response, since long tract signs are extremely uncommon in Alzheimer's disease (Koller et al, 1984). Some discretion on behalf of the observer as to what constitutes a focal sign is, of course, warranted. If the patient happens to have distal wasting, reflex loss and hypotonia, then this would be interpreted as evidence of coincidental peripheral nerve damage rather than a focal sign likely to help in the differentiation of MID from SDAT! When the sensory examination is considered, we use the term focal neurological sign to refer to any loss of sensation of central but non-cortical nature. Thus we would accept a hemisensory loss to pain and temperature perception, but not astereognosis or graphasthesia.

The various components making up the score are a distillation of the salient clinical features of MID. The numerical value attached to each feature is intended to reflect personal and reported experience. When the score is applied to a demented population, the group fractionates into two, with most subjects scoring less than four and a second group with ratings greater than seven (Hachinski et al, 1975; Harrison et al, 1979). It is in this latter group that further evidence of multiple infarctions can be obtained by EEG, CT scan and PET scan (Harrison et al, 1979; Loeb et al, 1983; Ladurner et al, 1982; Frackowiak et al, 1981). The score does not offer a linear scale of severity, and so a total of, say, the maximum of 18 does not necessarily imply that the dementia is any more severe or the diagnosis of MID any more certain than when the score is 8. This becomes clear when the various components are considered individually. Thus, retention of personality, emotional responsiveness, depression, nocturnal confusion and somatic complaints are all features which may even disappear as the disease progresses.

Rosen et al (1979) have confirmed the discriminant function of the scoring system in an autopsy study of 14 elderly demented subjects. Scores ranging from 2 to 5 were obtained from patients with SDAT, whereas subjects with MID and a combination of MID and SDAT had scores in the range of 7 to 14. They found that fluctuating course, nocturnal confusion and associated atherosclerosis did not help differentiate the two groups, and hence these were eliminated from their revised score. So, too, was 'relative preservation of personality', since data on previous personality was not available to the investigators. A similar study involving greater numbers would facilitate further refinement, since each parameter could be assessed independently and then weighted by discriminant function analysis.

Loeb & Gandolfo (1983) found that four features (abrupt onset, history of stroke, focal symptoms and focal signs) offered the best differentiation between SDAT and MID or MID plus SDAT in 94 subjects. However, their study did not include pathological data, and the final diagnosis was made on the basis of the CT appearance. Their observations, therefore, do no more than demonstrate that the four features of the modified score are associated with focal lesions on the CT. We do not know if the patients had SDAT, since there is no histological data. The subsequent suggestion that the score can be further improved by including scores for isolated and multiple ischaemic lesions on the CT completes the tautology.

Portera-Sanchez et al (1982) retrospectively analysed the discriminant value of 14 variables in differentiating MID from SDAT in 84 elderly patients with unexplained dementia. Again, there were no pathological data, but what emerged was that the group as a whole fractionated into two distinct subgroups (one presumed SDAT, the other MID and MID plus SDAT) on clinical grounds. Seven factors (hypertension, abrupt onset, previous history of stroke, focal motor disturbances, pyramidal signs, focal CT atrophy and focal EEG slowing) were of particular value, and when weighted by discriminant function analysis, by far the most important single entity was previous history of stroke.

The use of the ischaemic score in research has theoretical limitations, because it may not differentiate the purely vascular dementias from those in which multiple infarctions and SDAT coexist. Although widely used in this context, it requires further refinement and validation. Clinically the score is valuable, since it alerts the physician to the possibility that repeated strokes may be either causing or compounding the dementing process.

EVALUATION OF THE PATIENT WITH MID

A detailed history should be obtained from the patient and close relatives. Factors listed in the ischaemic score can be used to direct questions about the temporal evolution of the intellectual decline. Particular attention should be paid to previous strokes and/or episodes of transient ischaemia, because even if the final score suggests Alzheimer's disease, coincidental vascular disease may accelerate the dementing process. The family history may be important, not only because some 5% of Alzheimer's disease patients will have a close relative similarly afflicted (Cook et al, 1979), but also because several families have been reported in which MID has been inherited as a Mendelian dominant trait (Sourander & Walinder, 1977;

Sonninen et al, 1984). In these families, the disease appears in mid-adult life with recurrent strokes and progressive intellectual decline secondary to small vessel disease affecting the central grey and white matter.

The main consequence of dementia is an impaired ability to cope with the tasks of daily living, and it may be helpful to quantify this by applying a scale based on enquiry from the patient and relatives, listing such items as the ability to dress, perform household tasks, deal with small sums of money, etc. A convenient scale has been described by Blessed et al (1968) which also includes certain aspects of change in personality, interests and drive.

The general physical examination should be comprehensive, indeed especially so, since it is often not repeated once the diagnosis of dementia has been made. In the context of MID, particular attention should be paid to the cardiovascular system. Atrial fibrillation is now recognized as an independent risk factor for stroke (Wolf et al, 1983) and the pulse should be noted. Absent foot pulses, lower limb ischaemic changes and femoral bruits would suggest generalized atherosclerosis, a feature which appears on the ischaemic score. A carotid bruit would be important in this context and might have a direct bearing on the ischaemic process itself, since carotid artery disease is probably responsible for about half of cerebral infarctions. The blood pressure should be measured in both arms and the estimation repeated later on in the examination if it is abnormal.

Emboli arising from the heart are increasingly implicated in the pathogenesis of stroke, and careful auscultation may reveal hitherto undiagnosed abnormalities such as the systolic click and regurgitant murmur of a floppy mitral valve.

The neurological evaluation begins with an assessment of the patient's mental status. A depressed level of consciousness is not a feature of either Alzheimer's disease or MID, so its presence favours other diagnoses such as a toxic or metabolic encephalopathy. The patient's affect is noted and may prove diagnostically helpful. Lability of affect may be particularly prominent in patients with pseudobulbar palsy, a feature seen in MID. A depressive state, as adjudged by flatness of affect and the response to direct questions regarding mood, may occur in all types of dementia and is frequently present in MID. A common error is to misinterpret psychomotor retardation for depression, but the distinction needs to be made in patients with extrapyramidal and bilateral corticospinal dysfunction syndromes, since mood can not be inferred from the patients apathetic and retarded appearance.

Language function should be assessed before any other aspect of higher cortical function because a serious disturbance may affect the patient's ability to respond to other aspects of the examination. An impression of the patient's ability will have been gained from the spontaneous verbal output noted during the history-taking. Dysarthria implies a subcortical lesion and is unusual in Alzheimer's disease, whereas dysphasia is a prominent symptom in severe Alzheimer's disease. After noting how the patient uses language spontaneously, comprehension of spoken language, repetition of simple sentences and word-finding abilities are also assessed. Reading skills and handwriting should be evaluated.

Other aspects of higher cortical function can then be assessed and here a simple tool, such as the information-concentration-memory scale of Blessed et al (1968) or the Mini-Mental State Examination (Folstein et al, 1975; Dick et al, 1984), can provide semi-quantitative data on various aspects of cognitive function. Although no substitute for a full neuropsychological assessment, they are easy to apply, take no more than a few minutes and can be repeated frequently.

The examination then centres on the visual system, with attention being paid to the visual acuity, visual fields and fundoscopic appearances. Hemianopic field defects suggest MID, and the fundi may show changes consistent with sustained hypertension. Examination of the lower cranial nerves may reveal evidence of a pseudobulbar palsy (dysarthria, diminished gag reflex, slow tongue movements and brisk jaw jerk) which would again favour MID. In the limbs, signs of pyramidal tract involvement suggests MID. The sensory examination needs to be comprehensive and should include cortical aspects such as astereognosis, extinction and graphesthesia, since there may be abnormalities of these higher functions in Alzheimer's disease.

Dyspraxia and loss of constructional skills are prominent features of Alzheimer's disease and should be evaluated once the assessment of motor function is complete. The gait merits brief description, since certain features such as slowness, small steps and a tendency to fall are features characteristic of the lacunar state and other primarily subcortical dementias. It is at this stage that the ischaemic score can be completed and a clinical diagnosis offered. Ancillary investigations are then required to confirm the diagnosis and establish the pathogenesis of repeated strokes when the score suggests MID.

Baseline investigations

In almost all patients with dementia the following haematological and biochemical investigations can be justified: full blood count (including haematocrit and platelet count), a blood smear, erythrocyte sedimentation rate (ESR), serum urea and electrolytes, serum calcium, plasma protein electropheresis, thyroid function tests, serum and folate levels and a VDRL. Estimations such as the serum B_{12} and T_4 are required to exclude those rare causes of intellectual decline and can be considered as routine in the evaluation of any patient with dementia. The full blood count will exclude conditions such as polycythaemia rubra vera, a disease which may present with repeated strokes (Chievitz & Thiede, 1962). An ESR is performed because, in the elderly, temporal arteritis may present with recurrent episodes of cerebral ischaemia and, in the younger population, intellectual decline can be a feature of the generalized vasculitides which may accompany systemic lupus erythematosus and polyarteritis nodosa. If a collagen-vascular disease is suspected, then the anti-nuclear factor, LE cell preparation and DNA binding should be included in the evaluation. Recurrent strokes in a young subject can occur in the presence of lupus anticoagulant, so the PTT should be checked. Diabetes mellitus needs to be excluded by the appropriate tests in all patients with MID, since abnormal glucose tolerance is a potent risk factor for stroke. The VDRL remains mandatory in any type of either generalized or focal dementia, but is rarely positive nowadays.

A chest X-ray is always worth performing. Left ventricular enlargement would alert to the possibility of long-standing hypertension; metastases involving the brain often also appear in lungs.

The ECG remains a valuable investigation in patients with MID because of the frequent coexistence of ischaemic heart disease and cerebral infarction (Wolf et al, 1978). Disturbances of cardiac rhythm may be an important aetiological factor in some patients with stroke, so 24-hour Holter monitoring can prove useful. Two-dimensional echo cardiography with additional radio-isotope studies of wall motion may also be indicated in patients with recurrent strokes, since intracardiac sources of embolism (intraventricular clot, floppy mitral valve, etc.) can be evaluated by these methods.

Where facilities permit, a CT scan of the brain should be performed on all subjects with dementia. Occasionally, a treatable lesion such as a chronic subdural haematoma or subfrontal meningioma will declare itself. Lacunes may be visualised (Pullicino et al, 1980; Weisberg, 1982); the low white matter attenuation of Binswanger's disease has a characteristic appearance (Rosenburg et al, 1979), and larger cortical or subcortical infarcts are readily visualized. Multiple infarcts in various vascular territories may suggest cardiac embolism. An estimate of generalized atrophy can also be made. About 60% of patients with MID will have multiple infarcts visualized on CT scan (Ladurner et al, 1982). The CT scan may show generalized atrophy as the sole abnormality, even when the clinical picture and ischaemic score both suggest MID. This was the case in one patient described by Frackowiak et al (1981) where subsequent post-mortem examination confirmed multiple infarctions. Occasionally the converse, where the ischaemic score suggests Alzheimer's disease and the CT scan demonstrates focal pathology, also pertains. Thus, the CT and ischaemic score are not always in agreement, and the clinical diagnosis remains a matter of judgment. A degree of diagnostic uncertainty necessarily persists in the absence of pathological material, a fact which has considerable implications for research.

Focal or lateralizing e.e.g. abnormalities were found in almost half the demented patients with high ischaemic scores studied by Harrison et al

(1979). By contrast, similar changes were seen in less than 5% of their comparative group of dementia subjects in whom the ischaemia score results were low. Diffuse abnormalities were common in both groups. The EEG may thus have some discriminant value if it demonstrates focal slowing.

Cerebral angiography is occasionally indicated in the investigation of patients with MID. The prerequisite condition is that, if a surgically treatable lesion were discovered, then an operation would be undertaken. Considerations such as the patient's age and the extent of the dementing process will be part of that decision. Again it should be stressed that when vascular disease leads to dementia, the process is one of multiple infarcts and not the results of chronic flow retardation. This appears so even in patients with bilateral carotid occlusion where dementia may develop as a result of bilateral watershed infarctions (Fisher, 1968). The infarctions may be haemodynamically induced but, once they have occurred, surgery designed to improve flow (e.g. EC/IC bypass procedure) will rarely, if ever, lead to an improvement in dementia. The main rationale behind surgery is to remove potential sources of recurrent emboli and so prevent further deterioration rather than effect improvement.

One further cautionary note comes from the data reported by Harrison et al (1979). They found that the incidence of atheromatous carotid disease was no higher in demented patients with high ischaemic scores than in patients with low scores. Atherosclerosis is a common disease in the elderly and so is Alzheimer's disease, hence the two conditions often coexist.

Special investigations

Ever since Kety & Schmidt (1945) first introduced a technique for measuring cerebral blood flow in humans, considerable interest has focused on the organic dementias. It has emerged that global cerebral blood flow is reduced in dementia of all types (Freyhan et al, 1951; Lassen et al, 1957; Munk & Lassen, 1957; Obrist et al, 1970; Hachinski et al, 1975; Perez et al, 1977; Yamaguchi et al, 1980; Risberg & Gustafson, 1983; Barclay et al, 1984) and that the amplitude of the reduction seems to depend mainly on the severity of the dementia syndrome rather than the underlying aetiology (Gustafson & Risberg, 1974; Hagberg & Ingvar, 1976). There is some evidence, however, that patients with MID may have a greater decrease in CBF than patients with Alzheimer's disease of similar severity (O'Brien & Mallett, 1969; Hachinski et al, 1975), although a study by Simard et al (1971) has suggested the opposite. In the individual case, the size of the rate of change of CBF correlates with the degree of functional impairment as the dementia progresses (Risberg, 1980; Barclay et al, 1984).

Although global CBF may have little diagnostic significance, the pattern or regional CBF may help distinguish between Alzheimer's disease and MID. Most investigators have reported parietal, temporal and, in severe cases, frontal reductions in CBF in Alzheimer's disease (Gustafson &

Risberg, 1974; Risberg & Gustafson, 1983) whereas right–left asymmetries and spotty flow abnormalities are apparent in MID (Yamaguchi et al, 1980; Risberg & Gustafson, 1983).

In their early study on CBF in patients with MID, Hachinski et al (1975) demonstrated that the cerebral vessels respond in a normal way to reduction in PCO_2 brought about by hyperventilation. This implies that a coupling of CBF to the metabolic requirements of the brain remains intact, even though flow is generally reduced. The reduction can be explained by the fact that focal areas of cerebral tissue have been destroyed, whereas in areas of non-infarcted tissue flow is adequate to maintain neuronal structure and function. This concept of MID remained somewhat speculative until more advanced techniques of metabolic imaging became available.

PET scanning

In 1980, Frackowiak et al described a technique using oxygen-15 and a positron emission tomograph for the non-invasive measurement of regional CBF, regional cerebral metabolic consumption ($rCMRO_2$) and regional oxygen extraction fraction (rOER). The technique was then used in a study of 22 demented subjects, nine of whom were considered vascular and 13 degenerative (Frackowiak et al, 1981). Focal disturbances of rOER were not observed in either the degenerative or vascular dements, suggesting that the coupling of rCBF to $rCMRO_2$ remains intact in both groups. If chronic cerebral hypoperfusion were a primary event resulting in a secondary fall in $CMRO_2$, then an increase in OER would have been expected in patients with MID, and this was not found. In degenerative dementias, a more generalized depression of flow and metabolism was noted. The findings added further support to the hypothesis suggested by Fisher (1968) and argued by Hachinski et al (1974) that chronic global ischaemia is not a major pathogenic mechanism in dementia.

The case history of a patient recently investigated in the MRC cyclotron unit at the Hammersmith Hospital, London, may prove informative, and we are indebted to Dr R. Frackowiak for supplying details. The patient was a 37-year-old moderately demented woman who was found at age 28 years to have left ventricular hypertrophy, aortic and mitral valve incompetence and hypertension. She had possibly suffered from an episode of chorea aged 12 and there was no other significant past history. At the age of 33 years, she was noted to have a slurring dysarthria and a moderate dysnomia. A year later, a memory defect was noted. She required help with household duties. Her intellectual powers declined and two years later she developed dyspraxia of hand movements.

At the time of evaluation, she was emotionally incontinent and had a spastic dysarthria but was not considered dysphasic. She was perseverative, had a short-term memory deficit and was dyscalculic. She was right–left disorientated and had marked constructional and dressing dyspraxias.

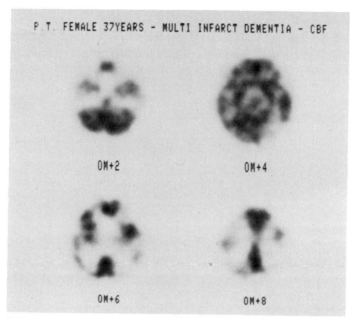

Fig. 12.1

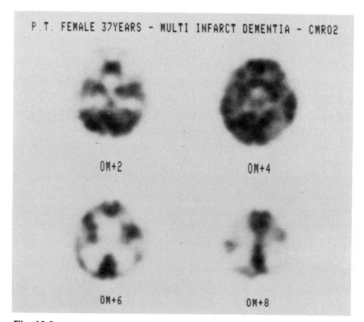

Fig. 12.2

Fig. 12.1 and **Fig. 12.2** CBF and CMRO$_2$ in four axial planes 2, 4, 6 and 8 cm above the orbito-meatal line. Note the similarity between the patchy areas or reduced CBF and CMRO$_2$ in multi-infarct dementia

Tongue movements were slow and she had a brisk jaw jerk. In the limbs, she had a mild spastic quadraparesis and dyspraxia. The deep reflexes were brisk and the plantars extensor. On the dementia scale describe by Blessed et al (1968) she scored 8, and 27 on the information-memory-concentration test. Her ischaemic score was 10. Fig. 12.1 shows the tomographs of CBF and $CMRO_2$ in four planes: 2, 4, 6 and 8 cm above the orbitomeatal line. Patchy foci of reduced CBF can be seen and the areas of low $CMRO_2$ have a similar distribution. In non-infarcted areas, values for CBF and $CMRO_2$ are within normal limits. These findings suggest that the clinical picture results from multiple infarction rather than a generalized reduction in CBF.

TREATMENT

The incidence of cerebrovascular disease is falling in most developed countries (Fratiglioni et al, 1983) partly because of the earlier recognition and more effective treatment of hypertension (Levy, 1979; Whisnant, 1984). It is now unusual to see patients with the lacunar state (Fisher, 1982), and the incidence of MID in general is almost certainly on the decline. However, it remains an important diagnosis because of the possibility of halting the dementing process by effective treatment.

Throughout this section we have emphasized that vascular disease, when it causes dementia, does so by multiple small and large infarcts. Assuming that the risk factors for single stroke also pertain to multiple strokes, which seems reasonable, then the treatment of the individual with MID should be along the same lines as those generally accepted for completed stroke. The aim is to prevent recurrence. Hypertension is the dominant predisposing factor for stroke, and the risk is directly related to the height of the elevation of the blood pressure (Kannel et al, 1970). Systolic pressure appears the more closely linked to the risk of stroke than the diastolic value and the effect does not diminish with increasing age. A number of clinical studies have now confirmed that the incidence of stroke declines when hypertension is treated (Veterans Administration Cooperative Study Group on Antihypertensive Agents, 1967, 1970).

Perhaps the second most important risk factor is cardiac disease, and included within this are patients with coronary heart disease, congestive failure, evidence of left ventricular hypertrophy and dysrhythmias, particularly atrial fibrillation, even in the absence of rheumatic heart disease (Wolf et al, 1983). A floppy mitral valve is now recognized as a potenial source of emboli destined for the cerebral circulation (Barnett et al, 1980). When a cardiac source of emboli is suspected, and perhaps confirmed by ancillary tests, then anticoagulation should be considered in an attempt to prevent further episodes.

Aspirin, 325 mg q.d.s. reduces the incidence of subsequent stroke in subjects who present with either transient episodes of cerebral ischaemia or completed stroke (Canadian Cooperative Study Group, 1978; Bousser et al, 1983) and, by analogy, may prove useful in preventing further strokes in patients with MID. Cerebral infarcts are common in patients with elevated haematocrit values (Tohgi et al, 1978), and patients with polycythaemia rubra vera frequently present with stroke (Chievitz & Thiede, 1962). There is good evidence to suggest that treatment designed to lower the haematocrit will reduce the incidence of subsequent stroke (Pearson & Wetherley-Mein, 1978) and it should certainly be considered in any patient with MID in whom the haematocrit value is over 50.

Diabetes mellitus is a key risk factor for stroke and is treatable, but whether this actually reduces the risk of subsequent stroke is uncertain. However, common sense dictates that, when diabetes is discovered, the blood sugar should be kept within acceptable limits, and support for this comes from the experimental observation that ischaemic brain damage is more extensive under hyperglycaemic than normoglycaemic conditions (Pulsinelli et al, 1982).

The rationale for using cerebrovasodilators has clearly come into question over the past decade. The naive assumption that cerebral vasodilatation can lead to improved neuronal function has become untenable in the light of the rCBF data suggesting normal coupling of cerebral metabolism and flow (Hachinski et al, 1975) and the failure to demonstrate chronic cerebral ischemia with the PET scanner (Frackowiak et al, 1981). Although some drug will certainly produce an increase in CBF in patients with MID (Merory et al, 1978), there is no reason to suppose that this will improve mental function or prevent further infarction.

The question of using ergot derivatives in dementia has been a subject of a recent review and remains controversial (Lancet, 1984). Co-dergocrine mesylate (Hydergine®) is widely prescribed in Europe for dementia in the elderly but its role remains uncertain. It was introduced some 30 years ago as a cerebral vasodilator at a time when dementia in the elderly was usually attributed to cerebral arteriosclerosis. As our understanding of the dementias has improved, this potential effect is no longer stressed and it seems unlikely that it has any role to play in MID (Fanchamps, 1983). Whether it has a place in AD remains uncertain despite numerous clinical trials (Lancet, 1984). Cyclandelate (Cyclospasmal®) and naftidrofuryl oxalate (Praxilene®) were also introduced as cerebrovasodilators likely to be efficacious in 'arteriosclerotic' dementia, but again the rationale seems illogical and there are no adequate clinical trials of treatment with either compound in MID.

CONCLUSION

All the available evidence suggests that when vascular disease causes dementia, it does so as a result of multiple large and small infarctions. Almost certainly it is still overdiagnosed as a cause of mental deterioration in the elderly, but this bias is in a sense welcome, since MID represents one of the few forms of dementia in which the intellectual decline may be halted by treatment. The clinical features which favour the diagnosis of MID have been distilled into an ischaemic score with which reasonable diagnostic accuracy can be achieved when used in conjunction with CT. Modern methods of cerebral metabolic imaging have undermined the rationale behind the use of cerebrovasodilators, cerebral oxygenators and other non-specific 'brain activators'. In the absence of empirical evidence of efficacy, they can not be recommended. Treatment is directed towards the prevention of further strokes and may involve hypotensive agents, antiplatelet drugs, oral anticoagulants and even vascular surgery, depending on the underlying mechanism for recurrent infarction.

REFERENCES

American Psychiatric Association 1980 Diagnostic and statistical manual of mental disorders, (DSM III) Criteria for dementia, 3rd edn. Washington DC

Arab A 1954 Plaques séniles et artériosclerose cérébrale: abscence de rapports de dépendance entre les deux processes. Étude statistique. Revue Neurologique 91: 22–36

Barclay L, Zemcov A, Blass J P, McDowell F 1984 Rates of decrease of cerebral blood flow in progressive dementias. Neurology 34: 1555–1560

Barnett H J M, Boughner D R, Taylor D W, Cooper P E, Kostuk W J, Nichol P M 1980 Further evidence relating mitral-valve prolapse to cerebral ischemic events. New England Journal of Medicine 302: 139–144

Benson D F, Cummings J L, Tsai S Y 1982 Angular gyrus syndrome simulating Alzheimer's disease. Archives of Neurology 39: 616–620

Blessed G, Tomlinson B E, Roth M 1968 The association between quantitative measures of dementia and of senile change in the cerebral grey matter of elderly subjects. British Journal of Psychiatry 114: 797–811

Bousser M G, Eschwege E, Haguenau M, Lefaucconnier J M, Thibult N, Touboul D, Touboul P J 1983 'AICLA' controlled trial of aspirin and dipyridamole in the secondary prevention of athero-thrombotic cerebral ischemia. Stroke 14: 5–16

Brust J C M 1983 Dementia and cerebrovascular disease. In Mayeux L, Rosen W G (eds) Advances in Neurology, Vol 38. The dementias. Raven Press, New York

Burger P C, Burch J G, Kunze U 1976 Subcortical arteriosclerotic encephalopathy. Stroke 7: 626–631

Canadian Cooperative Study Group 1978 A randomized trial of aspirin and sulphinpyrazone in threatened stroke. New England Journal of Medicine 299: 53–59

Caplan L R, Schoene W C 1978 Clinical features of subcortical arteriosclerotic encephalopathy (Binswanger's disease). Neurology 28: 1206–1215

Castaigne P, Buge A, Cambier J, Escourolle R, Brunet P, Degos J 1966 Démence thalamique d'origine vasculaire par ramollissement bilateral limité au territoire du pédicule retro-mammillaire (à propos de 2 observations anatomo-cliniques). Revue Neurologique 114: 89–108

Castaigne P, Lhemitte F, Buge A, Escourolle R, Hauw J J, Lyon-Caen O 1981 Paramedian thalamic and midbrain infarcts: clinical and neuropathological study. Annals of Neurology 10: 127–148

Chievitz E, Thiede T 1962 Complications and causes of death in polycythaemia vera. Acta Medica Scandinavica 172: 513–523

Cook R H, Bard B E, Austin J H 1979 Studies in aging of the brain. IV. Familial Alzheimer's disease: relation to transmissible dementia, aneuploidy and microtubular defects. Neurology 29: 1402–1412

Cummings J L, Benson D F 1983 Dementia. A clinical approach. Butterworth, Boston, p 5

Cummings J L, Benson D F 1984 Subcortical dementia: review of an emerging concept. Archives of Neurology 41: 874–879

Cummings J L, Benson D F, Loverme Jr S 1980 Reversible dementia. Journal of the American Medical Association 243: 2434–2439

De Reuk J, Crevits L, De Coster W, Sieben G, Vander Eecken H 1980 Pathogenesis of Binswanger's chronic progressive subcortical encephalopathy. Neurology 30: 920–928

Dick J P R, Guiloff R J, Stewart A, Blackstock J, Bielawska C, Paul E A, Marsden C D 1984 Mini-Mental State Examination in neurological patients. Journal of Neurology, Neurosurgery and Psychiatry 47: 496–499

Fanchamps A 1983 Dihydroergotoxine in senile cerebral insufficiency. In: Agnoli A, Crepaldi C, Spano D F, Trabucchi M (eds) Aging brain and ergot alkaloids. Aging, Vol 23. Raven Press, New York, p 311–322

Fisher C M 1967 A lacunar stroke. Neurology 17: 614–617

Fisher C M 1968 Dementia in cerebral vascular disease In Toole J F, Seikert R G, Whisnant J P (eds) Cerebral vascular diseases. 6th Princeton Conference. Grune & Stratton, New York, p 232

Fisher C M 1982 Lacunar strokes and infarcts : a review. Neurology 32: 871–876

Folstein M F, Folstein S E, McHugh P R 1975 'Mini-Mental State'. A practical method for grading the cognitive state of patients for the clinician. Journal of Psychiatric Research 12: 189–198

Frackowiak R S J, Lenzi G L, Jones T, Heather J D 1980 Quantitative measurement of regional cerebral blood flow and oxygen metabolism in man using oxygen-15 and positron emission tomography: theory, procedure and normal values. Journal of Computer Assisted Tomography 4: 727 736

Frackowiak R S J, Pozzilli I C, Legg N J, Du Boulay G H, Marshall J, Lenzi G L, Jones T 1981 Regional cerebral oxygen supply and utilisation in dementia: a clinical and physiological study with oxygen-15 and positron tomography. Brain 104: 753–778

Fratiglioni L, Massey E W, Schoenberg D G, Schoenberg B S 1983 Mortality from cerebrovascular disease: international comparisons and temporal trends. Neuroepidemiology 2: 101–116

Freyhan F A, Woodford R B, Kety S S 1951 Cerebral blood flow and metabolism in psychoses of senility. Journal of Nervous and Mental Disease 113: 449–459

Gilbert J J, Vinters H V 1983 Cerebral amyloid angiopathy: incidence and complications in the aging brain. Stroke 14: 915–923

Gilles C, Brucker J M, Khoubesserain P, Vanderhaeghen J J 1984 Cerebral amyloid angiopathy as a cause of multiple intracerebral hemorrhages. Neurology 34: 730–735

Graff-Radford N R, Eslinger P J, Damasio A R, Yamada T 1984 Nonhemorrhagic infarction of the thalamus: behavioral, anatomic and psychological correlates. Neurology 34: 14–23

Guberman A, Stuss D 1983 The syndrome of bilateral paramedian thalamic infarction. Neurology 33: 540–546

Gustafson L, Risberg J 1974 Regional cerebral blood flow related to psychiatric symptoms in dementia with onset in the presenile period. Acta Psychiatrica Scandinavica 50: 516–538

Hachinski V C, Iliff L D, Zilkha E, Du Boulay G H, McAllister V C, Marshall J M, Ross Russell R W, Symon L 1975 Cerebral blood flow in dementia. Archives of Neurology 32: 632–637

Hachinski V C, Lassen N A, Marshall J 1974 Multi-infarct dementia: a cause of mental deterioration in the elderly. Lancet 2: 207–209

Hagberg B, Ingvar D H 1976 Cognitive reduction in presenile dementia related to regional abnormalities in the cerebral blood flow. British Journal of Psychiatry 128: 209–222

Harrison M J G, Thomas D J, Du Boulay G H, Marshall J 1979 Multi- infarct dementia. Journal of Neurological Sciences 40: 97–103

Jellinger K 1976 Neuropathological aspects of dementias resulting from abnormal blood and cerebrospinal fluid dynamics. Acta Neurologica Belgica 76: 83–102

Kannel W B, Wolf P A, Verter J, McNamara P M 1970 Epidemiologic assessment of the role of blood pressure in stroke: the Framingham survey. Journal of the American Medical Association 214: 301–310

Kety S S, Schmidt C F 1945 The determination of cerebral blood flow in man by the use of nitrous oxide in low concentrations. American Journal of Physiology 143: 53–66

Kitagawa Y, Meyer J S, Tachibara H, Mortel K F, Rogers R L 1984 CT–CBF correlations of cognitive deficits in multi-infarct dementia. Stroke 15: 1000–1009

Koller W C, Wilson R S, Glatt S L, Fox J H 1984 Motor signs are infrequent in dementia of the Alzheimer type. Annals of Neurology 16: 514–516

Ladurner G, Iliff L D, Lechner H 1982 Clinical factors associated with dementia in ischaemic stroke. Journal of Neurology, Neurosurgery and Psychiatry 45: 97–101

Lancet Editorial 1984 Ergot for dementia? Lancet ii: 1313–1314

Lassen N A, Munk O, Tottey E R 1957 Mental function and cerebral oxygen consumption in organic dementia. Archives of Neurology and Psychiatry 77: 126–133

Levy R I 1979 Stroke decline: implications and prospects (editorial). New England Journal of Medicine 300:490

Loeb C, Gandolfo C 1983 Diagnostic evaluation of degenerative and vascular dementia. Stroke 14: 399–401

Mandybur T I, Stephen R D, Bates M B 1978 Fatal massive intracranial hemorrhage complicating cerebral amyloid angiopathy. Archives of Neurology 35: 266–268

Mayer-Gross W, Slater E, Roth M 1969 Clinical psychiatry, 3rd ed. Baillère Tindall, London

Merory J, Du Boulay G H, Marshall J, Morris J, Ross Russell R W, Symon L, Thomas D J 1978 Effect of tinofedrine (Homburg D 8955) on cerebral blood flow in multi-infact dementia. Journal of Neurology, Neurosurgery and Psychiatryt 41: 900–902

Munk O, Lassen N A 1957 Bilateral cerebral blood flow and O consumption in man by use of Krypton 85. Circulation Research 5: 163–168

O'Brien M D, Mallett B L 1970 Cerebral cortex perfusion rates in dementia. Journal of Neurosurgery and Psychiatry 33: 497–500

Obrist W, Chivian E, Cronqvist S, Ingvar D H 1970 Regional cerebral blood flow in senile and presenile dementia. Neurology 20: 315–322

Okazaki H, Reagan T J, Campbell R J 1979 Clinicopathological studies of primary cerebral amyloid angiopathy. Mayo Clinic Proceedings 54: 22–31

Pearson T C, Whetherley-Mein G 1978 Vascular occlusive episodes and venous haematocrit in primary proliferative polycythaemia. Lancet ii: 1219–1222

Perez F, Mathew N T, Stump D A, Meyer J S 1977 Regional cerebral blood flow, statistical patterns and psychological performance in multi-infarct dementia and Alzheimer's disease. Canadian Journal of Neurological Sciences 4: 53–62

Portera-Sanchez A, del Ser T, Bermejo F, Arredondo J M 1982 Clinical diagnosis of senile dementia of Alzheimer type and vascular dementia In: Terry R D, Bolis C L, Toffano G (eds) Neurological pathology. Aging, Vol 18. Raven Press, New York

Pullicino P, Nelson R F, Kendal B E, Marshall J 1980 Small deep infarcts diagnosed on computed tomography. Neurology 30: 1090–1096

Pulsinelli W A, Waldman S, Rawlinson D. Plum F 1982 Moderate hyperglycaemia augments ischemic brain damage: a neuropathologic study in the rat. Neurology 32: 1239–1246

Risberg J 1980 Regional cerebral blood flow measurements by 133-Xe inhalation: methodology and applications in neuropsychology and psychiatry. Brain and Language 9: 9–34

Risberg J, Gustafson L 1983 133-Xe cerebral blood flow in dementia and in neuro-psychiatric research In: Magistretti P L (ed) Functional radionuclide imaging of the brain. Raven Press, New York, p 151–159

Ron M A, Toone B K, Garralda M E, Lishman W A 1979 Diagnostic accuracy in presenile dementia. British Journal of Psychiatry 134: 161–168

Roth M 1981 The diagnosis of dementia in late and middle life. In: Mortimer J A, Shuman L M (eds) The epidemiology of dementia. Oxford University Press, New York, p 31–33

Rosen W G, Terry R D, Fuld P A, Katzman R, Peck A 1979 Pathologic verification of ischemic score in differentiation of dementias. Annals of Neurology 7: 486–488

Rosenburg G A, Kornfield M, Stovring J, Bicknell J M 1979 Subcortical arteriosclerotic encephalopathy (Binswanger): computerised tomography. Neurology 29: 1102–1106

Simard D, Olesen J, Paulson O B, Lassen N A, Skinhoj E 1971 Regional cerebral blood flow and its regulation in dementia. Brain 94: 273–288

Sonninen V H, Savontaus M L, Oksi J 1984 Hereditary multi-infarct dementia. Clinical, genetic and neuroradiological studies of one family. Acta Neurologia Scandinavica 69: (Suppl 98) 289–290

Sourander P, Walinder J 1977 Hereditary multi-infarct dementia. Morphological and clinical studies of a new disease. Acta Neuropathologica 39: 247–254

Tohgi H, Yamanouchi H, Murakami M, Kameyama M 1978 Importance of hematocrit as a risk factor in cerebral infarction. Stroke 9: 369–374

Tomlinson B E, Blessed G, Roth M 1970 Observations on the brains of demented old people. Journal of Neurological Science 11: 205–242

Veterans Administration Cooperative Study: Group on Antihypertensive Agents 1967 Effects of treatment on morbidity in hypertension. Journal of the American Medical Association 202: 1028–1034

Veterans Administration Cooperative Study: Group on Antihypertensive Agents 1970 Effects of treatment on morbidity in hypertension. Journal of the American Medical Association 312: 1143–1152

Vinters H V, Gilbert J J 1983 Cerebral amyloid angiopathy: the distribution of amyloid vascular changes. Stroke 14: 924–928

Weisberg L A 1982 Lacunar infarcts: clinical and computed tomographic correlations. Archives of Neurology 39: 37–40

Whisnant J P 1984 The decline of stroke. Stroke 15: 160–168

Wolf P A, Kannel W B, Dawber T R 1978 Heart disease as a precursor of stroke. In: Schoenberg B S (ed) Advances in neurology, Vol 19. Raven Press, New York, p 107

Wolf P A, Kannel W B, Verter J 1983 Current status of risk actors for stroke. Symposium on Cerebrovascular Disease. Neurologic Clinics 1: 317–343

Yamaguchi F, Meyer J S, Yamamoto M, Sakai F, Shaw T 1980 Noninvasive rCBF measurements in dementia. Archives of Neurology 37: 410–418

Dementia in disorders of movement

INTRODUCTION

Dementia has long been considered to be a clinical syndrome which arises from generalized brain disease principally affecting the cerebral cortex, as occurs in Alzheimer's disease and Pick's disease. In more recent times it has become apparent that neurological disorders which arise from pathological changes in subcortical structures in the brain may also be accompanied by changes in cognitive function. Such diseases include idiopathic Parkinson's disease, arteriosclerotic Parkinsonism, post-encephalitic Parkinsonism, Huntington's chorea and a number of rarer disorders. Although there is now good evidence that cognitive impairment can occur in disease of the basal ganglia, it is unclear whether these changes amount to dementias, what are the characteristic changes in cognitive function in each disorder, and whether they arise from the disease process in the basal ganglia alone or imply a more widespread pathology. The occurrence of cognitive impairment in disease of the basal ganglia is of great clinical importance, as patients may be much more disabled than seems to be justified by the severity of motor changes. If cognitive changes in these disorders are eventually shown to arise from lesions occurring other than in the cerebral cortex, knowledge of the normal function of the basal ganglia and other subcortical structures would be considerably advanced.

We will first consider changes in cognitive function in Parkinson's disease in some detail, then describe the changes found in Huntington's chorea more briefly and finally discuss the concept of subcortical dementia.

IMPAIRMENT OF COGNITIVE FUNCTION IN PARKINSON'S DISEASE

When James Parkinson (1817) first described the disease that later would bear his name. he specifically excluded intellectual changes from his description. Subsequent reports questioned this observation, and in recent years there has been an increasing awareness of the frequency of mental changes associated with the disease. The changes in cognitive function reported vary from minor disturbances in memory or intellectual function on the one hand, to frank dementias on the other. Some writers have considered these changes to be a reflection of the disease process taking place in the subcortical structures of the brain; others attribute them to the effects of drugs used in therapy, such as levodopa; and yet others have implicated concomitant disease processes of the cerebral cortex of a similar nature to that which occurs in Alzheimer's disease and Pick's disease. The occurrence of cognitive impairment in Parkinson's disease is not fully established to be a part of the self-same disease as the motor symptoms, and the characteristics of any impairment are unclear, as are the frequency and pathological causes of such decline. The issue is further complicated by the introduction of the concept of subcortical dementia (Albert et al, 1974). Although the syndrome of subcortical dementia is recognizable in some patients with Parkinson's disease, it is by no means clear whether it is a variant of global dementia, whether it arises purely from neuropathological changes in the basal ganglia, or, indeed, whether it has any neuropathological basis at all. In attempting to clarify these issues, we will review some of the present literature regarding the occurrence of dementia in Parkinson's disease and examine several possible aetiological processes.

THE PREVALENCE OF DEMENTIA IN PARKINSON'S DISEASE

Estimates of the prevalence of dementia in Parkinson's disease have varied widely, ranging from 2% to 77% (Mortimer et al, 1984). However, it is difficult to compare the reports of many studies of prevalence rates because of difference in patient selection, differences in methods of assessment, diverse criteria for the diagnosis of dementia and inconsistencies in diagnosis of Parkinson's disease itself. Consequently, whilst the vast majority of previous studies confirm the occurrence of dementia in a proportion of cases of Parkinson's disease, they are often difficult to interpret and do not provide accurate prevalence rates. The most acceptable method of obtaining a prevalence figure for dementia in Parkinson's disease would be to sample an entire population, including both hospitalized patients and those residing at home. To date, there have been reports of three major studies designed to estimate prevalence using this method. Pollock & Hornabrook (1966), in a study carried out in a defined area of New Zealand, found that overall incidence of patients with significant mental impairment in Parkinson's disease was 20%, with the majority of cases appearing among those cases where the patient was thought to have cerebrovascular disease. In a similar large-scale epidemiological study, carried out in Finland, Marttila & Rinne (1976) found that the overall prevalence of dementia in Parkinson's disease was 29%, with no significant differences in prevalence between idiopathic and cerebrovascular sub-groups. Finally, in a more recent American study, Rajput and colleagues (1984) reported a prevalence rate of dementia in Parkinson's disease of 31%.

Critical review of these three studies suggests that these fairly consistent prevalence rates should not be accepted at face value. As Brown & Marsden (1984) point out, the studies utilized different methods of assessment and different criteria for the diagnosis of dementia, and in consequence the figures quoted are difficult to evaluate. There is also the problem of the diagnosis of Parkinson's disease. The syndrome of Parkinsonism may be produced by many diseases other than the degenerative process found in the brain of subjects who have suffered from idiopathic Parkinson's disease, and as a result it is important to separate idiopathic Parkinson's disease from post-encephalitic Parkinsonism, or the so-called arteriosclerotic Parkinsonism, in many studies this distinction has not been made. Finally, none of the studies really attempts to compare the patient sample with a suitable control population, and so distinguish cognitive impairment in Parkinson's disease from dementia arising from the diverse causes that may be expected in the general population of that age.

In addition to the difficulties in establishing the prevalence of dementia, little agreement has been reached concerning the qualitative nature of intellectual impairment in Parkinson's disease. Some authors have described specific deficits of cognition, such as memory impairment, whilst others have emphasized a more pervasive, global decrement in intellectual functioning. In a neuropsychological analysis of cognitive functioning in Parkinson's disease, using age, sex and education-matched controls, Pirozzolo et al (1982) found that as many as 93% of patients with Parkinson's disease showed some evidence of cognitive impairment. In other words, 93% of patients with Parkinson's disease performed worse than their matched controls. Pirozzolo and her colleagues concluded that the neuropsychological performance of patients with Parkinson's disease falls along a continuum of impairment, and that consequently the assignment of a prevalence rate for dementia in the disease is likely to be misleading, because the diagnostic criteria usually employed will be arbitrary.

Cools and his colleagues (1984) suggest that patients suffering from disease of the basal ganglia exhibit characteristic neuropsychological changes with impairment of the capacity to change from one sphere of activity to another. Eighteen patients with Parkinson's disease and nineteen control patients were compared on test measuring 'shifting aptitude' at cognitive and motor levels (word production, sorting blocks, and finger pushing sequences) and they reported that patients with Parkinson's disease produced fewer different names of animals and professions in one minute than control patients, needed more trials for detecting a shift in sorting criteria, and produced fewer finger responses in a change of pushing sequence than controls. These workers conclude that these deficits are a characteristic feature of Parkinson's disease, but are not necessarily positively correlated with increasing degrees of severity of the motor symptoms and signs of Parkinsonism.

The relationship between symptom duration, severity of motor symptoms, age at onset and cognitive impairment have been studied by a number of investigators, and the results are also equivocal. Several studies have suggested a continued downward progression of cognitive, motor and social disabilities (Hoehn & Yahr, 1967), whereas other have only indicated a weak relationship between degree of intellectual impairment and the severity of motor symptoms and functional disablility (Loranger et al,1972). Whilst severity, as assessed by stage of the disease, has been shown to be related to increasing cognitive impairment (Loranger et al, 1972), there seems to be no relationship between disease duration and intellectual impairment (Riklan et al, 1976). There appears to be persuasive evidence that cognitive impairment is a frequent concomitant of Parkinson's disease, but there is no conclusive evidence that this impairment is a manifestation of the disease process which gives rise to the motor symptoms through its effects on the functioning of the basal ganglia.

THE RELATIONSHIP BETWEEN DEMENTIA AND MOOD

A great variety of affective symptoms have been described in patients suffering from Parkinson's disease. In a review of the literature, Mayeux (1982) reported that the prevalence rates for depression in Parkinson's disease varied from 40–50% of patients. Although consistently found, these symptoms appear to be unrelated to any other specific feature of the disease (Mayeux et al, 1981). The association between depression and intellectual impairment also appears to be weak. Memory, perception and attention are certainly impaired in a proportion of subjects suffering from primary depressive disorders (Folstein & McHugh, 1978), and frequently mislead the clinician when he/she is making a diagnosis. As a consequence, where the incidence of depression in Parkinson's disease is high, the intellectual capability of the patient may be diminished because of depression and add to the apparent prevalence of dementia. In these circumstances, depression of mood and intellectual deficits are likely to be reversed by antidepressant therepy, which makes the recognition of depression of mood in Parkinson's disease particularly important so that appropriate treatment may be given. Mayeux and his co-workers (1981) reported a low, but significant relationship between depression in Parkinson's disease and impaired intellectual, performance, whereas Mindham and his colleagues (1976) found no relationship between depression and intellectual performance. Taken together, the data from these studies suggest that the relationship between depression and intellectual impairment is weak, or non-existent, and that further research is required in order to determine whether the cognitive impairment found in Parkinson's disease is just another variant of the 'pseudodementia' seen in depressive states occurring in subjects with no evidence of organic brain disease.

THE ROLE OF DRUG TREATMENT IN COGNITIVE IMPAIRMENT

Few drugs have had as dramatic an impact on clinical neurology as levodopa. Despite a variety of unwanted effects, the drug is capable of reversing some of the most disabling symptoms of many patients with Parkinson's disease and is particularly effective in anergia, a symptom resistant to other forms of treatment. More recent experience indicates that this improvement is frequently not sustained indefinitely, presumably because dying cells are not longer able to metabolize levodopa to dopamine, even when the precursor is present in high concentrations. Several authors have suggested that the administration of levodopa reverses the cognitive deficits of the Parkinsonian patient, although, as in the case of motor symptoms, not indefinitely. For example, Loranger and his colleagues (1972), using the Wechsler Adult Intelligence Scale, the best standardized test of general intelligence, found an improvement in performance after eight months of levodopa treatment, but a return to baseline after three years of treatment. Bowen and associates (1975) suggest that levodopa improves 'vigilance', rather than increasing the patient's overall cognitive ability. On the other hand, Sweet and his colleagues (1976) described a group of patients with Parkinson's disease in whom protracted agitated confusion developed during treatment with levodopa and, furthermore, those patients with cognitive impairment before treatment with levodopa subsequently developed more severe cognitive impairment. These workers concluded that cognitive impairment is a feature of the Parkinsonian syndrome rather than a complication of levodopa therapy. Certainly, the beneficial effect of this medication on cognition appears to be relatively short-lived.

A wide variety of unwanted effects, including psychiatric syndromes, are reported to accompany treatment with levodopa. These disturbances range from agitation, restlessness and depression, to suicide attempts and overt psychosis. However, Mindham and associates (1976) point out that many of the patients who suffer depressive episodes during treatment with levodopa have a previous history of psychiatric disorder of the same type. The effect of levodopa in many of these patients appears to be the rekindling of a latent susceptibility to depressive illness. A history of previous depressive illness is one of the most important contra-indications to the use of levodopa in Parkinson's disease.

Various authors have examined the cognitive effects of the chronic administration of anticholinergic agents, which are known to cause cognitive deficits (Smith, 1984). For example, Syndulko and his colleagues (1981) examined the long-term effects of benzotropine mesylate on patients with idiopathic Parkinson's disease, with particularly reference to performance on test of verbal memory. In a double-blind trial, these workes showed that patients receiving the anticholinergic medication showed a statistically significant decrease in word acquisition on the test. De Smet and his colleagues (1982) suggest that anticholinergic medication should be avoided in patients with Parkinson's disease because the use of such medication may exacerbate already existing cognitive impairment.

DISORDERS OF MOVEMENT IN DEMENTING ILLNESS

Disorders of movement are regularly seen in a range of disorders in which the primary feature is a dementing process. The appearance of physical, as well as of mental, changes is due to the extension of the underlying disease process into those parts of the brain concerned with movement.

In Alzheimer's disease up to two-thirds of patients eventually show sign of Parkinsonism with disturbances of posture and gait, increased muscle tone, tremor and other features typical of the syndrome (Pearce & Miller, 1973). Similar changes are seen in dementias of the Alzheimer type of late onset. In Pick's disease the appearance of motor signs is much less frequent, but occasionally the typical clinical picture of Parkinsonism is seen. In these dementing illnesses, the motor signs follow the appearance of dementia by a considerable period, and are seen only when the dementing process is reaching an advanced stage. For these reasons the distinction from idiopathic Parkinson's disease does not usually present great difficulty.

Parkinsonism may also be seen in arteriosclerotic or multi-infarct dementia. Here again the syndrome follows the appearance of dementia, and the illness has all the characteristics of a disorder of the central nervous system arising from vascular disease. In the original description of 'arterio-sclerotic Parkinsonsm', dementia was regarded as a common feature (Critchley, 1929). There is clearly some likelihood of difficulty in separating a dementing illness due to vascular disease of the brain from an extrapyr-amidal syndrome of the same aetiology. The validity of the suggested relationship between cerebral vascular disease and Parkinsonism in the term 'arteriosclerotic Parkinsonism' has been questioned, and the status of the syndrome remains uncertain (Eadie & Sutherland, 1964).

A familial disease occurs in the Pacific island of Guam sometimes presents with amyotrophic lateral sclerosis and sometimes with a syndrome of Parkinsonism and dementia. A high proportion of the subjects presenting with one syndrome eventually develop the other, suggesting a close relation-ship between them (Elizan et al, 1966). This disease does not occur else-where in precisely the same form but is of considerable general interest; the distribution of pathological lesions resembles that in both Parkinson's disease and in cortical dementias; the disorder runs in families; and the levels of manganese in the soil and water may contribute to its appearance.

COGNITIVE CHANGES IN HUNTINGTON'S CHOREA

The relationship of cognitive impairment to the motor disorder is different in Huntington's chorea from that in Parkinson's disease. Here, cognitive impairment is regarded as such a major part of the syndrome that a diagnosis of Huntington's chorea is rarely made in its absence (Bruyn, 1968). Lieberman and associates (1979) suggest that as many as 90% of Huntington's chorea patients are demented, and that the interval between the onset of disease to onset of cognitive impairment is shorter in Huntington's chorea than in Parkinson's disease. Fedio and his colleagues (1979), in a brief review of the literature, suggest that cognitive impairment is not only widespread, but global, as is the case in the pre-senile dementias, although there appears to be an absence of disorientation in time and place, and a lack of focal symptoms. On the other hand, Wexler (1974) suggests that the early stages of deterioration in Huntington's chorea are characterized by specific deficits, primarily 'a failure in the capacity to recongnize and encode incoming stimuli'. As the disease progresses, further specific deficits in grammatical conceptualization, reduced word fluency and difficulty in dealing with competing stimuli seem to reflect problems in the integrity of mechanisms attributed to the frontal lobes.

In addition to cognitive impairment, patients with Huntington's chorea also commonly manifest emotional changes. When George Huntington (1872) first desribed the disease, he specifically mentioned ' a tendency to that insanity that leads to suicide' as one of the characteristics of the disease. Many research reports have subsequently documented the increased risk of psychiatric symptoms (Minski & Guttmann, 1983). For example, McHugh & Folstein (1975) report high incidence of schizophrenia and manic-depressive illness in patients with Huntington's chorea, and Folstein and associates (1979) report a high frequency and severity of emotional distress. A recent study, in which the frequency of a past history of depressive illness in Huntington's chorea and Alzheimer's disease was compared, has shown that the tendency to depressive episodes in Huntington's chorea cannot be simply regarded as a feature of dementia (Mindham et al, 1986).

Consequently, whilst there are fairly clear clinical, pathological and biochemical differences between the motor disorders of Parkinson's disease and Huntington's disease, there are similarities. Cognitive impairment is common in both syndromes, as is the psychiatric symptomatology associated with the two diseases. Lieberman and his colleagues (1979) suggest that it is reasonable to assume that both disorders begin in the basal ganglia, and may later be characterized by cortical changes, and that they have common clinical overlapping features, both in terms of the nature of the cognitive impairment and emotional disturbance.

THE CONCEPT OF SUBCORTICAL DEMENTIA

The most characteristic global dementias are seen in Alzheimer's disease and Pick's disease, each showing striking and characteristic neuropsychological changes which are attributed to widespread disease of the cerebral cortex. Albert and colleagues (1974) described clinical differences between such 'cortical dementia', and the cognitive deterioration observed in progressive supranuclear palsy, a neurological syndrome associated with neuropathological changes in the rostral brain stem, red nucleus, thalamus and basal ganglia, all subcortical structures, which they dubbed 'subcortical dementia'. Four cardinal features were proposed as characterizing subcortical dementia: forgetfulness, slowness of the mental processes, affective changes (particularly depression of mood), and intellectual deficits characterized by impaired ability to manipulate acquired knowledge. However, the distinctive abnormalities seen in the global dementias and known to be associated with cortical lesions, the dysphasias, agnosias and apraxias, are not apparent in patients with 'subcortical' dementia.

In 1975, McHugh & Folstein suggested that cognitive impairment in Huntington's chorea shared many of the same clinical features observed in progressive supranuclear palsy, and they suggested that this cognitive impairment was also of subcortical origin. On the basis of accumulated research evidence, it appears that a majority of patients with Parkinson's disease exhibit some neuropsychological impairment. If the characteristics of this impairment are similar to those found in Alzheimer's disease, it would be necessary to demonstrate a number of relationships before attributing the clinical features to lesions in similar sites in the brain. Firstly, it would be crucial to demonstrate that neuropsychological deficits observed in Parkinson's disease *are* the same, or similar to those found in Alzheimer's disease. Secondly, it would be necessary to show that the type of cognitive impairment found in Alzheimer's disease is more common in Parkinson's disease than could be expected by chance in an ageing population. Finally, pathological studies would need to show similar neuropathological changes in both syndromes.

The clinical features of cognitive impairment in Parkinson's disease, in many respects, resemble those identified in progressive supranuclear palsy. However, as there have been no direct comparisons of neuropsychological profiles of patients with Parkinson's disease, or Alzheimer's disease, or progressive supranuclear palsy, neuropathological and neurochemical findings provide the only clues as to whether the three syndromes share similar characteristics, or whether Parkinson's disease can by regarded as a disease of subcortical origin.

An examination of the present literature on the neurochemistry of dementing illness seems to suggest no common ground between Parkinson's disease and Alzheimer's disease. The major neurochemical change reported in Parkinson's disease is a loss of dopamine from the nigrostriatal pathways and the ventrotegmental area (Hornykiewicz, 1982), whereas in Alzheimer's disease the cholinergic system is thought to be disturbed, with changes in enzymes concerned in the metabolism of acetylcholine showing the greatest reduction in concentration in the cerebral cortex (Carlsson et al, 1980). Neuropathologically, the cause of cognitive deficits in Parkinson's disease is controversial, Hakim & Mathieson (1979) suggested that the dementia observed in Parkinson's disease is attributable to a coexisting Alzheimer's disease. Their conclusion is based on the finding that senile plaques and neurofibrillary tangles, characteristic neuropathological findings in Alzheimer's disease, are present in the cerebral cortex of patients with Parkinson's disease. However, this conclusion has been criticized because plaques and tangles also increase in the brains of normal elderly people, and consequently their occurrence may not be sufficient to be diagnostic of Alzheimer's disease. In order to confirm Hakim and Mathieson's view, one would have to demonstrate that the concentration of plaques and tangles in the cerebral cortex in Parkinson's disease exceeds that in the brain of the normal ageing subject.

The concept of subcortical dementia has recently become more complicated, with the suggestion that subcortical dysfunction may contribute to the dementia of Alzheimer's disease and possibly other 'cortical dementias'. Whitehouse and associates (1982) have demonstrate a profound loss neurones from the nucleus basalis of Meynert in Alzheimer's disease. This discovery poses questions as the specificity of the findings to Alzheimer's disease. It has even been suggested that lesions in subcortical structures are the primary changes in dementia and to be found in all varieties to the syndrome.

There is a need in the future for studies to examine in greater detail the qualitative nature of intellectual impairment in both Parkinson's disease and Alzheimer's disease, so that comparisons can be made, and furthermore these findings should be evaluated in the light of neuropathological changes in both diseases. It would also be useful if future studies reported what intellectual skills are *intact* in both syndromes, in order to allow fuller comparisons to be made between them. Attention to these issues should help to define the relative roles of cortical and subcortical structures in neuropsychological function, and provide further insight into the role of different neuroanatomical structures in intellectual functioning. Mayeux and his co-workers (1983) suggest that the whole concept of subcortical dementia may be misleading, as current evidence suggests that cognitive impairment in Alzheimer's disease, Parkinson's disease and Huntington's chorea may relate to a combination of cortical and subcortical degeneration. As a consequence of these uncertainties, until further neuropsychological and neuropathological research is carried out, the concept of subcortical dementia must be regarded as provisional (Cummings & Benson, 1984).

CONCLUSIONS

Impairment of cognitive function is known to accompany several disorders where the cause of motor disorder is known to reside in subcortical structures. Although some of the characteristics of cognitive impairment in these disorders are known, it is not yet possible to characterize fully the changes observed nor to assess to what extent they arise from the same pathological changes as the motor symptoms and signs. The dementing illnesses in which the more severe stages of the dementing processes are accompanied by motor signs are more fully understood; the development of motor signs is likely to be due to an extension of the pathological process into subcortical structures.

The appearance of impairment of cognitive function in patients with movement disorders has serious implications for the patient: self-confidence may be greatly reduced, and disability may be much greater than seems to be justified by the severity of motor symptoms. In such patients the relationship between cognitive impairment and mood should be carefully explored. 'Pseudodementia' secondary to depression of mood is usually readily treated, and mood change is frequently seen in both Parkinson's disease and Huntington's chorea.

The concept of subcortical dementia, whilst still of uncertain status, has served to bring new thinking to the relationship between neuropathological changes and impairment of cognitive functions. Although the situation is at present confused, clarification of this relationship is likely to lead to a better understanding of the role of subcortical structures in cognition and brain mechanism more widely.

Further study of cognitive impairment in disorders affecting the basal ganglia is clearly needed. Whilst there is an expanding literature of biochemical and neuropathological investigations of the basal ganglia, these are usually conducted in the absence of detailed and standardized neuropsychological assessments. Very few studies have considered the full range of aetiologies which may explain cognitive impairment in disorders of the basal ganglia, let alone measured them objectively and quantitatively. To answer the question of whether dementia does occur in disorders of the basal ganglia, neuropsychological testing of a sizeable group of patients with Parkinson's disease and Huntington's chorea must be carried out, and the profiles compared with Alzheimer's disease. These changes should then be considered in the light of neuropathological findings. Preliminary work on this task has already started in several centres but is likely to require several years to be brought to fruition.

REFERENCES

Albert M L, Feldman R, Wills A L 1974 The 'subcortical dementia' of progressive supranuclear palsy, Journal of Neurology, Neurosurgery and Psychiatry 37: 121–130
Bowen E P, Kamienny R S, Burns M M, Yahr M D 1975 Parkinsonism: effects of levodopa treatment on concept formation, Neurology 25: 701–704
Brown R G, Marsden C D 1984 How common is dementia in Parkinson's disease? Lancet 1st December: 1262–1265
Bruyn G 1968 Huntington's chorea: historical, clinical and laboratory synopsis. In: Vinken P, Bruyn G, Amsterdam (eds) Handbook of clinical neurology, vol 6. Disease of the basal ganglia. Elsevier
Carlsson A, Gottfries C G, Svennerholm L 1980 Neurotransmitters in human brain analysis post mortem: Changes in normal aging, senile dementia and chronic alcoholism. In: (eds)

Parkinson's disease: current progress, problems and management. Rinne U K, Klinger M, Stamm G, Elsevier, New York

Cools A R, Van Den Bercken J H L, Hurstink M W I, Van Spaendonck K P M, Berger H J C 1984 Cognitive and motor shifting aptitutde disorder in Parkinson's disease. Journal of Neurology, Neurosurgery and Psychiatry 47: 433–453

Critchley M 1929 Arteriosclerotic Parkinsonism. Brain 52: 23–83

Cummings J L, Benson D F 1984 Subcortical dementia: review of an emerging concept. Archives of Neurology 41: 874–879

De Smet Y, Ruberg M, Serdaru M, Dubois B, Lhermitte F, Agid Y 1982 Confusion, dementia and anticholinergics in Parkinson's disease. Journal of Neurology, Nerosurgery and Psychiatry 45: 1161–1164

Eadie M J, Sutherland J M 1964 Arteriosclerosis in Parkinsonism. Journal of Neurology, Neurosurgery and Psychiatry 27: 237–240

Elizan T S, Hirano A, Abrams B 1966 Amyotrophic lateral sclerosis and parkinsonism dementia complex of Guam. Archives of Neurology 14: 356–368

Fedio P, Cox C S, Neophytides A, Canal-Frederick G, Chase T N 1979 Neuropsychological profile of Huntington's disease: patients and those at risk . In: Chase T N, Wexler N S Barbeau A (eds) Advances in neurology, vol. 23. Huntington's disease. Raven Press, New York

Folstein M F, McHugh P R 1978 Dementia, syndrome of depression. In: (eds) Katzman R, Terry R D, Bick K L, Alzheimer's disease: senile dementia and related disorders. Aging, vol 7. Raven Press, New York

Folstein M F, McHugh P R 1979 Psychiatric syndromes in Huntington's disease. In:(eds) Chase T N, Wexler N S, Barbeau A , Advances in neurology, vol 23: Huntington's disease. Raven Press, New York

Hakim A M, Mathieson G 1979 Dementia in Parkinson's disease: a neuropathologic study. Neurology 29: 1209–1214

Hoehn M M, Yahr M D 1967 Parkinsonism: onset, progression and mortality.Neurology (Minneap) 17: 427–442

Hornykiewicz O 1982 Brain neurotransmitter changes in Parkinson's disease. In: (eds) Marsden C D, Fahn S. Movement disorders. Butterworth, Boston

Lieberman A, Dziatolowski M, Neophytides A, Kupersmith M, Aleksic S, Serby M, Korein J, Goldstein M 1979 Dementia of Huntington's and Parkinson's disease. In: (eds) Chase T N, Wexler N S, Barbeau A, Advances in neurology, vol. 23. Huntington's disease. Raven Press, New York

Loranger A W, Goodell H, Lee J E, McDowell F 1972 Levodopa treatment of Parkinson's syndrome. Archives of General Psychiatry 26: 163–167

McHugh P R, Folstein M F 1975 Psychiatry syndromes of Huntington's chorea: a clinical and phenomenologic study. In: (eds) Benson D F, Blumer D. Psychiatric aspects of neurologic disorder Grune & Stratton New York

Martilla R J, Rinne U K 1976 Dementia in Parkinson's disease, Acta Neurologic Scandinavica 54: 431–441

Mayeux R 1982 In: (eds) Marsden C D, Fahn, Movement disorders Butterworth, London p: 75–95

Mayeux R, Stern Y, Rosen J, Leventhal J, 1981 Depression, intellectual impairment and Parkinson's disease. Neurology (N Y) 31: 645–650

Mayeux R, Stern Y, Rosen J, Benson D F 1983 Is 'subcortical dementia' a recognisable clinical entity? Annals of Neurology 14, 3: 278–283

Mindham R H S, Marsden C D, Parkes J D 1976 Psychiatric symptoms during L-dopa therapy for Parkinson's disease and their relationship to psysical disability. Psychological Medicine 6: 23–37

Mindham R H S, Steele C, Folstein M F, Lucas J 1986 A comparison of the frequency of major affective disorder in Huntington's disease and Alzheimer's disease. Journal of Neurology, Neurosurgery and Psychiatry (in press)

Minski L, Guttmann E, 1938 Huntington's chorea: a study of 34 families. Journal of Mental Science 84: 21–96

Mortimer J A, Christenson M A, Webster D D 1984 Parkinsonian dementia. In: Handbook of clinical neurology, vol 46. Neurobehavioural disorder. Raven Press, New York

Parkinson J, 1817 An essay on the shaking palsy. Sherwood, Neely & Jones, London

Pearce J, Miller E 1973 Clinical aspects of dementia. Baillière Tindall, London

Pirozzolo F J, Hansch E C, Mortimer D A, Webster D D, Kuskowski M A 1982 Dementia in Parkinson's disease. A neuropsychological analysis. Brain and Cognition 1: 71–83

Pollock M, Hornabrook R W 1966 The prevalence, natural history and dementia of Parkinson's disease. prain 89: 429–448

Rajput A H, Offord K, Beard M C, Burland N T 1984 Epidemiological survey of dementia in parkinsonism and control population. In: Hassler R G, Christ J J (eds) Parkinson-specific motor and mental disorders: role of the pallidum; pathophysiological, bichemical and therapeutic aspects. Advances in neurology, vol 40. Raven Press, New York

Riklan M, Whelihan W, Cullinan T 1976 Levo-dopa and psychometric test performance in Parkinsonism 5 years later. Neurology 26: 173–179

Smith R J 1984 Cognitive effects of general anaesthesia in young and elderly patients. Unpublished M.Phil. thesis, University of Bradford

Sweet R D, McDowell F H, Feigenson J S, Loranger A W, Goodell M 1976 Mental symptoms in Parkinson's disease during chronic treatment with levodopa, Neurology 26: 305–310

Syndulko M, Gildon E R, Hansch E C, Potvin A R, Tourtellotte I M, Potvin J M 1981 Decreased verbal memory associated with anticholnergic treatment in Parkinson's disease patients. International Journal of Neuroscience 14: 61–66

Wexler N 1974 Perceptual-motor, cognitive and emotional characteristics of persons at risk for Huntington's disease. Unpublished doctoral disseration, University of Michigan

Whitehouse P J, Price D L, Struble R G 1982 Alzheimer's disease and senile dementia: loss of neurons in the basal forebrain. Science 215: 1237–1239

Delirium and dementia

INTRODUCTION

Delirium shares many of the cardinal features of dementia. Both are confusional states, with impairment of recent memory and disorientation (though impaired consciousness may contribute as much to disorientation in delirium as dysmnesia). There are characteristic features of the mental state in delirium which may help to distinguish it from dementia, but they are not so pathognomonic nor so univerally present that the diagnosis can confidently be made by them alone. A history from a reliable informant is far more enlightening, and if that is not available it is the course and outcome of the disorder which finally makes the distinction.

How different, fundamentally, are delirium and dementia? There was a move by British geriatricians (Anderson & Carlton-Ashton, 1977) to replace the terms by 'acute' and 'chronic' 'brain failure', suggesting an analogy with other organ failures (heart, liver, kidney) and a continuity between the two states. Implicit in this approach is the hope of reversibility at any stage if the cause (e.g. intermittent heart-block, Livesley, 1977) can be identified and remedied.

In DSM 111 (1980) on the other hand, the Americans seem to have moved in the opposite direction, by replacing the former 'acute' and 'chronic' 'brain syndromes' with 'delirium' and 'dementia', thus espousing a greater differentiation of the two conditions.

How superficial, then, are the similarities between delirium and dementia, and how basic and considerable are the differences? Are these differences qualitative or only quantitive? What is the relationship between two conditions? How wholly reversible is dementia in those who survive? Does delirium sometimes lead directly into dementia, and if so, does it happen more often than by chance, or more often than, say, depressive illness ends in dementia? Or is dementia premonitory of later dementia? Does delirium in old age differ from that in those who are younger? Are there predisposing as well as precipitating factors in delirium? Is dementia itself one of these? Are neurobiochemical differences between the two clinical states known? Do the means whereby delirium is reversed point to similar remedies for dementia? In the rest of this chapter answers to most of these questions will be sought.

CLINICAL COMPARISONS

Roth (1985) has helpfully contrasted the features of delirium and dementia, and his guidelines are used to start this section.

1. Onset: This is always acute in delirium, so that the duration can be stated with some precision to within a day or two, whereas dementia develops so insidiously that it is very hard indeed to know just when normal ageing gave way to pathological deterioration. True, traumatic and anoxic (associated with anaesthetic disaster) dementias start acutely, but degenerative dementia always begins very gradually.

2. Duration: In delirium this is a matter of days, weeks or perhaps one or two months, whereas by the time the demented old person presents as a patient, it is usually apparent that the disorder has been developing over the course of a year or more.

Marsden's (1978) succinct definition of dementia as 'global mental impairment of more than three months' duration in an alert patient' effectively eliminates delirium by its not lasting so long, as wll as by the relative lack of alertness.

3. Variability: Roth makes the point that the level of consciousness fluctuates in delirium, and traditionally what Lipowski (1980) refers to as 'disordered wakefulness' is more evident in morning drowsiness and nocturnal vigilance (though sometimes, perhaps, the effects of the delirium are compounded by the use of tranquillizers and hypnotics, which may not sedate the patient until the end of the night, thus contributing to disruption of the sleep–wake cycle). Variability in the clinical picture characterizes multi-infarct dementia (Hachinski, 1975 — see also Chapter 12) in which confusion tends to be greatest towards evening (the 'sundown' phenomenon) and often least in the middle of a good day. Roth's point, though, is that it is specifically the level of consciousness which fluctuates in delirium.

4. Perceptual disorders: The propensity to illusions and hallucinations is greater in delirium than in dementia. Visual hallucinations predominate over auditory, but auditory hallucinations (e.g. those which plagued Mr Pinfold in Evelyn Waugh's story of his ordeal) and illusions may be troublesome in delirium, whereas in dementia they are negligible. Delirious hallucinations are classically vivid and disturbing (though probably less so in the elderly). Visual hallucinations is the demented are generally more fleeting and less troublesome, but not always; sometimes a regular tendency to twilight apparitions is a bothersome phase in dementia. (In the writer's experience such hallucinations often emanate from the television screen.)

5. Orientation: The demented rarely know the time, day or month, are often ignorant of where they are (beyond 'here') and occasionally fail to

recognize their nearest and dearest, while greeting those they have never met before as family and old friends. Disorientation in delirium is more intermittent — at times the patient knows exactly where he is, whereas at others he is 'all at sea' — and, according to Roth, misidentifications are more colourful and richer.

6. Emotional disorder: Classically the delirious patient is by turns distraught, enraged and euphoric. Perplexity may be painful, fear may turn to terror, and agitation may be extreme. The demented, on the other hand, are apathetic, vacuous, shallow, off-hand or tetchy. The contrast between the two states may, however, be diminished in old age, when the drama of, say, delirium tremens in younger adults is subdued, and composure, or no more than abstracted bemusement, is compatible with acute confusion.

7. Affect: While blunting of affect and disinhibition are associated with Alzheimer's disease, and a rather labile, even mercurial emotionalism with multi- infarct dementia, the affect which surfaces from the clouded consciousness of delirium is pretty normal.

8. Memory: In delirium, registration and recent memory are impaired, but long-term memory is intact. In dementia, while at first there is obedience to Ribot's law ('last in, first out'), in the later stages memory for the more remote past is lost too.

9. Intellectual cohesion: In delirium this is generally preserved, whereas its loss is a cardinal feature of dementia; however, the cohesion can hardly be recognized when the delirium is at its height, but in lucid moments reasoning and problem-solving may be found to be quite well preserved.

10. Response to questions: According to Roth, the tendency in dementia is for errors to be random, while in dementia they tend to be more of commission than omission, with a richer and more extensive confabulation.

Returning now to DSM III (1980), the diagnostic criteria for delirium are:

a. Clouding of consciousness (reduced clarity of awareness of the environment) with reduced capacity to shift, focus and sustain attention to environmental stimuli.

b. At least two of the following:
   (i) Perceptual disturbance — misinterpretations, illusions or hallucinations.
   (ii) Speech at times incoherent.
   (iii) Disturbance of the sleep–waking cycle, with insomnia or daytime drowsiness.
   (iv) Increased of decreased psychomotor activity.

c. Disorientation and memory impariment (if testable).

d. Clinical features that develop over a short period of time (usually hours to days) and tend to fluctuate over the course of a day.

e. Evidence from the history, physical examination or laboratory tests, of a specific arganic factor judged to be aetiologically related to the disturbance.

These criteria will now be scrutinized for their specificity for delirium.

a. Clouding of consciousness is the cardinal feature of the mental state of the delirious. Rabins & Folstein (1982), rating patients on a continuum from accessible to inaccessible, used it alone as their means of classifying cognitively impaired patients as delirious or demented, and the different outcomes of the two groups validated their distinction. However, the sensitivity of this sign must be doubted, for it is by no means always present in confused old people who on other grounds are deemed more likely to be delirious than demented. Even the absolute specificity of the sign may be questioned, at least to be extent that demented patients have often been subjected to tranquillizers and sedatives. And, as Roth states, clouding may be hard to evaluate in the presence of the gross cognitive deficits of severe dementia.

b. None of the four forms of disorder listed, i.e. perceptual disturbance, incoherent speech, disorder of the sleep–waking cycle, altered psychosomatic activity — is confined to delirium. All, to a greater or lesser extent, are also found in dementia.

c. Disorientation and memory impairment are virtually always found in dementia.

d. No underlying organic factor is detected in a substantial minority (say 25%) of confusional states in the elderly which prove reversible. Lipowski (1983) draws attention to the term 'pseudodelirium', proposed by Goldney (1979) to cover the confusional features of some acute functional mental disorders apparently unrelated to bodily illness. Mania in old age, for example, may mimic delirium in the early stages. This phenomenon is not confined to the elderly, but is characteristic of puerperal psychoses (Jansson, 1964). A somatic factor may well be operating here, but it is not manifest as somatic illness.

Quite a few old people, however, show no functional mental illness as well as no bodily malady underlying their acute confusion. A small cerebral infarct is often invoked, but neurological signs are fleeting or absent.

Finally, it is 'd', the short history, which undoubtedly should distinguish delirium from dementia. It is not only the short course but the acute onset which separates the two. But it is not quite clear that this is a qualitative rather than a quantitative difference.

UNDERLYING ABNORMALITIES

In both states the clinical condition reflects neuronal dysfunction, presumably neurotransmitter depletion and other neurobiochemical changes. There must be differences in the nature of the factors which occasion delirium and the state of the brain which they afflict, and the factors and state of the brain in dementia, but are these differences in kind rather than degree? The answer is not self-evident.

We know less of the pathology of the brain of someone who has died in delirium than of the demented brain, and there are problems in distinguishing what is intrinsic to the delirium itself from what has caused it.

The electroencephalograph is of some little help. In both disorders it is deranged, and though slowing in delirium is generally more striking than in dementia, where occasionally recordings are normal, the differences are, again, quantitative rather than qualitative. Pro & Wells (1977) make the point that, while diffuse slowing is a feature of delirium in severely ill patients with reduced awareness and arousal, it may not be if the patient is overactive (as in delirium tremens). Rabins & Folstein (1982) found diffusely slow EEGs in 81% of their delirious elderly subjects and in only 33% of their delirious — a highly significant difference; but a third is a not inconsiderable minority.

Incidentally, they also found a comparably significant difference in body temperature, the delirious being feverish whereas the demented were not, and in pulse rate, which was higher in the delirious. These findings seem likely to be due to the illness causing the delirium, but the authors argue that they could reflect a primary brain disturbance.

Computerized axial tomography is of limited value. One might expect little or no abnormality in delirium (unless the cause is a cerebral infarct or space-occupying lesion), while cortical atrophy is usual in dementia. But 10% of the elderly demented have normal CT scans (Jacoby & Levy, 1980), 10% of seemingly normal old people have cortical atrophy, and as delirium occurs most readily in those already demented, there may be cortical atrophy and ventricular dilatation reflecting an underlying dementia.

Positron emission tomography, though never likely to be widely available and difficult in any case to use on a restless delirious patient, has research potential in elucidating differences in regional blood flow and oxygen and glucose utilization in the two (or two sorts of) disorders (Friedman et al, 1983; Possilli et al, 1982).

REVERSIBILITY

While it is generally true that delirious patients who survive make a full mental recovery while the demented do not, this is not invariably so. Delirium due to cerebral hypoxia during hypotensive surgery, following cardiac arrest or carbon monoxide poisoning or associated with meningitis or encephalitis (admittedly, not so very common in the elderly), may go on to dementia, and the dysmnesic Korsakow's syndrome follows Wernicke's encephalopathy.

Prognostic studies of delirium are unfortunately few and far between. That by Rabins & Folstein (1982) looked at survival a year after case identification (finding a much higher mortality in the delirious than in the demented) but not at mental state. Bedford (1959), however, found that 5%

of the two-thirds of delirious elderly patients who did not die within a month remained confused after six months, so many have become (or already have been) demented. The Pearces (1979) noted that 48% of elderly patients referred to a neurology service, compared with 13% of presenile patients, had presented with a 'toxic-confusional state', but concluded than an underlying dementia had been triggered by anoxia, infection, cardiac failure or some comparable physical affliction. It is unclear that delirium unmasks or arouses a dormant dementia, but it is commonly observed that when care shifts from home to hospital in an old person whose disabilities, though unlabelled dementia, have been burdensome discharge may be resisted, and the diagnosis is then made part of the process of obtaining continuing institutional care.

There seems therefore to be a need for up-to-date prospective prognostic studies which will determine how fully delirious old people recover, relating outcome to the severity, duration and cause of the delirium, and whether delirium is, sooner or later, a risk factor for subsequent dementia as dementia is known to be for delirium (Royal College of Physicians, London, 1981).

AGE AS A RISK FACTOR

It is often stated that the very young as well as the very old are liable to delirium, and this is many parents' experience, but it might be an aspect of the suspectibility of children to infectious diseases which today's adults in developed countries are generally spared. Their forebears, of course, subject to typhoid, cholera, smallpox and pneumonia without recourse to antibiotics, knew delirium, sometimes as a prelude to their deaths, and it has been suggested that this almost universal experience contributed to the imagery of the literature of those times: the alleged heightened sensibility and creativity of the tuberculous might have been in part the consequence of sub-acute or intermittent delirium.

An important factor in the apparently higher morbidity for delirium of the elderly (noted in a third of those over 65 admitted to hospital in Hodkinson's 1973 study) might be their greater morbidity for serious physical illness. However, Burrows et al (1985) have demonstrated that mental impairment after cataract extraction is significantly greater (though transitory) in an older group (41 elderly with a mean age of 74) than a younger (9 with a mean age of 50). Sorting shapes, recall of an address after ten minutes, digit span and random reaction time were all significantly worse in the elderly on post-operative days 1–3. It is, too, common knowledge that old people are more liable to post-operative delirium than young. This greater morbidity for delirium in the elderly is matched, of course, by a greater morbidity for dementia, increasing with advancing age over 65 (Kay et al, 1970).

DELIRIUM IN OLD AGE

The chief risk factor for delirium in younger adults in the developing countries (and, indeed, an important factor in dementia in the same population) is alcoholism, through the direct effects of alcohol upon the brain, thiamine deficiency and the failure of the cirrhotic liver. Classical delirium tremens in this age-group is unlike delirium in the elderly in several ways. It is more acute, dramatic and frightening, with richer imagery and heightened activity and arousal rather than clouding of consciousness. The EEG does not show diffuse slow activity (Allahyari et al, 1976). The picture may reflect increased central noradrenergic activity.

This vivid picture is not typical in old age, however, when delirium may have to be looked for under circumstances when it might be expected, as it does not boldly declare itself. Pitt & Silver (1980) found that, in patients admitted to a joint geriatric:shpsychiatric unit in a general teaching hospital, delirium had often been missed by the registrars (residents) in internal geriatric medicine, This may help to explain why, as Lipowski (1983) has demonstrated, delirium has been neglected as a topic for research: in comparison with dementia, it is transitory and too often unobtrusive, overshadowed by physical illness.

MECHANISMS

There is evidence that the final common pathway of those stresses and strains which end in delirium is an impaired central cholinergic system. Blass & Plum (1983) have suggested that impairment of cerebral oxidative metabolism especially affects the synthesis of acetyl choline, and Stephens (1967), Kounis (1974), Heiser & Wilbert (1974), Summers (1978), Tune et al (1981) and Blazer et al (1983) have shown how readily delirium is induced by anticholinergic drugs used as eye drops, in anaesthesia, by anti-Parkinsonian drugs and by antidepressants. Grimley Evans (1982) sees delirium as an exacerbation of neural noise, against which inputs from the world outside are distorted, with effects upon perception, memory and attention. Ultimately this increase in noise is due to disordered neurotransmitter activity from anoxic or toxic effects on neurones. He suggests that in the elderly neural noise is already somewhat increased anyway, and that blood–brain barrier to some noxious substances is impaired.

Delirium induced by anticholinergic drugs may be temporarily reversed by the anticholinesterase physostigmine (Duvoisin & Katz, 1968; Greene, 1971; Baldessarini, 1975; Summers & Reich, 1979) while Lipowski (1980) reports its effectiveness in alcohol and cimetidine-induced delirium too. Smith & Swash (1979) incidentally, noted a transitory amelioration of intrusion errors in dementia from the use of physostigmine.

Itil & Fink (1966) proposed that imbalance of central cholinergic and adrenergic mechanisms underlies delirium, and increased noradrenergic activity has been found in delirium tremens during alcohol withdrawal

(Giacobini et al, 1960; Hawley et al, 1981), while Banks & Vojnik (1978) have also implicated serotonin in the disorder. Petrie & Ban (1977) have reported relief of delirium in some old people by the administration of propranolol, presumably exerting its beta-adrenergic blocking effect centrally. While acetylcholine is the neurotransmitter most deranged in Alzheimer's disease, there are significant impairments in other neurotransmitter systems, notably the noradrenergic, too (Rosser, 1982; see also Chapter 8).

Lipowski (1980) describes 'disorder of wakefulness' as the second core feature of delirium (the first being disorder of cognition) and points not only to the similarity of the sense of unreality, illusions and hallucinations in the delirious to the dreamer awake, but also to the reversals of the sleep–waking cycle, with sleepiness by day and restless insomnia at night. The waking dream has been related to stage-1 REM sleep from malfunction of serotonergic neurones in the raphe nuclei and/or noradrenergic neurones in the locus caeruleus (Hishikawa et al, 1981). These structures are selectively damaged in Alzheimer's disease (see Chapter 7) and to this has been attributed the phenomenon of nocturnal delirium in dementia. Reversal of the sleep–waking cycle is commonplace in dementia, as many nurses and family carers will attest, and is not wholly to be explained by the delayed action of hypnotics, with long half-lives, administered too late. Here then is another characteristic shared by delirium and dementia, differing perhaps in degree and duration but not in kind.

Delirium is not wholly to be explained by the central or systemic disorder which has brought it about. While it is as true that given enough trauma, toxaemia or metabolic upset anyone could become delirious as that anyone under certain circumstances will have a fit, thresholds vary widely, and age alone cannot be the critical factor. It is sometimes as interesting to speculate why one very old lady with, say, a severe urinary tract infection does not become delirious as to observe how another, of like age or younger, with no more severe on infection, does. Do the other factors involved have a bearing on dementia too? A prospective study of old people about to undergo major surgery might elucidate these factors.

Finally, the clinical picture of delirium can be produced by a wide variety of diseases and disorders, but does not vary much according to aetiology: it is a 'final common pathway' phenonenon. Likewise it is known that dementia is not the consequence of a single pathology, and it is now postulated that there are two forms of Alzheimer's disease (Roth, 1985). But may it too not be a 'final common pathway' disorder? A variety of factors — genetic, degenerative, environmental, infective, immunological, metabolic, endocrine, possibly even psychological — may then act together in diverse proportions and degrees ultimately to present clinically as the dementia when a certain threshold of neurological (neuronal) damage has been exceeded. Delirium may thus present a kind of model of dementia, and there may be more profit in studying the similarities between the two forms of confusional state than in emphasizing the difference.

CONCLUSION AND SUMMARY

It is most important to recognize delirium and to distinguish it from dementia. The identification and energetic treatment of the disorder underlying the delirium may make all the difference to the prognosis. But to achieve a greater understanding of dementia, the many close resemblances between the two confusional syndromes should be noted. Clinically, apart from the short history and the level of consciousness, they are rather alike, and though diffuse slowing on the EEG tachycardia and a raised body temperature are more often associated with delirium, they do not absolutely distinguish it from dementia. The mental state of both is largely determined by impairment of neurotransmitter systems, chiefly but not exclusively the cholinergic, and though the neurones are more likely to survive in delirium, and there is no marked excess of senile plaques and neurofibrillary tangles in that disorder, not all the delirious who survive the acute illness recover normal mental function, nor are all dementias irreversible. Dementia patients are especially susceptible to delirium, and the delirious may be to the development, sooner or later, of dementia: prognostic studies are needed. Delirium is a 'final common pathway' phenomenon with a variety of aetiologies. So, by analogy, may be Alzheimer's disease.

REFERENCES

Allahyari H, Deisenhammer E, Weiser G 1976 CSF levels of norepinephrine during alcohol withdrawal. Psychiatry Clinic., (Basel) 9: 21–31
Anderson W F and Carlton-Ashton J R (eds) 1977 Brain failure in old age. Age and Ageing supplement
Banks C M, Vojnik M 1978 Comparative simultaneous measurement of CSF 5-hydroxyindoleacetic acid and blood serotinin levels in delirium tremens and clozapine-induced delirious reaction. Journal of Neurology, Neurosurgery and Psychiatry 41: 420–424
Bedford P D 1959 General medical aspects of confusional states in elderly people. British Medical Journal ii: 185–188
Blass J P, Plum F 1983 Metabolic encephalopathies. In: Katzman R, Terry R D (eds) The neurology of ageing. Davis, Philadelphia
Blazer D G, Federspiel C F, Ray W A The risk of anticholinergic toxicity in the elderly: a study of prescribing practices in two populations. Journal of Gerontology 38: 31–35
Burrows J, Briggs R S, Elkington A R 1985 Cataract extraction and confusion in elderly patients. Journal of Clinical and Experimental Gerontology 7: 51–70
Diagnostic and Statistical Manual Of Mental Disorders 3rd edn, 1980 Americal Psychiatric Association, Washington DC
Duvoisin R C, Katz 1968 Reversal of central anticholinergic syndrome in man by physostigmine. Journal of the American Medical Association 290: 1963–5
Friedland R P 1983 Regional cerebral metabolic alterations in dementia of the Alzheimer type: positron emission tomography with [18F] fluorodeoxyglucose. Journal of Computer Assisted Tomography 7: 590
Giacobini E, Izikowitz S, Wegmann A 1960 Urinary norepinephrine and epinephrine excretion in delirium tremens. Archives of General Psychiatry 3: 289–296
Goldney R 1979 Pseudodelirium. Medical Journal of Australia 1: 630
Granacher R P, Baldessarini R J 1975 Physostigmine. Its use in acute anticholinergic syndrome with antidepressant and antiparkinsonian drugs. Archives of General Psychiatry 32: 375–380
Greene L T 1971 Physostigmine treatment of anticholinergic drug delirium in post-operative patients. Anaesthesia and Analgesia 50: 222–226

Grimley Evans J 1982 The psychiatric aspects of physical disease. In: Levy R, Post F (eds) The psychiatry of late life. Blackwell, Oxford

Hachinski V C 1975 Cerebral blood flow in dementia. Archives of Neurology 32: 632–637

Hawley R J 1981 CSF levels of norepinephrine during alcohol withrawal. Archives of Neurology 38: 289–292

Heiser J F, Wilbert D A 1974 Reversal of delirium induced by tricyclic antidepressant drugs with physostigmine. American Journal of Psychiatry 131: 1275–7

Hishikawa Y 1981 A dissociated sleep state 'stage 1-REM' and its relation to delirium. In: Baldy-Moulinier M (eds) Actualités en médicine expérimentale. Euromed, Montpellier

Hodkinson H M 1973 Mental impairment in the elderly. Journal of the Royal College of Physicians, London 7: 305–317

Itil T, Fink M 1966 Anticholinergic drug-induced delirium: experimental modification, quantitative EEG and behavioural correlations. Journal of Nervous and Mental Disorders 143: 492–507

Jacoby R J, Levy R 1980 Computed tomography in the elderly: 2. Senile dementia: diagnosis and functional impairment. British Journal of Psychiatry 136: 256–259

Jansson B 1964 Psychic insufficiencies associated with childbearing. Acta Psychiatrica Scandinarica Suppl 172

Kay D W K, Bergmann K, Foster E M, Mckechnie A A, Roth M 1970 Mental illness and hospital usage in the elderly: a random sample followed up. Comprehensive Psychiatry 2: 1

Kounis N G 1974 Atropine dye-drops delirium. Canadian Medical Association Journal 110: 759

Lipowski Z J 1983 Transient cognitive disorders (delirium, acute confusional states) in the elderly. American Journal of Psychiatry 140: 1426–1434

Livesley B 1977 The pathogenesis of brain failure in old age. In: Anderson W F, Carlton-Ashton J R (eds) Brain failure in old age. Age and Ageing supplement

Mardsen C 1978 The diagnosis of dementia. In: Isaacs A and Post F (eds) Studies in geriatric psychiatry. Wiley, New York

Pearce J M S, Pearce I 1979 The nosology of Alzheimer's disease, early recognition of potentially reversible deficits. In: Glen A I M, Whalley L J (eds) Churchill Livingstone, Edinburgh

Petrie W M, Ban T A 1981 Propanolol in organic agitation. Lancet i:324

Pitt B, Silver C P S 1980 The combined approach to geriatrics and psychiatry: evaluation of a joint unit in a teaching hospital district. Age and Ageing 9: 9–16

Pozzilli C 1982 Positron emission tomography in vascular dementia: a study with the 0–15 inhalation technique. Journal of Neurological Science 26:93

Pro J D, Wells C E 1977 The use of EEG in diagnosis of delirium. Diseases of the Nervous System 38: 804–808

Rabins P V, Folstein M 1982 Delirium and dementia: diagnostic criteria and fatality rates. British Journal Psychiatry 140: 149–153

Rossor M 1982 Neurotransmitter in CNS disease: dementia. Lancet ii: 1200–04

Roth M 1985 Convergence and cohesion of recent neurobiological findings in relation to Alzheimer's disease and their bearing on its aetiological basis. In: Bergener M, Ermini M, Stahlein H B (eds) Thresholds in ageing. Academic Press, London

Roth M 1985 Correlation of neuropathological and clinical findings in dementia. Lecture given at 13th International Congress of Gerontology, New York

Royal college of Physicians Of London 1981 Organic mental impairment in the elderly: implications for research, education and the provision of services

Smith C M, Swash M 1979 Possible biochemical basis of memory disorder in Alzheimer's disease. Age and Ageing 8: 289–293

Stephens D A 1976 Psychotoxic effects of benzhexol hydrochloride (Artane®). British Journal of Psychiatry 113: 213–218

Summers W K, 1978 A clinical method of estimating risk of drug-induced delirium. Life Sciences 22: 1511–1516

Summers W K, Reich T C 1979 Delirium after cataract surgery: review of 2 cases. American Journal of Psychiatry 136: 386–391

Tune L E, Holland A, Folstein M, Damlouji N F, Gardner T J, Coyle L T 1981 Association of post-operative delirium with raised serum levels of anticholinergic drugs. Lancet ii 651–653

Depression and dementia

INTRODUCTION

The relationship of depression and dementia has become a subject of increasing in recent years. Diagnostic difficulties are presented by patients who have both affective disorder and memory impairment, seen both in depression and dementia, and evidence from the current literature suggests that the relationship between these two disorders is complex (Feinberg, 1984; Post, 1975). This chapter has been divided into four sections: the first reviews recent findings regarding cognitive deficits in depression; the second examines current conceptions of the clinical phenomenon of pseudodementia; the third presents the latest themes regarding cerebral changes occurring in the depressed elderly; and the final section presents recent findings relevant to depression in the course of dementia.

COGNITIVE DEFICITS IN DEPRESSION

Depression is accompanied by a number of alterations in cognitive function. In the clinical setting, these alterations are similar to, and sometimes indistinguishable from, the changes produced by the progressive dementias (Caine, 1981; Weingartner et al, 1981). There is a growing literature documenting the deficits in cognition exhibited by patients with depression, although at present there is insufficient evidence to support either the notion that these deficits have a characteristic pattern or that they can be reliably distinguished from the cognitive deficits of dementia (McAllister, 1981).

A number of studies have assessed the effects of depression on verbal learning and memory. Henry et al (1973) studied memory function in a group of patients with affective disorder and found depressed patients showed impaired performance on serial and free-recall verbal learning tasks. They also found that depressives had no impairment in short-term memory (STM) and concluded that, because these patients had intact STM but impaired serial learning ability, the memory deficit was best viewed as an inability to shift information from short- to long-term memory storage.

251

He did not compare learning in depressives to that in dements and therefore did not draw conclusions about the difference between the two groups.

Sternberg & Jarvik (1976) studied a group of hospitalized depressed patients before and after recovery to try to clarify the nature of memory deficit in depression. Unlike Henry et al (1973), they found that depressed patients had impairment of short-term memory improved as the depressed state remitted.

Whitehead (1973) tried to distinguish between the learning and memory impairment of depression and dementia by comparing results of learning and memory tests. Depressed patients, while both actively depressed and when assessed following recovery, scored significantly higher on tests of verbal learning than did demented patients. Depressed patients did better on rote memory, logical memory and retrieval by learning tests. There was no difference in depressed and demented patients on tests of digit span and delayed recall. Recovered depressives scored better than actively depressed patients on the rote memory tasks. Whitehead found that depressed patients made different types of errors from demented patients. In particular, she found that while depressives made more transposition errors, dements made more random and false positive errors. Omission errors occurred at about the same frequency in both groups. Whitehead felt that her data supported the idea that verbal learning impairment, though present in both depression and dementia, is of different origin in the two diseases.

Cavanaugh & Wettstein (1983) administered the Beck Depression Inventory, a depression scale, and the Mini-Mental State (MMS) examination, a brief scale used to assess cognitive impairment, to 289 randomly selected medical inpatients. In contrast to the studies cited above, they found no significant relationship between the severity of depression and cognitive dysfunction as measured by their scales, although the moderately to severely depressed group scored lower on the MMS exam than normals. They concluded that one should not assume that measurable cognitive deficits in a depressed person are necessarily caused by depression. Their study suggests the limitations of relying upon the MMS examination alone to assess the cognitive deficits of depression.

Some recent investigations have sought to study the nature of cognitive impairment in depression. Weingartner et al (1981) attempted to assess how depressed patients process and organize information. Using a series of word-learning and recall tests, they found that depressed subjects had difficulty learning minimally structured information and using information encoding strategies that would aid in later recall. On the other hand, they found that when subjects were presented with more structured information, the depressives were able to learn and recall in an essentially normal way. Weingartner et al concluded that depressed patients suffer an encoding impairment that results in incomplete and unstable learning, and reported that these changes are similar to those seen in Alzheimer's disease and in normal ageing.

Cohen et al (1982) used motor and memory tasks to assess motivational factors in depressive learning. They found that the degree of motor and cognitive deficits a patient exhibited correlated with severity of depression, and they found the greatest impairment involved motor and memory tasks requiring sustained effort. They felt that their results challenged the notion that there were specific memory deficits in depression that were separate from deficits of motivation, drive and attention. They hypothesized that depressed patients exhibit an impairment of a 'central motivational state'.

One additional factor complicating both research and clinical evaluation of the elderly depressed patient is a recent report suggesting that elderly depressives with prior history of electroconvulsive therapy (ECT) may demonstrate worse cognitive functioning when depression recurs than elderly depressives who have never received ECT. Pettinati & Bonner (1984) retrospectively assessed the cognitive status of 61 patients with major depressive disorder and schizoaffective disorder. Twenty patients were age 65 or greater (mean age 69.7 years), and 41 patients were under 65 (mean age 41.7 years). Using the Train Making B test from the Halstead Reitan Neuropsychological Battery, they found that elderly depressed patients with a history of ECT were more likely to show cognitive impairment than either elderly depressives without a history of ECT or younger patients with or without an ECT history. Their findings suggest that the cognitive dysfunction of depression in the elderly may sometimes result from past treatment for depression as well as from current depression. Thus one should carefully inquire into a cognitively impaired elderly patient's history of past psychiatric treatment as well as into his/her past psychiatric history in order to adequately assess the probability that a patient's memory deficits are due to depression.

PSEUDODEMENTIA

The concept of 'pseudodementia' has appeared increasingly in the literature of psychiatry over the past thirty years. The first use of the term is usually ascribed to Madden et al (1952) who, in describing a series of older persons with non-dementing psychoses, noted that 10% of 300 patients ages 45 and older in their psychiatric unit had 'pseudodementia'. The pseudodementia he described was characterized by disorientation and impaired recent memory retention, calculation and judgment. Madden et al noted that the pseudodementia picture disappeared following short-term intensive treatment.

Nine years later, Kiloh (1961) presented a series of 10 patients with a variety of psychiatric disorders whom he described as pseudodemented.

Four of the patients he described carried diagnoses of 'Ganser state' or 'hysteria' of one sort or another and did not demonstrate deficits that would have been mistaken for dementia by a knowledgeable psychiatrist. The other 6 patients had affective disorders: 3 had endogenous depression, 1 had 'depression as a symptom of paraphrenia', 1 had mania and 2 had uncertain diagnoses (though in retrospect they appear to have had major depression with psychotic features). Kiloh made no distinctions between the pseudo-dementia of the first and second groups of patients. Indeed, his paper seems to have been intended primarily as a series of case presentations intended to illustrate a curious symptom, rather than an attempt to describe defini-tively pseudodementia as presently conceived.

Since the 1970s, however, the term pseudodementia has come to be used primarily to designate a clinical picture in which a psychiatric disorder produces symptoms that simulate dementia caused by structural change in the brain. The emphasis has been on understanding how to distinguish patients with symptoms amenable to psychiatric treatment from patients whose dementias have a toxic, metabolic or aetiologically uncertain but progressive dementia (McAllister, 1983; Caine, 1981; Wells, 1979). The focus has shifted away from the factitious or hysteria-based pseudodementia.

Pseudodementia, though most commonly associated with depression in elderly patients, has been described in a number of different psychiatric disorders, including mania, hypomania, dissociative reaction, conversion reaction, Ganser's syndrome, post-traumatic neurosis, personality disorders and schizophrenia (Caine, 1981; Good, 1981; Wells, 1979; Kiloh, 1962). Though 'pseudodementia' is used to mean different things by different authors, a reasonable and clear definition has been offered by Caine (1981), who defined the syndrome as one in which: 1. there is intellectual impair-ment of a patient with a psychiatric disorder; 2. a patient exhibits deficits on neuropsychological testing similar to those seen in neuropathologically-based dementias; and 3. the impairment is reversible and there is no evidence that a structural neurological change is responsible for the impair-ment. This definition, though not universally accepted, is a useful one.

Nonetheless, the term pseudodementia has become increasingly contro-versial (McAllister, 1983; Shraberg, 1979; Folstein & McHugh, 1978). As used by some, pseudodementia defines the condition of patients who have a psychiatric disorder and appear demented because of the conscious or unconscious desire of the patient to present as having a psychiatric disorder. The term is also applied to the condition of individuals with psychiatric disorders who appear demented because of inattentiveness and apathy, as well as to those who reveal significant impairment of cognitive function on objective psychological testing, but whose impairment resolves with treat-ment of the underlying psychiatric disorder.

Studies of the reliability of the clinical diagnosis of dementia have indi-cated that depression and dementia are frequently confused. They show that a significant number of patients with affective disorder are misdiagnosed as having a degenerative or vascular dementia. Nott and Fleminger retrospectively examined 35 patients who had received a diagnosis of presenile dementia. Of this group, 20 did not prove to have degenerative dementia on follow-up 5–23 years after the original diagnosis, and all of the 20 patients had psychiatric disorders of some type. Three (9%) of the original group were depressed. The others carried diagnoses of anxiety state, somatic symptoms without organic basis, hysterical reaction and paranoid reaction. Psychometric testing and electroencephalography (EEG) did not accurately predict who would deteriorate and who would not. Only pneumoencephalograms correlated with future deterioration.

Ron et al (1979) retrospectively followed up a group of 52 patients ages 42–64 discharged from the hospital with a diagnosis of presenile dementia. Sixteen patients, or 31% of the original group, had been misdiagnosed on follow-up 5 to 15 years later. Retrospective diagnoses were made on the misdiagnosed patients, and 5 (31% of the misdiagnosed patients) appeared to have had affective disorders, and additional 2 (13%) appeared to have had mixed affective disorders and dementia. Two other patients were retrospectively diagnosed as having had paranoid psychosis or schizophrenia disorders.

Marsden & Harrison (1972), in their study of 106 patients referred to a neurological hospital with a presumptive diagnosis of dementia, found that 15 (14%) had no demonstrable intellectual impairment on psychological testing, and of these 15, 8 (53% of patients without intellectual impairment) were depressed. Smith & Kiloh (1981), reported that, of 200 patients referred to a neuropsychiatric institute, 20 (10%) had psychiatric disorders. Of these, one half had depressions that had produced impaired concentration and lack of interest, 2 patients were hypomanic, 7 were schizophrenic and 2 carried uncertain psychiatric diagnoses. Garcia et al (1981) reported that 26 of 100 patients referred to their outpatient dementia clinic by family physicians had been misdiagnosed, and that of these patients 15 (57% of misdiagnosed patients) were depressed.

There are regional variations in the misdiagnosis of progressive dementias as well. Duckworth & Ross (1975) demonstrated that psychiatrists in the Queens district of New York tended to heavily overdiagnose organic mental disorders in elderly patients with affective disorder that could be diagnosed by a standardized diagnostic instrument. This tendency toward overdiagnosing dementia was not present when diagnostic patterns of the Queens physicians were compared to that of their counterparts in Toronto and London.

Wells (1979) identified a series of clinical features that help to distinguish pseudodementia from dementia, organizing them under the headings of clinical course, complaints and clinical behaviour, and memory and intellectual deficits. Typical of the course, Wells wrote, are: a fairly distinct date of onset, short duration of symptoms prior to clinical presentation, rapid progression, previous psychiatric history, and an intense awareness by the family of the severity of the patient's impairment. Complaints and clinical behaviour of pseudodemented patients are characterized by detailed accounts of intellectual decline, poor effort on psychological testing, affective change, early loss of social skills and lack of nocturnal exacerbation of dementia ('sundowning'). On memory testing, patients commonly give 'don't know' answers, exhibit equally severe recent and remote memory loss, have memory gaps for particular events or times, and exhibit variability in performance on psychological testing.

Though the above features are helpful in distinguishing pseudodementia from dementia, a number of investigators have shown that there is virtually no clinical finding that will inevitably distinguish between dementia and pseudodementia. In contrast to the general impression that pseudodementia patients generally have an abrupt onset of symptoms, Wells (1979) noted that only 1 in 10 of the patients he studied had an abrupt onset of symptoms; the others had symptoms of insidious onset that were slowly progressive. His patients exhibited disorientation, confusion about the purpose of their hospital stay, poor concentration, distractibility and inability to recall familiar pieces of information. McAllister et al (1982b) have described 4 patients, 2 with coexisting dementia and 2 without, who presented with depressive pseudodementia that was virtually indistinguishable from progressive dementia. In all 4 of their cases, the primary reason for suspecting psychiatric disorder was the short duration of symptoms and a past history of psychiatric disorder, clinical features which Wells (1979) & Good (1981) found were not invariably present in pseudodementia patients. The cases McAllister et al reported did not have pronounced affective change, did not reply with 'don't know' answers, did not have good attention span, and did not exhibit inconsistencies in the mental status exam.

Thus, although certain features of clinical presentation can help the clinician to distinguish dementia of neurological dysfunction from pseudodementia, no single clinical symptom or sign is invariably present, and the clinician must therefore maintain a suspicion of the presence of pseudodementia in order to diagnose correctly the condition at an early point in the course of the disorder.

CEREBRAL CHANGES IN DEPRESSION

The issue of whether are similarities in the nature of depression and dementia that account for the dementia-like syndrome of depression remains open. There are two major questions about cerebral changes in depression. First, are there brain changes in depression that parallel those present in the progressive dementias? And, second, can the current understanding of the biological basis of depression be used to distinguish between depressive and vascular or degenerative dementias where the clinical presentation is difficult to interpret?

The question of how organic brain changes in elderly patients are related to the emergence of affective disorders in late life is old and as yet unsettled. Kay (1955) looked at a large group of patients with affective disorders of both early (prior to age 60) and late (after age 60) onset and found no evidence to support an aetiological association between 'cerebral degeneration' and late-onset affective disorder. Post (1962) found that a large number of the 96 elderly depressives he studied had cerebrovascular disorders, but he concluded that, though the cerebral disease was a precipitating factor for affective disorder, there was no evidence that affective disorder and brain disease were otherwise aetiologically linked. More specifically, he affirmed that on the basis of his evidence there was no evidence that 'depression of old age might be a prodromal symptom of an otherwise as yet sub-clinical process'.

In the same year that Post's study was published, another paper by Kay (1962) reported follow-up of 154 elderly patients with either early or late-onset affective disorder or paraphrenia. He examined the course of their illness from 1931–1937 until 1956 or their death, whichever came first. He concluded that cerebrovascular disease may play a part in the onset of affective illness in a minority of cases of late affective disorder and that it might precipitate a relapse in manic depressive disorder.

More recent studies have continued to produce diverse conclusions. Cawley et al (1973) studied a group of depressed elderly patients who were challenged with a barbiturate to assess their sedation threshold. Working under the assumption that patients with a lower sedation threshold (a value determined by the amount of intravenous amobarbital needed to cause the patient to exhibit specified symptoms of sedation) have decreased cortical arousability, they found that the older a patient was at the time of onset of affective disorder, the lower was his/her threshold as compared to age-matched controls, and the smaller was the increase in threshold following treatment for depression. They felt their results lent weight to the notion that cerebral functioning in the aged is impaired and therefore the aged are more prone to depression.

A similar study by Davies et al (1978) compared the sedation threshold in depressed and demented patients. Although they found a major difference in the sedation threshold of demented and depressed patients, they were unable to confirm the association of lower threshold with late-onset depression. Neither was there a significant change in pre- and post-treatment thresholds for depressed patients — thus calling into question this piece of evidence for a change in cerebral arousal during depression.

Computerized tomography (CT) has provided evidence supporting the notion that some depressed patients have organic changes of aetiological significance. Jacoby et al (1980) studied clinical and CT scan data in series of 41 elderly depressives in comparison with 50 age, sex and social status matched controls. They isolated a subgroup of patients with late-onset depression who had large ventricular size. The authors viewed their findings as evidence of a relationship between depression and cerebral atrophy in non-demented patients. A follow-up study of the same patient group by Jacoby et al (1981) found increased mortality among the subgroup of depressives with ventricular enlargement. Jacoby et al (1983) also found that the depressed subgroup with ventricular dilatation had a high incidence of low Hounsfield Units (HU), a CT numerical figure thought to be related to tissue density. This finding of low HU in a subgroup of depressed patients also lends weight to the idea that, in some elderly depressed patients without progressive dementia, a structural change is associated with the emergence of depression.

Can we use our knowledge of cerebral changes in depression to distinguish between depression and dementia? Several approaches have been taken. A number of investigators have attempted to use the dexamethasone suppression test (DST), a neuroendocrine measure, to distinguish between depression and dementia, though its usefulness of the DST for this purpose is as yet unsettled.

McAllister et al (1982a) described two patients, ages 75 and 72, who presented with marked cognitive deficits. Both had recent onset of mental status change, and both had previous psychiatric histories. In both patients, a DST revealed cortisol non-suppression. The patients both received e.c.t. and improved markedly in affective and cognitive state. In one case, post-DST cortisol values returned to normal after treatment. In the other they did not.

Two other reports published the same year, however, challenged the usefulness of the DST in distinguishing depression from degenerative dementia. Spar & Gerner (1982) administered the DST to 17 consecutive demented patients at their facility. None met DSM-III criteria for major depressive episode, none had 'prominent and relatively dysphoric mood', and only one had a history of depression. All but one carried a diagnosis of vascular or degenerative dementia; the exception had Parkinson's disease with dementia. The patients were drug-free except for haloperidol, and none had any of the medical exclusion criteria that would invalidate the DST. Nine of 17 patients had 4 pm cortisol values greater than the 5.0 nmol/l, said to be characteristic of melancholia, a result which casts doubt on the specificity of the DST for depression in patients who are demented.

Following this report was a similar one by Raskind (1982) in which the DST results of 15 non-depressed patients carrying a diagnosis of primary degenerative dementia were compared to those of 15 age and sex-matched controls. Using a higher than required cortisol cut-off value for non-suppression (6.0 nmol/l), Raskind et al found that 7 of 15 dementia patients and no controls were non-suppressors, a finding that reached statistical significance. All of Raskind's demented subjects, however, had had dementia of long duration (mean duration 7.4 years) and had severe intellectual impairment.

In spite of the above studies, however, Carnes et al (1983) reported that in their examination of DST results in 7 elderly non-depressed demented patients, none had abnormal DST results. Carnes accounted for discrepancies from earlier studies by suggesting that her subjects were outpatients or were less severely demented than those in the previous studies.

Similarly, Jenike & Albert (1984) studied 18 non-depressed patients with dementia and found that a group of 13 patients with less severe dementia produced an abnormal DST result in only one instance, while a group of five patients with more severe dementia produced an abnormal DST result in four or five instances. They concluded that the DST could be used to discriminate between depression and dementia in mildly but not in severely impaired demented patients. But Jenike et al did not report the duration of dementia in the 'moderate to severe' impairment group and used a different measure for rating the severity of dementia than other investigators, thus leaving in question the value of DST in distinguishing affective from degenerative dementias.

Several studies have also looked at the way in which depression and dementia affect event related potentials (ERPs). Buchsbaum et al (1971) suggested that, on the basis of their study of average evoked responses (AERs) to visual stimuli, patients with unipolar depression tended to show decreases in AER amplitude with increasing stimulus intensity and therefore tended to be 'stimulus reducers'. They were thus distinguishable from both normal and bipolar patients on the basis of AER.

In 1971 Levy measured evoked potentials in elderly demented and depressed patients and found that demented subjects tended to have prolonged latencies of AER to somatosensory stimuli. In 1979, Levy and his co-workers (Henderson et al, 1979) published a study comparing auditory and somatosensory AERs in depressed, demented, mixed depressed and demented, and normal subjects. They found that demented patients had significantly longer AER latency to auditory stimuli than controls. They also found that depressed patients had response latencies in a range between that of demented and narmal patients, but that their response latencies persisted even after the depression had remitted clinically. They suggested that their results could be interpreted as indicating either that depression in the elderly produces subtle but irreversible brain changes, or alternatively, that some elderly depressives have impairment of brain functioning prior to the depressive episode. A third possibility not mentioned is that AER latency may be a function of depression that persists longer than the clinical picture of depression, and consequently the return of depressed patients to normal AER latency was not picked up by the authors on their 6–8 week follow-up examination. However, the somatosensory and auditory AERs are not sufficiently distinct in depressed and demented patients to be clinically useful as yet.

In addition to the AER studies described above, Brown et al (1982) have studied the ERP component P300 in depression and dementia. They found that P300 could be used to help distinguish some demented from depressed patients. Prolonged P300 latency appeared in most of their demented, but in none of their depressed subjects. They concluded that a prolonged P300 latency is diagnostic of dementia, although the absence of prolonged latency does not rule out dementia.

Another strategy for addressing the question of how to use brain changes to differentiate between dementia and depression has been the use of sleep studies. A number of studies have demonstrated significant changes in the sleep pattern of depressives as measured by polysomnography. The most predictable and specific finding is shortened rapid eye movement (REM) sleep latency. Sleep changes also occur in normal elderly subjects, and these changes are similar to those that occur in depressives. They include shortened REM sleep latency, increasing number of nightly arousals, and diminished stage 3 and 4 sleep (Kupfer & Reynolds, 1983). Reynolds et al (1983) studied 18 patients with a mean age of 65.4, of whom half were depressed and half demented. They found that in comparison to demented patients, patients with depression had more sleep continuity disturbance, more REM activity, shorter REM latency and a different temporal distribution of REM density during periods of REM sleep. They suggested that e.e.g. sleep studies may be able to differentiate between depressed and demented patients. Thus, even though the normal changes in sleep with ageing are similar to changes in sleep seen in younger depressed patients, preliminary evidence suggests that differentiation of depression from dementia on the basis of sleep studies is possible.

DEPRESSION IN THE COURSE OF DEMENTIA

The coexistence of depression and dementia is a subject receiving increased attention in the psychiatric literature. A number of reports have indicated that depression occurs relatively commonly in demented patients. Sim & Sussman (1962) found depressive symptoms in 24 of 46 patients with presenile dementia, 33 of whom had histologically demonstrated disease. They noted that in patients with Alzheimer's disease, affective symptoms were present early in the disease, but later became obscured by the dementing process. Liston (1977) retrospectively examined the records of 50 patients who met his criteria for presenile dementia and found that, of these, 30 (60%) exhibited dysphoric mood prior to the diagnosis of presenile dementia. His findings highlight the frequent existence of depression early in the course of presenile dementia. Ron et al, in a study of diagnostic accuracy in presenile dementia mentioned above, found that even though the presence of a history of affective illness and of current depressive affect distinguished significantly between demented and non-demented patients, 10 of 33 demented patients (30%) nonetheless had 'depressive mood' at the time of hospital admission.

Results from the investigation of depression in senile dementia are similar. Reifler et al (1982) studied 88 cognitively impaired elderly out-patients (mean age 78 years) and found that depression was superimposed upon dementia in 17 (19%) of the 88 cognitively impaired patients they studied. Patients with greater cognitive impairment exhibited less depression. Their work suggests that coexistence of these two disorders is a relatively common occurrence in the elderly and, like other studies, it indicates that depression, when it occurs, generally appears early in the course of dementia.

In contrast, a recent report by Knesevich et al (1983) suggested that depression appears *less* commonly than is frequently supposed in the course of Alzheimer's disease. They administered Hamilton and Zung scales to 30 mildly demented Alzheimer's disease patients and 30 controls both at the time of initial evaluation and then 12 months later. The investigators excluded at the beginning of their study all patients with current evidence of depression, as well as patients with a history of depression at any time in their lives, in order to avoid the possibility of misdiagnosing patients with cognitive impairment on the basis of depression. They found that the mean depression scores of patients remained unchanged at the end of the 12-month period on both the Hamilton and Zung depression rating scales. They concluded, somewhat tenuously, that their results suggested the possibility that patients with Alzheimer's dementia rarely develop a depressive syndrome, and that if a depressive syndrome appears in these patients, it should be viewed as an unrelated affective disorder that deserves vigorous treatment. While few clinicians would dispute that depression in the course of dementia should be treated, these results are compromised because depressed patients were excluded from the study in its early stages, i.e., the frequency of depression in the course of dementia is based on a sample skewed heavily and intentionally in the direction of non-depression.

The question of whether affective symptoms are more common in some types of dementia than in others remains unsettled. Ehrentheil, (1957) summarizing the findings of 22 previous studies, suggested that 'arteriosclerotic psychosis' was characterized by emotional lability, 'senile dementia' by the existence of depression and agitation in some patients, and Alzheimer's disease (which he distinguished from senile dementia by the early appearance and prominence of microscopic changes) by irritable mood and restless behavior.

Roth (1983) has noted that the onset of a depressive syndrome for the first time in late life is particularly common in the initial phases of multi-infarct dementia (MID); approximately 25% of cases are affected. In the rest of MID cases, he reports ideas of guilt, pessimism and a labile affect to be frequent. Hachinski (1975) lists depression as one of the symptoms which distinguishes MID from Alzheimer's disease.

One study conducted by Bucht et al (1984), however, examining clinical features that might distinguish Alzheimer's disease from MID, was not able to confirm distinctive affective symptoms in MID. These investigators found that the Alzheimer's disease patients had 'more pronounced signs of depression' than MID patients. Whether patients fulfilled DSM-III or RDC criteria for major depression was not stated. Bucht et al concluded that, while their results confirmed previous reports of the coexistence of depression and mild to moderate dementia, they failed to confirm the presence of emotional lability in MID patients.

SUMMARY

The relationship of depression and dementia is multifaceted. Current research has provided increased clarification of the nature of cognitive deficits during depression and has begun to refine the concept of pseudodementia. Nonetheless, our understanding of the changes in the brain that lead to the onset of first-time late-life depression remains imprecise as does our knowledge of the cause, course, and therapy of depression during dementia. The relationship of depression and dementia is still fertile ground for future psychiatric research.

REFERENCE

Breen A R, Larson E B, Reifler B V, Vitaliano P P, Lawrence G L 1984 Cognitive performance and functional competence in coexisting dementia and depression. Journal of the American Geriatric Society 32: 132–137
Brown W S, Marsh J T, LaRue A 1982 Event-related potentials in psychiatry: differentiating depression and dementia in the elderly. Bulletin of the Los Angeles Neurologic Society 47: 91–107
Bucht G, Adolfsson R, Winblad B 1984 Dementia of the Alzheimer type and multi-infarct dementia: a clinical description and diagnostic problems. Journal of the American Geriatric Society 32: 491–498
Buchsbaum M, Goodwin F K, Murphy D, Borge G 1971 A E R in affective disorders. American Journal of Psychiatry 128: 19–25
Caine E D 1981 Pseudodementia: current concepts and future directions. Archives of General Psychiatry 38: 1359–1364
Carnes M, Smith J C, Kalin N H, Bauwens S F 1983 Effects of chronic medical illness and dementia on the dexamethasone suppression test. Journal of American Geriatric Society 31: 269–271
Cohen R M, Weingartner H, Smallberg S A, Pickar D, Murphy D L 1982 Effort and cognition in depression. Archives of General Psychiatry 39: 593–597
Cawley R H, Post F, Whitehead A 1973 Barbiturate tolerance and psychological functioning in elderly depressed patients. Psychological Medicine 3: 39–52
Cavanaugh S V A, Wettson R 1983 The relationship between severity of depression, cognitive dysfunction and age in medical inpatients. American Journal of Psychiatry 140: 495–496
Davies, G Hamilton S, Hendrickson D E, Levy R, Post F 1978 Psychological test performance and sedation thresholds of elderly dements, depressives and depressives with incipient brain change. Psychological Medicine 8: 103–109
Duckworth G S, Ross H 1975 Diagnostic differences in psychogeriatric patients in Toronto, New York, and London, England. Canadian Medical Association Journal 112: 847–851
Ehrentheil O 1957 Differential diagnosis of organic dementias and affective disorders in aged patients. Geriatrics 12:426
Feinberg T, Goodman B 1984 Affective illness, dementia and pseudodementia. Journal of Chinical Psychiatry 45: 99–103

Folstein M F, McHugh P R 1978 Dementia, syndrome of depression Alzheimer's disease: senile dementia and related disorders. Aging 7: 87–93

Garcia C, Reding M J, Blass J P 1981 Overdiagnosis of dementia. Journal of the American Geriatric Society 29: 407–410

Good M I 1981 Pseudodementia and physical findings masking significant psychopathology. American Journal of Psychiatry 138: 811–814

Hachinski V C et al 1975 Cerebral blood flow in dementia. Archives of Neurology 32: 632–637

Hendrickson E, Raymond L, Post F 1979 Averaged evoked responses in relation on cognitive and affective state of elderly psychiatric patients. British Journal of Psychiatry 134: 494–501

Henry G M, Weingartner H, Murphy D L 1973 Influence of affective states and psychoactive drugs on verbal learning and memory. American Journal of Psychiatry 130: 966–970

Jacoby R J, Levy R, Bird J M 1981 Computed tomography and the outcome of affective disorder: a follow-up study of elderly depressives. British Journal of Psychiatry 139: 288–292

Jacoby R J, Levy R 1980 Computed tomograhpy in the elderly. 3. Affective disorder. British Journal of Psychiatry 136: 270–275

Jacoby R J, Dolan J D, Levy R, Baldy R 1983 Quantitative computed tomography in elderly depressed patients. British Journal of Psychiatry 143: 124–127

Jenike M A, Albert M S 1984 The dexamethasone suppression test in patients with presenile and senile dementia of the Alzheimer's type. Journal of the American Geriatric Society 32: 441–444

Kahn R L, Zarit S H, Hilbert N M, Niederehe G 1975 Memory complaint and impairment in the aged: the effect of depression and altered brain function. Archives of General Psychiatry 32: 1569–1573

Kay D W K, Roth M, Hopkins B 1955 Affective disorders arising in the senium: 1. their association with organic cerebral degeneration. Journal of Mental Science 101: 302–316

Kay D W K 1962 Outcome and cause of death in mental disorders of ald age: a long-term follow-up of functional and organic psychoses. Acta Psychiatrica Scandinarica 38: 249–276

Knesevich J W, Martin R L, Berg L, Danziger W 1983 Preliminary report on affective symptoms in the early stages of senile dementia of the Alzheimer type. American Journal of Psychiatry 140: 233–235

Kiloh, L G 1961 Pseudo-dementia. Acta Psychiatrica Scandinavica 37: 336–351

Kupfer D J, Reynolds C F 1983 Electroencephalographic sleep changes in psychiatric patients. In: Hughs J R, Wilson W P (eds) EEG and evoked potentials in psychiatry and behavioral neurology. Butterworth, Boston, ch 7

Liston E H 1977 Occult presenile dementia. Journal of Nervous and Mental Diseases 164: 263–267

Madden J J, Luhan J A, Kaplan L A, Manfredi H M 1952 Nondementing psychoses in older persons. Journal of the American Medical Association 150: 1567–1570

Marsden C D, Harrison M J G 1972 Outcome of investigation of patients with presenile dementia. British Medical Journal 2: 249–252

McAllister T W 1983 Overview: pseudodementia. American Journal of Psychiatry 140: 528–533

McAllister T W 1981 Cognitive functioning in the affective disorders. Comprehensive Psychiatry 22: 572–586

McAllister T W, Ferrell R B, Price T R P, Neville M B 1982a The dexamethasone suppression test in two patients with severe depressive pseudodementia. American Journal of Psychiatry 139: 479–481

McAllister T W, Price T R P 1982b Severe depressive pseudodementia with and without dementia. American Journal of Psychiatry 139: 626–629

Nott P N, Fleminger J J 1975 Presenile dementia: the difficulties of early diagnosis. Acta Psychiatrica Scandinavica 51: 210–217

Post, F 1975 Dementia, depression and pseudodementia. In: Benson F, Blumer D (eds) Psychiatric aspects of neurological disease. Grune & Stratton, New York, ch 6

Post F 1962 The significance of affective symptoms in old age. Oxford University Press, London

Raskind M, Peskind E, Rivard M-F, Veith R, Barnes R 1982 Dexamethasone suppression test and cortisol circadian rhythm in primary degenerative dementia. American Journal of Psychiatry 139: 1468–1471

Reifler B V, Larson E, Hanley R 1982 Coexistence of cognitive impairment and depression in geriatric outpatients. American Journal of Psychiatry 39: 623–626

Reynolds C F, Spiker D G, Hanin I, Kupfer D J 1983 Electroencephalographic sleep, aging and psychopathology: new data and state of the art. Biological Psychiatry 18: 139–155

Ron M A, Toone B K, Garralda M E, Lishman W A 1979 Diagnostic accuracy in presenile dementia. British Journal of Psychiatry 134: 161–168

Roth M Depression and affective disorders in later life. In: Angst (ed) The origins of depression: current concepts and approaches. Springer, New York, p 39–76

Sim M, Sussman I 1962 Alzheimer's disease: its natural history and differential diagnosis. Journal of Nervous and Mental Diseases 134: 489–499

Smith, J Stanley, Kiloh, L G 1981 The investigation of dementia: results in 200 consecutive admissions. Lancet 1: 824–827

Sternberg D E, Jarvik M 1976 Memory functions in depression: improvement with antidepressant medication. Archives of General Psychiatry 33: 219–224

Wells C E 1979 Pseudodementia. American Journal of Psychiatry 136: 895–900

Weingartner H, Cohen R M, Murphy D L, Martello J, Gerdt C 1981 Cognitive processes in depression. Archives of General Psychiatry 38: 42–47

Whitehead A 1973 Verbal learning and memory in elderly depressives. British Journal of Psychiatry 123: 203–8

Drugs for dementia

The treatment of dementia poses problems which are quite different from those posed by most other disorders. Dementia of the Alzheimer type (DAT) probably develops over a long period of time and is the end result of a process or series of processes which are at best poorly understood. A logical approach to therapy is therefore difficult, perhaps at this time impossible. However, since an increasing proportion of the population is elderly and dementia is relatively common in this age group, the need for treatment of some kind is very great. The combination of aetiological uncertainty together with the magnitude of the potential patient population must make the development of a method of prevention or some form of treatment the greatest therapeutic challenge for today and tomorrow.

The answers to some of the questions about the management of Alzheimer's disease may come over the next decade or so. The patients who need treatment are with us now. Faced with this situation the psychiatrist or the geriatrician might turn either to textbooks or to the literature. Unfortunately most textbooks read by undergraduates do not include the word 'dementia' in their index sections. The potential therapist who then turns to the literature finds that it is extensive, confusing and completely unhelpful in the sense that it fails to provide useful guidelines. It contains reports of many different drugs which are said to work in a variety of different ways. Some work to some extent, some of the time. It would be possible to read the literature and decide that a few drugs are effective in that they can be 'shown' to improve certain clinical features of patients with Alzheimer's disease. It would also be possible to study the same publications and conclude that there is no convincing evidence that any drug can effectively reverse the dementing process in DAT. Both views are unsatisfactory, since both uncritical acceptance of the results of poor trials and total nihilism will hinder progress.

Faced with the difficulties outlined above, the aim of this chapter will be to try to take an analytical and critical view of the problem rather than simply to catalogue the drugs which are available. Throughout, the emphasis will be on Alzheimer's disease, and the starting point is to consider the numerous ways in which drugs may assist or adversely affect a demented patient.

POTENTIAL EFFECTS OF DRUGS IN DEMENTIA

The drugs being taken by an apparently demented patient may be:
1. One of the causes of the patients condition
2. Having a non-specific beneficial effect
3. Treating another or coexisting type of dementia
4. Correcting one of the basic defects of Alzheimer's disease, or
5. Ameliorating symptoms or modifying secondary factors
6. Having a placebo effect on the patient, the relatives, the staff of the institution or the doctor in charge.

These different possibilities will now be considered briefly in turn.

1. The depressant effect of drugs on the central nervous system is well known. Nevertheless, all doctors need to be reminded of the fact that patients may be made worse by drugs prescribed by them, or by a previous doctor or obtained elsewhere. In this context sedatives, antidepressants or antihistamines are relevant. Other drugs may be making things worse by, for example, a metabolic effect, by causing hypothyroidism or by reducing cerebral blood flow.

2. The assessment of drugs in dementia relies largely on observing the patients' ability to answer questions and perform simple tasks. Many non-demented individuals would perform better after coffee if they were feeling 'low' or perhaps after a beta-blocker if they were feeling tense and over-anxious. People with organic illnesses would probably do better if infections were controlled, anaemia treated or pains relieved. Care must therefore be taken not to confuse non-specific and perhaps short-term effects, which drugs or other factors may have on performance, with the hoped-for long-term improvement in memory and intelligence.

3. If the patient has dementia secondary to some treatable disorder, then correcting that disorder should improve the situation. Thyroxine for myxoe-dema is an obvious example. Patients with Alzheimer's disease may also have other coexisting disorders which may be remedied.

4. The major aim, with the primary dementias, is to determine the basic mechanism and to correct or modify the underlying defect. For some time the hope has been that Alzheimer's disease could be ascribed to a deficiency in one of the cerebral neurotransmitter systems which might be corrected. To this end a number of trials on precursors of acetyl choline, anticholin-esterases and cholinomimetic agents have been performed and will be considered later. Other deficiencies may be found which could be corrected by drugs.

5. Patients with dementia may also have treatable symptoms which are a manifestation of the underlying dementia or may develop as a consequence of inability to do things or remember what they have done. Insomnia, anxiety and depression, for example, may respond to suitable medication. This may improve the situation both for the patients and for relatives and/or attendants, but these measures would not be expected materially to improve intellectual function nor the long-term prognosis.

6. In almost any clinical trial situation the possibility of a drug having a placebo effect on the patient or the observers has to be considered. This is particularly important when there is no objective end-point. The demented patient admitted to have treatment given by people, who are hoping for a response, presents the classical situation for a good placebo response.

The doctor who treats dementia may well be grateful for any drug which improves the patient by whatever mechanism. However, we are more likely to make progress in this vitally important area if we can analyse and understand what we are doing and how we are doing it. With this in mind we should also remember that, just because a drug increases serotonin levels or blocks alpha-2 receptors, we cannot conclude that this is necessarily the way it is modifying the mental process in our patient.

DRUG ASSESSMENT

The literature on the treatment of dementia makes worrying reading for clinical pharmacologists. The standards of clinical trials methodology are usually very much lower than would be tolerated in other areas of therapeutics. This is largely due to the difficulties encountered by the investigators, which are considerable. Nevertheless sensible decisions on drug efficacy depend on reasonably sound clinical trials. We should therefore set ourselves some requirements and be ready to ask pertinent questions when presented with information about a new drug which may appear to help patients with DAT.

The drug

a. How does it work?

As part of the information on the drug, it would help to know how the drug is supposed to work and to have some evidence that it can achieve its effect. If it is supposed to elevate cortical choline concentrations — does it? If it mobilizes glucose or improves glucose utilization — has this ever been demonstrated in any way? Further, if there is a known pharmacological action, it will almost certainly produce some predictable side-effects and a dose-response curve.

b. Can it reach the site of action?

The drug which is used can only be effective if it reaches its presumed site of action in concentrations sufficient to achieve the hoped-for pharmacological effect. To improve mental function we should require evidence that the drug is reasonably well absorbed and then crosses the blood-brain barrier. It should be sufficiently lipid-soluble to pass into the brain substance and 'adequate' concentrations in the brain should be maintained for most of the time. Therapeutic peaks achieved twice daily for 10–15 minutes are unlikely to correct a persistent, progressive defect.

c. Pharmaceutical and pharmacological considerations

We must also ask some questions about the drug's pharmaceutical and pharmacological characteristics. The nature of a disease should modify the requirements we make of any drug to be used in treatment. Alzheimer's disease is a common chronic dementing disorder which radically reduces the quality of life for both patients and relatives and leads eventually to the patient's death. Since the numbers affected are large and the treatment will probably need to be prolonged, it should be relatively cheap and reasonably well tolerated. It must not only be effective but also be relatively simple to administer. This means once or twice daily by mouth or at longer intervals by injection.

Unpleasant symptoms such as headache, nausea or vomiting would not be acceptable, and any drug which caused insomnia or disturbed or aggressive behaviour would be most undesirable. On the other hand, a drug which might occasionally cause renal damage or bone marrow suppression, which are normally regarded as very serious adverse effects, would be quite acceptable in the treatment of a terminal disabling disease. Similarly, the risk of addiction need not be a serious contra-indication.

Clinical trials

In a clinical trial we should expect an adequate number of patients with the disease. Studies on fewer than 15 patients are often of doubtful relevance unless a clear-cut objective result is expected, such as a 10 mm fall in blood pressure. The disease must be defined and criteria for inclusion and exclusion must be specified. These patients must then be given, or it must be fairly certain that they have taken, the supposedly active agent for a reasonable period of time. Since dementia is usually a slowly developing process, recovery, if it takes place, is likely to take months rather than days or weeks.

We turn next to clinical trial design. Whilst there is no doubt that open trials on small groups may indicate whether the drug is having an effect, they do not provide evidence of efficacy. The strong possibility of a placebo effect means that only the results of double-blind controlled trials can be used as evidence that a drug works. In this area scrupulous attention to detail is vital. The state of the home, hospital or other institution, the food, the weather, the time of day, concommitant therapy and coexisting medical disorders may all materially affect performance. The clinical trial reader has to ask, 'Was the drug the only factor which could have produced the effect?' and the clinical trial designer and performer must be ready for this question.

Methods of assessing patients are considered in other chapters. In relation to the drug trial, we should consider how objective the assessments are and to what extent they could be influenced by observer bias or could have occurred by chance. This latter aspect is particularly important in situations where a number of different variables are included. Statistically significant ($P > 0.05$) means that there is a less than 1 in 20 likelihood of that observation occurring by chance. Studies on demented patients often involve repeated assessments using many different measures of cognitive function and behaviour patterns. In the vast number of results obtained, it is only too easy to find some chance differences which are reported as being 'statistically significant' but they are clinically irrelevant. If there really is a statistically significant improvement, was the patient's lifestyle or mental performance really any better? If it was, was the improvement maintained?

Ethical considerations

In clinical trials ethical considerations are concerned with maintaining the balance between the need of the community to acquire knowledge and the right of the patient to be protected from unnecessary harm. This has rightly become a vital aspect of the planning of any clinical trial.

Under 'normal' circumstances, when a drug is being assessed in a group of adults with a particular disease, it is relatively easy to conduct the trial ethically. This involves giving an adequate explanation of what is involved in the trial and what effects the drug or drugs may have, and thereafter obtaining the patient's informed consent, given willingly, preferably in the presence of an independent witness. The demented patient is unlikely to be able to understand much of any explanation and cannot give informed consent. Under these circumstances it is necessary to develop a new set of guidelines. These can be based on some of the normal considerations which suggest that the investigator should consider the following when planning his or her trial:

1. The trial should be capable of providing useful information which cannot be obtained in other ways

2. The anticipated results should justify the disturbance to the patient, his/her family or attendants

3. All physical and mental suffering should be kept to a minimum

4. Preparations should be made and adequate facilities provided to cope with any adverse effects

5. Those who conduct the trial shall exercise the highest degree of skill and care and be appropriately qualified

6. The investigator must terminate the trial if its continuation would be in any way detrimental to the patient.

Having considered the above, the investigator must submit the protocol to an established ethical committee. This committee should be quite independent, with no links with the investigator, and ideally it should contain:

1. a doctor experienced in clinical research, 2. a psychiatrist or geriatrician knowledgeable about dementia, 3. a senior nurse and, 4. a lay person. If this committee approves the protocol, then consent should be obtained from an appropriate relative. This carries more weight if the relative is given a brief description of the project (its nature, purpose and risks) in writing, which he or she then signs on behalf of the patient.

Trials which have not been performed without due care being paid to the above ethical considerations are not only likely to be morally wrong but cast doubt on the whole professional integrity of the investigators. The trial reader must demand ethical standards of the trial performer.

DRUG TREATMENT — THERAPEUTIC

In this section drugs, which are believed by some to have a therapeutic role in that they are supposed to correct some real or imagined defect, will be reviewed. These are set out in Table 16.1. Inevitably the list is incomplete, as the number of drugs which have been tried is legion and a single agent may be considered experimental, therapeutic or obsolescent by different investigators.

Table 16.1   Drugs believed to have a therapeutic role

A. Drugs given to correct a neurotransmitter deficiency
   1. Cholinergic system
      a. Precursors: choline, lecithin, deanol
      b. Anticholinesterases: physostigmine
      c. Cholinomimetics: arecoline, bethanecol, RS 86
   2. Other neurotransmitters
B. Cerebral vasodilators
C. Cerebroactive substances
D. Miscellaneous
      a. Peptides
      b. Naloxone
      c. Others

A. Drugs given to correct neurotransmitter deficiencies

1. The cholinergic system

The role of a possible defect in the cholinergic system in the aetiology of Alzheimer's disease has been discussed extensively and is reviewed elsewhere in this book (Chapter 8). It is therefore inappropriate to discuss this subject further here. However, the fact that a deficiency in the cholinergic system is considered by many to the most plausible aetiological mechanism to explain the deficiencies found in Alzheimer's disease deserves emphasis. Accordingly, efforts to rectify the defect in this system are considered by many to be the most likely way of achieving therapeutic progress.

Three ways of trying to correct the adverse consequences of cerebral acetyl choline deficiency have been suggested and tried. These are to:

(i) increase the availability of suitable precursors by providing choline, lecithin or deanol.

(ii) decrease the breakdown of the acetyl choline which is formed by giving acetyl cholinesterases, particularly physostigmine.

(iii) supplement the effects of acetyl choline by administering other cholinomimetic agents which will stimulate the post-ganglionic receptors. Arecoline has been given with this aim.

a. Precursors Precursors have been given in the, perhaps mistaken, belief that by providing an excess of substrate the deficiency of acetyl choline can be corrected. To be effective, the material administered by mouth would have to be absorbed, to attain sufficient concentrations first in the blood and thereafter in the central nervous system and not cause any adverse effects. The enzyme system in the brain would then have to be able to utilize the chemical provided. In the hope that this may be possible various salts of choline, lecithin (phosphatidylcholine) and deanol (2-dimethyl aminoethanol) have been given to groups of patients with Alzheimer's disease.

Choline has been assessed by a number of different investigators. As with most treatments for Alzheimer's disease, the trials can be criticized. Usually the substance is given to a small group of patients for a short time and assessed without using a double-blind technique. Although animal studies suggest that brain concentrations of choline can be increased, the clinical data which is available does not suggest that choline has any useful therapeutic effect (Thal et al, 1981; Blass & Weksler, 1983) though the trials could not be said to prove that choline is ineffective. It does produce a fishy odour and can cause gastrointestinal upsets.

Lecithin, which is rapidly converted into choline (Etienne et al, 1981), is difficult to obtain in a pure form, and preparations containing a high concentration of lecithin are expensive. Nevertheless this substance has been investigated more extensively than choline. The overall impression, however, is one of disappointment (Etienne et al, 1981; Dysken et al, 1982; Canter et al, 1982; Blass & Weksler, 1983) though again the lack of efficacy could be ascribed to some extent to the inadequacy of the trials. One longer study using larger doses of lecithin yielded some more promising early results (Levy et al, 1983) but evidence of long-term, clinically relevant improvement is lacking.

The third precursor which has been the subject of a number of investigations is deanol. The literature on this agent contains a number of papers based on small groups of patients using open techniques which show some improvements in one or more measures of cognitive function or behaviour. In more carefully controlled investigations of greater duration it seems that adverse effects can be a problem, particularly as the dose is increased, and evidence of an overall improvement is not found (Fishman et al, 1981).

6. Anticholinesterases To the neuropharmacologist, the concept of compensating for a relative lack of acetylcholine in the brain, by providing an inhibitor to delay its breakdown, seems eminently satisfactory. The gratifying effects of anticholinesterases in patients with myasthenia gravis are well known. However, there are a number of problems associated with this group of agents. Some anticholinesterases have been developed specifically for their toxic effects and have been used as nerve gases and pesticides. Further, the effects of taking an overdose of one of the therapeutic agents are alarming (nausea, vomiting, confusion, cramping abdominal pain, bronchospasm, convulsions, etc). Add to this that (a) some anticholinesterases do not enter the brain, (b) most are relatively short-acting, and (c) acetylcholinesterases are widely distributed in the body. It would seem at first sight, therefore, that treatment with these agents would require a complicated regimen with a considerable risk of producing adverse effects. However the theoretical possibility of developing a long-acting preparation of an agent with good brain penetration and possibly some selectivity of action towards the relevant cortical cholinergic system must be seen as a major challenge for researchers working on Alzheimer's disease.

Physostigmine does penetrate into the central nervous system, and early trials with this drug have yielded some encouraging results. Whereas anticholinergic agents may cause an impairment of recognition memory function, physostigmine given intravenously has been shown to produce an improvement both in normal subjects (Davis et al, 1978) and in patients with Alzheimer's disease (Davis & Mohs, 1982). Techniques used to assess drug effects on memory have been reviewed by Brinkman & Gershon (1983). The demonstration that there appears to be a dose-response effect is intellectually satisfying, since this is what one would predict if a defect is being corrected pharmacologically. It is also of interest that the combination of lecithin with physostigmine appeared to be preferable to physostigmine alone in a small group of patients with Alzheimer's disease (Peters & Levin, 1979).

Having established that physostigmine may have a role in improving memory function in both controls and demented patients, the next step was to assess the effects of orally administered physostogmine. Thal & Fuld (1983), after performing a dose-finding study, have shown that 8 of 12 patients given oral physostigmine with lecithin did appear to improve. Similarly, Davis and colleagues (1983), also after determining the optimal dose, have demonstrated an improvement using a double-blind technique in a small group of patients with Alzheimer's disease given oral physostigmine alone.

Although we are a long way from curing or preventing Alzheimer's disease, the apparent beneficial effects of modifying and trying to correct one of the systems thought to be defective is an encouraging observation in an area of therapeutic uncertainty.

C. Cholinomimetic agents An increased effect on cholinergic receptors could also be achieved by the administration of muscarinic agonists. Agents like arecholine have been tried and may produce modest improvements in learning and memory, but the problem of systemic side-effects caused by the generalized cholinergic actions remains (Christie et al, 1981). One way of overcoming this problem is to use an implanted pump system and infuse a cholinomimetic such as bethanechol directly into the CSF. After studies in animals, Harbaugh and colleagues (1984) tried this technique in four patients with biopsy-proven Alzheimer's disease. Though this was a feasibility study rather than a clinical trial, improvements were noted which were reversed or not noted during placebo infusions. Double-blind techniques were used and the infusions were maintained for several months. This interesting study must be seen as most encouraging for all those researching the therapeutic implications of the cholinergic defect theory of the aetiology of DAT.

Further progress would be greatly assisted if a more specific agonist for the cholinergic system which is defective in DAT could be found. The observations of Hammer and colleagues (1980) that pirenzipine has a selective antimuscarinic effect with a greater affinity for receptors in glandular tissue than for muscarinic receptors in heart and smooth muscle gives hope that cholinergic receptors in different tissues may be pharmacologically recognizably different. This possibility has been advanced by the finding that in mice pirenzipine has the ability selectively to impair avoidance learning as opposed to other CNS functions (Caulfield et al, 1983). A selective agonist for the learnng, muscarinic, pirenzipine receptors may be an effective way of treating dementia. RS 86 may be one of a new group of more selective muscarinic agents (Wettstein & Spiegel, 1984).

2. Other neurotransmitter systems

There is evidence that other neurotransmitter systems may be defective in DAT. However, it would be difficult to present a case that modification of dopa, 5HT, noradrenaline or their receptors can effectively help patients with DAT.

B. Cerebral vasodilators

A variety of vasodilators have been tried by many different investigators seeking to help patients with DAT. Although there appear to be some reports of benefit in the literature, there are considerably more suggesting that as a group these agents are not effective. Before approaching the extensive literature, it may be helpful to consider the following. If a cerebral vasodilator is shown to be effective, we must assume that:

(i) impaired blood supply to the relevant part of the brain is an important aetiological factor.

(ii) the disease affecting the blood vessels is reversible.

(iii) the drug will specifically improve the blood flow to the underperfused part of the brain and will not steal blood to the more normal areas in which the disease-free vessels might be expected to be more responsive to dilators. A general vasodilator usually causes postural hypotension and may reduce cerebral blood flow when the subject is upright.

(iv) the result could not have occurred by chance or be a placebo response.

An apparent effect noted in patients on a so-called cerebral vasodilator might be caused by another action of the drug. Some agents are also classed as cerebroactive and these will be considered in the next section.

Cook & James (1981a, 1981b) reviewed cerebral vasodilators in 1981 and produced a classification given in Table 16.2. Only two drugs, Hydergine® and naftidrofuryl, probably working in other ways, were found to have some beneficial effects. All vasodilators were considered able to reduce blood flow to ischaemic areas. In conclusion, therefore, it would seem that there is no good evidence that any group of patients with Alzheimer's disease have been materially helped by an agent which has improved the blood supply to the defective area of the brain. Further information may be obtained from a number of useful reviews (Yesavage et al, 1979; Goodnick & Gershon, 1984).

Table 16.2 Cerebral vasodilators (based on Cook & James, 1981)

1. Direct-acting vasodilators
   Papaverine
   Cyclandelate
   Naftidrofuryl (Nafronyl)
2. Drugs acting on adrenoreceptors
   Isoxsuprine (alpha antagonist, beta agonist)
   Nylidrin (buphenine) (beta agonist)
   Co-dergorine (hydergine®) (alpha antagonist)
3. Drugs acting on histamine receptors
   Betahistine
4. Miscellaneous
   Vincamine
   Niacin derivatives
   Cinnarizine

C. Cerebroactive substances

There are a number of drugs which are described as being cerebroactive. This means that they are believed to reverse a defect, often of cerebral glucose utilization, which is thought to be contributing to patients' dementia. Suggested actions include metabolic or neuronal activation, increased energy utilization, neurotransmitter modulation or substitution, and membrane modification. It would be easy to dismiss this group of agents, since there is little evidence that a metabolic defect is a major aetiological factor in DAT and almost no evidence that these agents have a measurable, pharmacological effect which might be expected to produce a clinical improvement. However, there is an enormous literature on cerebroacative drugs and for some, particularly Hydergine®, the overall evidence suggests that the drug has some positive therapeutic effects (Yesavage et al, 1979; Spagnoli & Tognoni, 1983; Branconnier, 1983).

It is not really possible to classify this group of drugs in a meaningful way. In Table 16.3 they are presented in three groups: 1. Co-dergocrine, which is most widely used and extensively studied, 2. drugs which are fairly well documented and 3. drugs whose cerebroactive function is not clearly defined and whose efficacy is completety unproven. Modes of action given in this table are at best a rough guide. Further information can be obtained from the review of Spagnoli & Tognoni (1983).

Table 16.3   Cerebroactive drugs (based on Spagnoli & Tognoni, 1983)

Drug	Drug Type	Modes of action[1]
GROUP 1		
Co-dergocrine (Hydergine®, dehydroergotoxine)	Ergot derivative mixture	Diverse actions — affecting neurotransmitters, oxygen utilization, vasodilatation
GROUP 2		
Nafronyl	Complex acid ester of diethylaminoethanol	Vasodilator, promotes glucose utilization and oxidative metabolism
Piracetam	Cylic derivative of GABA	Increases cerebral ATP, effect on phospholipases
GROUP 3		
Cinnarizine	Piperazine-type antihistamine	Calcium antagonism
Vincamine and vinburnine	Plant alkaloid derivatives	Vasolidator
Oxpentifylline	Xanthine derivative	Vasolidator

[1] Modes of action — this is given as a guide only. For some drugs there are many suggested, often unproven, modes of action.

Co-dergocrine (Hydergine®)

Co-dergocrine consists of four ergopeptine derivatives: dihydroergocornine, dihydroergocristine, dihydro-α-ergocryptine and dihydro-β-ergocryptine in a ratio of 3:3:2:1. This mixture of ergot derivatives was first promoted as a cerbral vasodilator. It has now been reclassified among the drugs with mixed effects or the cerebroactive agents. It has been extensively investigated and is one of the most widely used of all drugs.

Hydergine® appears capable of modifying many different cerebral functions. It is supposed to increase certain enzymes involved in intermediary metabolism in ganglion cells, alter glucose stores in astrocytes; enhance oxygen utilization and increase e.e.g. amplitude. In addition, because of its chemical similarity to a number of neurotransmitters, it may act at receptor sites specific for noradrenaline, dopamine and serotonin, possibly as an antagonist at the first and an agonist at the latter two. As a result of these and many other actions, demonstrated in animals, Hydergine® can be shown to have diverse effects on neurotransmission, hormone release and many other cerebral functions.

The clinically relevant question is: does Hydergine® delay the progress or reverse the decline in intellectual performance seen in patients with Alzheimer's disease? The sceptical reader of the literature would simply answer no. However, this might be considered an oversimplication. The large number of trials have been carefully studied by a number of different groups (Yesavage et al, 1979; Spagnoli & Tognoni, 1981; McDonald, 1982; Branconnier, 1983), and those which meet certain criteria have been selected for further analysis. The conclusions that are reached are that Hydergine® (a) appears able to improve, often significantly, a proportion of the tests of cognitive function and behaviour, (b) performs better in these tests than placebo or a simple vasodilator using double-blind techniques, but (c) fails to produce an overall, clinically meaningful, improvement. Many would conclude that it is the best agent currently available and use it. In a dose of 3–4.5 mg daily it appears to be well tolerated and safe.

A study of the literature reveals several reasons for the uncertainty over the efficacy of Hydergine®. Firstly, only a small and probably very variable amount of drug reaches the brain. It is not well absorbed, there is a marked first-pass loss and it has difficulty crossing the blood-brain barrier (Woodcock et al, 1982; Castleden, 1984). Secondly, Hydergine® has many actions rather than a major effect on a relevant dysfunction. Thirdly, its overall effect appears to be predominantly on mood and responsiveness rather than on memory/cognitive function which is the basic clinical defect in Alzheimer's disease. Finally, most assessments are based on observer-scoring systems, which tends to make them subjective and not very reliable or reproducible.

Naftidrofuryl

This agent is also called nafronyl. Chemically it is an acid oxalate of ethyl-n-diethyl-amino-2-(naphthyl-1)-3-(tetrahydrofurfuryl-2-) propionate. It is a direct-acting vaasodilator which is also supposed to increase brain utilization of glucose and accelerates aerobic brain metabolism in rats (Branconnier, 1983; Goodnick & Gershon, 1984) and oxidative metabolism in humans (Shaw & Johnson, 1975). It is given orally 100 mg three times daily, but may cause nausea, epigastric pain, diarrhoea, headache and dizziness.

This drug has a low bioavailability and uncertain penetration into the central nervous system. It can be shown to produce some metabolic effects and may improve some parameters on the commonly-used rating scales. However, convincing evidence of a reliable clinical improvement in patients with Alzheimer's disease is lacking.

Piracetam

Piracetam (2-oxo-1-pyrolidine acetamide) is a cyclic derivative of gamma-aminobutyric acid (GABA). It is claimed to enhance the efficiency of telencephalic integrative activities. This sort of claim is based on various observations made in animal models. Clinical trials which have involved large numbers of patients have not shown evidence of convincing therapeutic efficacy (Wittenborn, 1981; McDonald, 1982; Branconnier, 1983).

Other cerebroactive agents

There are several other drugs which are classified as cerebroactive and brief details are given in Table 16.3. Further information can be obtained from reviews (Yesavage et al, 1979; Spagnoli & Tognoni, 1983; Goodnick & Gershon, 1984). None seem to have established themselves as reputable therapeutic agents. Most have actions which are ill-understood and effects which have been inadequately investigated. The optimist could consider that the group of cerebroactive agents may contain a close relative to an active agent or at least a clue for further work on mechanisms. The realist must conclude that at present they are a group of drugs of doubtful clinical relevance.

D. Miscellaneous

In addition to the three main groups of drugs discussed above, there are a number of other substances which have been considered as possible therapeutic agents for patients with DAT.

a. Peptides

ACTH, vasopressin and various fractions and analogues have been administered in the hope of modifying mental function. This concept has arisen from the observations of de Wied (1964) on the influence of anterior pituitary on avoidance learning and escape behaviour in rats. Short-term studies on memory function and attention have yielded some positive results (Gold et al, 1979; Galliard & Varey, 1979; Weingarter et al, 1981; Goodnick & Gershon, 1984) which are of considerable interest. However, attempts to demonstrate long-term benefit in patients with DAT have so far not proved very successful (Collins et al, 1981; Durso et al, 1982; Goodnick & Gershon, 1984).

6. Naloxone

Reisberg and colleagues (1983) have suggested that opioid antagonists may have a role to play in the treatment of dementia. This is because endorphins are believed to contribute to physiological amnesia, and encephalins may exert an inhibitory role over various neurotransmitter functions. In a placebo-controlled, double-blind trial of three doses of intravenous naloxone (1 mg, 5 mg and 10 mg), some statistically significant improvements were noted in a small group of patients with DAT. Furthermore, the effects lasted for up to 2 weeks. This must be seen as an interesting observation and the results of further studies using the oral analogue, naltrexone, are awaited.

c. Others

Other agents which have been considered worth assessing include alpha-2 agonists (Reisberg et al, 1983), anticonvulsants (Reisberg et al, 1983) and levodopa (Goodnick & Gershon, 1984). An alternative approach may lead to an increase in somatostatin which, like the cholinergic system, appears to be defective in DAT (Davies et al, 1980).

DRUG TREATMENT — SUPPORTIVE

Since the various approaches described above do not yet offer a convincing way of controlling or preventing the intellectual decline in Alzheimer's disease, alternative measures must be employed. In a chapter on the drug treatment of Alzheimer's disease, these may be subdivided into non-pharmacological and pharmacological.

Non-pharmacological management involves all the care and support, physical, psychological and social, given to the patient and, equally important, to his or her family. This aspect will not be discussed further, but it is important to emphasize that drug treatment is only part of the management of any medical problem. In a patient with Alzheimer's disease, it is only a small part. The care and support given by doctors, nurses and many other paramedical workers is obviously vital.

Under the heading 'pharmacological', we return to the thoughts on the possible effects of drugs set out at the beginning of the chapter. Therefore in addition to considering the drugs set out in the previous section, the doctor looking after a demented patient must ask at least three questions:

1. Is the patient taking any drugs which could conceivably be making the situation worse, i.e. any kind of sedative or other cerebral depressant?

2. Does the patient have any coexistent disease which could be improved by appropriate therapy, e.g. infection, anaemia, hypothyroidism or Parkinson's disease?

3. Are any of the patient's or relatives' problems caused by, or coexisting with the DAT, treatable? Insomnia, depression, confusion, incontinence and defective vision or hearing should be evaluated and if possible treated in the normal way. Obviously some of the drugs used may necessarily have a sedative effect, which is one of the things we wished to avoid. However, this may be a price which has to be paid to allow the other patients or relatives to sleep and to give them respite from the problems caused by the patient. Careful prescribing of short-acting hypnotics and the titration of mild sedatives to achieve a measurable balance will probably be required.

REFERENCES

Blass J P, Weksler M E 1983 Toward an effective treatment of Alzheimer's disease. Annals of Internal Medicine 98: 251–253

Branconnier R J 1983 The efficacy of the cerebral metabolic enhancers in the treatment of senile dementia. Psychopharmacology Bulletin 19: 212–219

Brinkman S D, Gershon S 1983 Measurement of cholinergic drug effects on memory in Alzheimer's disease. Neurobiology of Aging 4: 139–145

Canter N L, Hallett M, Growden J H 1982 Lecithin does not affect EEG spectral analysis or P300 in Alzheimer's disease. Neurology (NY) 32: 1260–1266

Castleden C M 1984 Therapeutic possibilities in patients with senile dementia. Journal of the Royal College of Physicians, London 18: 28–31

Caulfield M P, Higgins G A, Straughan D W 1983 Central administration of the muscarinic receptor subtype — selective antagonist pirenzipine selectively impairs possible avoidance learning in the mouse. Journal of Pharmacy and Pharmacology 35: 131–132

Christie J E, Shering A, Ferguson J, Glen A I M 1981 Physostigmine and arecoline: effects of intravenous infusions in Alzheimer pre-senile dementia. British Journal of Psychiatry 138: 46–50

Collins G B, Marzewski D J, Rollins M M 1981 Paranoid psychosis after DDAVP therapy for Alzheimer's disease. Lancet ii: 808

Cook P, James I 1981a Drug therapy: cerebral vasodilators. New England Journal of Medicine 305: 1508–1513

Cook P, James I 1981b Drug therapy: cerebral vasodilators. New England Journal of Medicine 305: 1560–1564

Davies P, Katzman R, Terry R D 1980 Reduced somatostatin-like immunoreactivity in cerebral cortex from cases of Alzheimer's disease and Alzheimer senile dementia. Nature 288: 279–280

Davis K L, Mohs R C, Rosen W G, Greenwald B S, Levy M I, Horvath T B 1983 Memory enhancement with oral physostigmine in Alzheimer's Disease. New England Journal of Medicine 308:721

Davis K L, Mohs R C, Tinklenberg J R, Pfefferbaum A, Hollister L E, Kopell B S 1978 Physostigmine: improvement of long term memory processes in normal humans. Science 201: 272–274

Davis K L, Mohs R C 1982 Enhancement of memory processes in Alzheimer's disease with multiple dose intravenous physostigmine. American Journal of Psychiatry 139: 1421–1424

de Wied D 1964 Influence of anterior pituitary on avoidance learning and escape behaviour. American Journal of Physiology 207: 255–259

Durso R, Fedio P, Brouwers P et al 1982 Lysine-vasopressin in Alzheimer's disease. Neurology (NY) 32: 674–677

Dysken M W, Fovall P, Harris C M, Davis J M 1982 Lecithin administration in Alzheimer dementia. Neurology (NY) 32: 1203–1204

Etienne P, Dastoor D, Gauthier S, Ludwick R, Collier B 1981 Alzheimer's disease: lack of effect of lecithin treatment for 3 months. Neurology (N7) 31: 1552–1554

Fisman M, Mersky H, Helmes E 1981 Double blind trial of 2, dimethylaminoethanol in Alzheimer's disease. American Journal of Psychiatry 138: 970–972

Gaillard A W K, Varey C A 1979 Some effects of an ACTH 4–9 analog (Org 2766) on human performance. Physiology and Behaviour 1979 23: 79–84

Gold P W, Weingarter H, Ballenger J C, Goodwin F K, Post R M 1979 Effects of 1-desamo-8-D-arginine vasopressin on behaviour and cognition in primary affective disorder. Lancet ii: 992–996

Goodnick P, Gershon S 1984 Chemotherapy of cognitive disorder in geriatic subjects. Journal of Clinical Psychiatry 45: 196–209

Hammer R, Berrie C P, Birdsall N J M, Burgen A S V, Hulme E C 1980 Pirenzepine distinguishes between different subclasses of muscarinic receptors. Nature 283: 90–92

Harbaugh R E, Roberts D W, Coombs D W, Saunders R L, Reeder T M 1984 Preliminary report: intracranial cholinergic drug infusion in patients with Alzheimer's disease. Neurosurgery 15: 514–518

Levy R, Little A, Chuaqui P, Reith M 1983 Early results from double blind, placebo controlled trial of high dose phosphatidylcholine in Alzheimer's disease. Lancet i: 987–988

McDonald R J 1982 Drug treatment of senile dementia. In: Wheatley D (ed) Psychopharmacology of old age. Oxford University Press, Oxford

Peters B H, Levin H S 1979 Effects of physostigmine and lecithin on memory in Alzheimer's disease. Annals of Neurology 6: 219–222

Reisberg B, London E, Ferris S H, Anand R, de Leon M J 1983 Novel pharmacologoic approaches to the treatment of senile dementia of the Alzheimer's type (SDAT). Psychopharmacology Bulletin 19: 220–225

Shaw S W J, Johnson R H 1975 The effect of naftidrofuryl on the metabolic response to exercise in man. Acta Neurologica Scandinavica 52: 231–237

Spagnoli A, Tognoni G 1983 'Cerebroactive' drugs. Clinical pharmacology and therapeutic role in cerebrovascular disorders. Drugs 26: 44–69

Thal L J, Fuld P A 1983 Memory enhancement with oral physostigmine in Alzheimer's disease. New England Journal of Medicine 308:720

Thal L J, Rosen W, Sharpless N J, Crystal H 1981 Choline chloride in Alzheimer's disease. Annals of Neurology 10:580

Weingarter H, Gold P, Bellenger J P et al 1981 Effects of vasopressin on human memory functions. Science 211: 601–603

Wettstein A, Spiegel R 1984 Clinical trials with the cholinergic drug RS 86 in Alzheimer's disease (AD) and senile dementia of Alzheimer's type (SDAT). Psychopharmacology 84: 572–573

Wittenborn J R 1981 Pharmacotherapy for age related behavioural deficiencies. Journal of Nervous and Mental Disease 169: 139–156

Woodcock B G, Loh W, Habedank W-O, Rietbrock N 1982 Dihydroergotoxine kinetics in healthy men after intravenous and oral administration. Clinical Pharmacology and Therapeutics 32: 622–627

Yesavage J M, Tinklenberg J R, Hollister L E, Berger P A 1979 Vasodilators in senile dementias. Archives of General Psychiatry 36: 220–223

Psychological management of dementia

INTRODUCTION

The major manifestations of dementia are usually psychological. Memory, reasoning and thinking ability show impairment and lead to problems in self-care and independent living. Psychological approaches have been applied to dementia for at least 30 years. At times they have been described as 'treatments' or 'therapies'. Here the word 'management' is used deliberately to emphasize that it is not cures for dementia, but long-term strategies for working with the dementing person that are being considered. This is akin to the situation with many other disabilities. In dementia, the natural history of progressive deterioration means there will usually not be a stable level of ability to work from and develop, but a variable, probably declining, pattern of abilities.

The belief that euthanasia is the appropriate response to dementia is not uncommon. Or it is argued that the person's poor memory and awareness mean that only basic physical care to keep the person alive need be given. They are not aware of their surroundings, so why try to improve the environment? They will not remember a conversation 5 minutes later, so why talk to them? A psychological approach, on the other hand, has as its basis that the dementing person is to be treated as a person — not as an object or as a vegetable. If people are to live, then they must be allowed to have life of the highest quality, with psychological needs met as well as the more basic physical needs.

Psychological needs are not so simple to fulfil as providing food, drink, shelter and warmth. They are less easy to define or to monitor. Dementing people vary greatly in their awareness, periods of relative lucidity and appreciation of their surroundings. They may lack 'insight' in the strict sense, but many do express awareness of loss of memory, of reduced grasp on reality. Even those who emphatically deny their problems or seem totally withdrawn from their surroundings may indeed be adopting ways of reducing the stress of loss of function that dementia brings. They cope by protecting themselves from the full enormity of what is happening to them.

The morale of carers is often low. They are often under great stress themselves, whether they are relatives or care-attendants in an old people's home, or hospital staff. Psychological approaches may help to increase their sense of value and self-respect in the difficult work they are undertaking — whether from love, duty or financial considerations.

It is important for our society as a whole that those unfortunate enough to suffer from these or any other disabilities receive the best possible care. It could be important for our own future, for none are safe from the scourge of this tragic condition. The term 'quality of life' is much used these days; it is difficult to define or to measure, but it is in this area where the ultimate test of psychological approaches will be made. Do they improve the quality of life for the dementing person and/or their carers? This must be the focus for the psychological management of dementia.

ATTITUDES

The attitudes and values underlying any psychological approach are crucial to its utility (Woods & Britton, 1977). Some attitudes can lead to more harm being done than good. For example, if a psychological approach succeeded in helping staff talk more to patients, it would not be helpful if in fact these interactions were devaluing and demeaning, or supporting the patients' helplessness. Holden & Woods (1982) argue that staff attitudes must allow the elderly person individuality as an adult, dignity, self-respect, choice and independence. With dementing people, achieving these attitudes is not seen as an easy task. Dementing people are *not* able to make choices or to be as independent as if they did not have the dementia. Dignity and self-respect are hard to retain when basic physical nursing care is needed. Individuality is difficult when you share an old people's 'home' with a number of others, or where some of the features that made you an individual are taken away by the dementia. These are aims to grapple with. We need to work out ways in which some choice, some independence, some individuality can be attained and how this can be maximized.

Normalization

This is an approach that has had considerable impact on the quality of life of mentally handicapped and physically disabled people. It is also relevant to dementia. It sets forward a vision of care at least as demanding — if not more so — as the attitudes outlined above. It does not mean making the person 'normal', or forcing conformity to a norm, or denying choice and forcing people to do 'normal' things. A definition of normalization in fact would emphasize the use of means valued in our society in order to develop and support personal behaviour, experiences and characteristics which are likewise valued. It is not then what is normal in society but that which is valued which is given attention.

Among the implications of this approach are:

1. Dementing people should be accorded full respect and dignity as people with human worth and rights.

2. Dementing people should be treated appropriately to their actual age.

3. Dementing people should be helped to participate in good social relationships in the ordinary community.

Applying this approach is challenging. Current services fall far short of this ideal. Whether the dementing people are in an institution or at home, they are bound to be cut off to some extent from previous social relationships. The problems of allowing full human dignity have been already mentioned. Treating people appropriately to their actual age presents difficulties when as a society we devalue normal elderly people, let alone those with cognitive difficulties. When society's values are varied, whose values are to be the guide? With dementing people at least we have the evidence of the person's previous lifestyle, interests, beliefs and choices as an indication of how they might deal with their present situation.

Who should be the arbiter of the dementing person's viewpoint? Can this task be safely left to the multidisciplinary team or to the person's relatives? Both groups may have vested interests conflicting with those of the patient. The system of advocacy that has been developed in the mental handicap field is attractive. An independent lay person befriends the patient, spends time in getting to know them as an individual and tries to ensure that their perspective is considered by all concerned. Even if this system cannot be achieved for all patients, maintaining services that are open to the public eye, that welcome external comments and feedback, should be a priority.

There is an emphasis here on the importance of experiences. Whether the person remembers the event is seen as unimportant — the enjoyment of it at the time is what counts. This is a particularly relevant attitude in work with dementing people, where almost anything (including, regrettably, physical abuse) can be and has been excused on the grounds that the dementing person will not remember anyway.

Can dementing people learn?

The final aspect of the normalization approach that should be mentioned here is the commitment it contains to development being possible, that the disabled person can change, learn and develop new skills. How does this apply to dementia where new learning is particularly impaired, and where deterioration rather than development is usually seen as the norm? This is best viewed as a refusal to 'write off' a person simply because the label 'dementia' has been attached to them. Every person is seen as having potential at any point in time, even though in dementia the overall outlook may be progressive decline.

From a behavioural perspective, what the person actually does is an interaction between their own skills and abilities and environmental influences. Changing the person's behaviour can then be achieved either by changing the person's environment or by teaching the person new skills, or by a combination of both. The emphasis with dementing elderly people must be on changing the environment, simply because the nature of dementia makes skill-learning difficult. Dementing people can learn some new skills (see Holden & Woods, 1982), but it is important to reserve this ability for those areas of function where the patient will benefit most from new learning.

One of the major problems with the outcome literature in this field is that there has been an implicit assumption that the dementing person will show intrinsic changes, rather than looking for changes in the person's function in a particular situational context. Some of the environmental changes discussed involve the elderly person in a little new learning. Many seek to use the person's remaining skills and abilities and their overlearned knowledge to elicit appropriate behaviour. Always this person — environment interaction is operating to produce the observed behaviour.

SPECIAL NEEDS OF DEMENTING PEOPLE

Dementing elderly people, like any group of disabled people, have a number of special needs that must also be considered. For most dementing people this will include, firstly, repeated failures at tasks that are transparently of low difficulty level, such as self-care and simple activities. Secondly, being lost, in the sense of not knowing where they are, who the people around them are, where significant people in their life are, at which stage of life they are currently. Thirdly, difficulties in communicating with other people. Poor memory leads to 'crossed wires', or the person assumes the listener has more information than they in fact have (cf. Hutchinson & Jensen, 1980) or there may be gross language difficulties. Problems of behavioural excess may occur — shouting or screaming continually, wandering, showing lack of social control (e.g. undressing in public). Some patients accuse other people of stealing their possessions, when they themselves have mislaid them. Some patients may be extremely resistive to the help they need with personal hygiene. Often it is these aspects of the person's behaviour which lead to problems for carers, necessitating a more restrictive placement than the person's actual lack of skills.

How to meet the person's special needs

Individual care-planning

A consequence of the above basic attitudes is that psychological management must be individual-centred. Where a number of individuals have similar needs there may be a case for ward-wide programmes. It is imperative to avoid trying to fit patients to programmes rather than vice versa. An excellent way of tackling the individual's management is for all concerned to be involved in drawing up an individual care-plan. This must cover physical, medical and social aspects as well as psychological concerns. Divisions between these areas are artificial, and the person's interests are best served if all are considered together. A multidisciplinary team is the ideal setting for these plans to be made with patients and their carers.

A thorough assessment of the person and their situation is the first stage in drawing up a care-plan. The views and wishes of the elderly person and their supporters need to be taken into account at the outset. Tensions may arise when the wishes of patient and carers do not coincide. Or it may be hard to evaluate the wishes of a severely demented person who has great difficulty in communicating. Occasionally, the patient's goal might be difficult to accept; some patients, with well-preserved insight, might even say they want to die. Complying with the patient's and/or carers' wishes will not always be possible. Establishing what these views are, and why they are held, is fundamental to understanding the individual patient and his/her unique situation.

The next stage is to identify the person's resources, strengths and abilities in each area to be considered. These are the building blocks from which any attempts to improve the person's quality of life must be constructed. Simply drawing up a list of problems, of negatives to be removed, is of little help if no positive aspects to be developed can be identified to occupy the remaining void. Having listed strengths, only then should a (shorter) list of problems, needs and difficulties be made. A care plan is then drawn up from the strengths and needs lists. It should attempt to meet some of the person's needs and to develop and utilize more of the patient's strengths. Those of most relevance to the person's quality of life should be initially selected. Goals must be specific and state exactly who is to do what, when and with whom, under what conditions. The goal must then be divided into a number of smaller steps, and means devised for assessing progress through the sub-goals to the main goal. The team should regularly review goals and progress. When goals are achieved, fresh goals can be set. If progress is not forthcoming, then smaller steps need to be created, or alternative means of tackling the same function devised.

A useful way of facilitating care-planning is to have a designated staff member (key worker) responsible for ensuring that a particular patient's care-plan is kept up to date, implemented appropriately and reviewed regularly. With training and support, most care staff can carry out care-planning and find it satisfying. Davies & Crisp (1980) and Holden & Woods (1982, ch. 10) give further details of this approach.

Although widely used in mental handicap, few evaluations of this approach with the elderly are available. The report by Brody et al (1971, 1974) of a multidisciplinary individualized treatment programme for elderly mentally impaired patients with 'excess disabilities' is relevant. During a one-year treatment period, patients showed improvements in areas directly tackled by the treatment programme, improving more than matched controls. Nine months later, when the treatment had been discontinued, these gains were lost. Continuous and consistent implementation is clearly important if such methods are to have any lasting impact.

There *is* documented evidence for behavioural change in dementing people, where a particular area of behaviour has been focused upon. A number of these specific areas, relating to dementing people's special needs, are discussed below.

Increasing activity

Several studies have specifically included dementing elderly people. Jenkins et al (1977) reported that activity levels in an old people's home lounge increased when the dementing residents were prompted to choose an activity from a selection offered, and then encouraged frequently to continue the activity. Burton (1980) showed that when hospital staff in group activity sessions consistently prompted and reinforced the patients' use of activity materials, then patients were indeed more often appropriately engaged. They were also less likely to sleep during the session! Melin & Gotestam (1981) showed that after staff had encouraged dementing patients to use activity materials on the ward for one week, they remained more active, without further encouragement, for at least a week compared with patients who had received no prompting at all. Reorganizing the environment to allow residents to participate more in activities with a clear, relevant purpose is a major feature of the group-living approach. Residents live in small groups, and are given more responsibility for the daily domestic routine. Rothwell et al (1983) found an increase in purposeful activity among residents (many suffering from dementia) in a home where this approach was introduced.

Self-care

Often nurses complain of being so busy helping dementing patients with their basic self-care that there is no time for activity sessions! Is any improvement possible? Rinke et al (1978) addressed 'self-bathing' in six elderly dementing nursing-home residents. Five components of self-bathing — undressing, soaping, rinsing, drying and dressing — were examined. Two control patients showed little systematic change, whereas the four remaining residents showed improvement (to near maximum levels) when each component was specifically prompted and reinforced. Prompting included verbal directions or a physical prompt, such as handing the resident the towel. Reinforcements used in this study included verbal praise, a wall chart for visual feedback on progress, and a choice of bathing luxuries (e.g. talcum powder or lotion) as a reward for a set level of response. The respective contributions of prompting and reinforcement were not elucidated, and it is not clear what level of intervention was needed to maintain the improvement. Possibly in some cases either prompting or reinforcement alone might have been sufficient to bring about or maintain the observed changes.

There is certainly a great deal of evidence that dependence in self-care is actually encouraged in many settings caring for dementing elderly people (e.g. Baltes et al, 1980, 1983). Perhaps skills are not being relearnt, but rather the environment is being restructured to elicit the person's remaining skills. A further example would be Melin & Gotestam's (1981) report of improved eating skills in hospitalized dementing patients when they were given unlimited time to feed themselves, and a freer choice of food and accompaniments. Previously patients had little choice, and if slow were fed by the staff. Many dementing patients may have more self-care skills than they are actually allowed to display.

Toiletting

The loss of toiletting skills — incontinence — is often described as a major problem in the care of dementing people, influencing placement, physical health and quality of life. Of psychogeriatric patients, 40–50% may be incontinent (Gilleard, 1981). Behavioural methods have been successful in reducing incontinence in children, mentally handicapped people and elderly chronic schizophrenic patients, but results with dementing people have been mixed. Some of the negative findings (e.g. Grosicki, 1968; Pollock & Liberman, 1974) may be attributed to lack of detailed behavioural analysis of the individual's toiletting difficulty (see Hodge, 1984). Certainly, Collins & Plaska (1975) had some success with the 'bell and pad' method for nocturnal incontinence. Patients were awoken and toiletted whenever the alarm on the bed sounded indicating they had begun to urinate. They showed a small reduction in bed-wetting compared with control subjects, who were awoken and toiletted as often during the night.

Toiletting programmes that take account of an individual's micturition pattern and encourage dryness, rather than accepting wetness as the norm, may enjoy success in settings where dementing patients have not previously been encouraged or prompted to remain continent. Note that this aim — keeping patients dry — is at a lower level than the independent toiletting that is the usual target of behavioural programmes in other fields. Sanavio (1981) reports the application of an independent toiletting programme with a 60-year-old dementing patient, previously incontinent day and night for two years. Wetting accidents decreased rapidly, whilst independent toiletting increased dramatically from its previous zero level. The improvements demonstrably related to the therapeutic procedures employed, and were maintained eight weeks later.

This level of independence may not be universally attainable — particularly where physical disabilities or greater degrees of cognitive deterioration are present. When toiletting is unavoidable, increasing the proportion of 'successful' visits to the toilet, whilst keeping accidents to a minimum, is desirable. Schnelle et al (1983) report a study with 21 dementing patients, none able to walk independently. The programme aimed to teach patients to ask for help from staff when the need to void occurred. Training involved prompting, social reinforcement for toileting requests and for being dry, and social disapproval for being wet. The frequency of correct toileting rose by approximately 45%. Incontinence decreased and appropriate toileting requests increased compared with controls. Similar results were obtained in two different nursing homes. The authors conclude from the rapidity of the changes observed (on the first day of intervention) that 'nursing home incontinence is more a staff–patient management problem than a patient relearning problem'. A patient requesting to be taken to the toilet is insufficient; staff must fulfil the request when it is made.

Independent toileting is a complex set of skills, including dressing/undressing, mobility, finding the toilet, recognizing the toilet as such, social awareness and planning ahead. Each individual case requires a thorough behavioural analysis, to identify exactly which aspects are causing difficulty (Hodge, 1984; Turner, 1980). The analysis needs to be multi-modal and also take into account environmental aspects, institutional factors and the relevant medical and nutritional variables. Incontinence is certainly not an area where therapeutic pessimism is justified.

Orientation

Disorientation, of some degree, is a virtually universal consequence of dementia. Verbal orientation (the ability to answer questions relating to orientation for time, person and place) has attracted more research than behavioural orientation (the ability to find the way from place to place without getting lost). Most of the relevant research comes from studies of reality orientation (RO). This approach has many components and facets, but an emphasis on encouraging correct verbal orientation, and discouraging disorientation, is usually apparent.

In the earlier studies there were hopes that improvements in orientation might lead to other behavioural changes, perhaps mediated through increased self-esteem. Unfortunately, this straightforward generalization of improvement from one area of function to others has not generally been supported in controlled studies of RO — despite many anecdotal accounts. A number of recent reviews of RO research are available (e.g. Holden & Woods, 1982; Greene, 1984; Hanley, 1984; Woods & Britton, 1985). Improvements in verbal orientation are well documented (e.g. Woods, 1979; Hanley et al, 1981; Johnson et al, 1981; Zepelin et al, 1981). Changes in other aspects of behaviour are reported much less frequently (e.g. Brook et al, 1975; Reeve & Ivison, 1985).

Two major aspects of RO are usually described. 24-hour RO is intended to be a continuous process. Staff encourage correct orientation in every contact with the dementing person, reinforced by memory aids (clocks, calendars, direction signs etc.) that clearly, unambiguously and accurately give useful and appropriate information. RO group sessions are the second component. These involve three to five patients meeting with one or two staff for 30 minutes or so at least twice a week. The content of the session varies according to the abilities and interests of group members, but would include discussion of current events and material aimed at correctly orientating group members, perhaps making links with past, well-learned knowledge. Group sessions usually utilize visual or auditory aids. Group activities enable members to enjoy some success and contact with other group members. In some places the group atmosphere has been more formal (the RO classroom). Elsewhere, social aspects have been emphasized — to the extent of having a pub setting for the RO session, complete with appropriate beverages! Certainly, best results are most likely when the person does not feel pressured, tense or afraid of failure.

There have been few attempts to evaluate the relative contributions of 24-hour RO and RO sessions. Some studies have included both, others only RO sessions. Hanley (1984) comments that evidence that staff trained to carry out 24-hour RO actually put it into practice is lacking, whereas RO sessions *have* been demonstrated to be carried out as planned (Holden & Woods, 1982). Reeve & Ivison (1985) suggest that RO sessions may add to the efficacy of 24-hour RO.

Several studies have isolated particular components of RO. Hanley et al (1981) showed that a relatively simple training procedure increased dementing patients' ability to find their way around their ward. RO sessions alone, of course, had no impact on this ability. It appears that a combination of signposting the ward and training using these signposts is most effective in bringing about and maintaining these improvements in behavioural orientation (Hanley, 1981; Gilleard et al, 1981). Signposts alone are not generally sufficient — staff need to point them out to the patients, and use them in orientating the patient around the ward.

Similarly, structured verbal orientation training programmes (including personalized information) have been examined using single-case methodology. Greene et at (1979) reported three case studies showing a clear learning effect in the phases where the items were taught; there was some generalization to performance in OT settings, but none to ratings of social behaviour in OT. Woods (1983) used a multiple-baseline design with one patient and showed that learning was largely confined to items specifically taught. Patterson (1982), as part of a much larger study of behavioural methods with the elderly, used a similar procedure with four dementing patients, who again showed a specific learning effect. This specificity does not necessarily imply that only rote learning is occurring — many items of current information (e.g. day, date and time) cannot be learnt simply by repeating what was taught in a previous session!

RO should not be seen in itself as the only psychological approach to work with dementing people. Despite recent critiques (e.g. Burton, 1982;

Schwenk, 1981; Powell-Proctor & Miller, 1982), it can make a valuable contribution to an overall approach to the dementing person. Learning — behavioural and verbal — has been demonstrated, and is most evident with material that has been specifically taught.

Social interaction and reminiscence

Relatively simple environmental changes will increase the amount of interaction between elderly patients. For example, Davies & Snaith (1980) showed that patients talked much more to each other at mealtimes if their chairs were grouped around tables — instead of being in lines along the walls! Efforts were made to reduce background noise levels, and to increase the social atmosphere of the meal. Similar changes have been reported in day-room sitting areas. Interaction increases when chairs are placed in small groups around coffee tables. This places more people within comfortable speaking distance and at a comfortable angle than the traditional round-the-walls arrangement (e.g. Peterson et al, 1977).

A shared task is important for a meaningful interaction. Melin & Gotestam (1981) used afternoon coffee to provide a focus. Previously, coffee had been served to patients in their seats, with sugar and cream already added. The effects of laying out coffee, cups, sugar, cream and cake on tables in a separate room were evaluated. From being passive recipients, patients now had to fend for themselves (or each other), as no staff were present. Social interaction increased dramatically, accompanying this opportunity for increased independence from staff and increased choice.

Other studies have attempted to increase social interaction in a small group setting. Linsk et al (1975) report that the group leader's use of behavioural methods (prompting and social reinforcement) increased talking in such a group. Gray & Stevenson (1980) showed positive feedback could help increase social interaction between group members. Having visual aids or other prompts is important in eliciting social behaviour to be reinforced. Experience of leading such groups suggests that good conversation stimulators include music, pets, children and reminders of the group members' younger days. As yet there is little evidence to back up such clinical impressions.

Interest is growing rapidly in the use of aids to reminiscence. Their use has often been elevated to the status of a therapy — Reminiscence or Life Review Therapy. Here a small group discuss topics prompted by reminiscence aids — old pictures, music and archive material from the past, mementoes etc. A good description of its implementation with dementing patients is provided by Norris & Abu El Eileh (1982). In the UK, Help the Aged (1981) have produced 'Recall', a set of six tape–slide sequences depicting events and experiences relevant to current elderly people, spanning approximately the years from 1900 to the present. Other materials are also becoming available (e.g. Holden, 1984).

Research on reminiscence with dementing people is scarce; what there is (e.g. Kiernat, 1979) is of a preliminary nature. Reminiscence, like many popular ideas, is in danger of being devalued because of its lack of focus. Thus the effects of reminiscence on depressed, unhappy elderly people may be quite different from its effects with dementing people. Research — modelled on the early RO research — that examines whether it can reduce disorientation and improve behaviour in dementing people is less likely to be productive than research assessing spontaneity and enjoyment in group sessions and improvements in relationships with staff (who are helped to know the patients better). Could reminiscence be harmful in encouraging patients to live more in the past? Clinical experience suggests this does not occur, but again research evidence is lacking.

Reminiscence is attractive — it enables the dementing person to be in the position of the expert, the authority. They were there, the staff member was not. It helps place the person in the context of his or her whole life, not simply the dementing shell now apparent. It is an age-appropriate activity, enjoyed by normal elderly people. It is most probably a valuable means of facilitating communication with dementing people. This alone would make it an important part of the overall approach.

Behaviour problems

Dealing with problem behaviours must be based on a thorough analysis of the problem, its frequency and intensity, what leads up to it, in what situations it is more and less probable and what consequences follow it. A constructional behavioural approach emphasizes the building up of appropriate behaviour — as has been described in the preceding sections — to replace the problem behaviour with something appropriate, not simply to eliminate it. Thus, Seidel & Hodgkinson (1979) report a case where a 74-year-old dementing patient was a considerable fire risk, being careless with cigarettes. They report increasing *safe* smoking behaviour.

Shouting and screaming are among the most difficult problem behaviours for staff (and other patients) to live with. Unfortunately, few successful interventions have been reported. Birchmore & Clague (1983) reduced the frequency of shouting of a 70-year-old blind lady by providing reinforcement when she was quiet. Finding an effective means of reward can be difficult; in this report several were tried, with touch — rubbing the patient's back — proving most helpful. Here the behavioural analysis had suggested that the shouting was a form of self-stimulation (for a lady receiving little sensory input). In other cases, pain, fear and a desire for contact with staff can be important factors.

Hussian (1981) reports a reduction in a patient's self-stimulatory stereotyped vocalizations when reinforcement was given for ten-second periods without any noise being made. Similar success was achieved in reducing stereotyped pulling at clothes and other objects within reach, when patients were reinforced for the similar (but appropriate) behaviour of clay moulding. In each of these cases, the potency of the intervention has been greatly increased by the use of 'artificial discriminative cues' — brightly coloured large cardboard shapes, specifically paired with reinforcement in brief training sessions. For example, a 62-year-old male nursing-home resident frequently masturbated in public. A large orange disc was used as the artificial discriminative cue, and was placed in the resident's room and in the bathroom. Elsewhere if he was observed publicly masturbating he was taken to his room, so that he could masturbate in private. The size of the cue was gradually reduced, as the frequency of masturbating in public decreased. The patient appeared to learn, with the aid of the artificial cue, to discriminate between places where the behaviour was acceptable and those where it was not. Hussian has also applied these cues to wandering, placing cues paired with positive reinforcement in safe areas. Cues paired with noxious stimuli (a loud hand-clap) were placed in hazardous areas — stairs, exits etc. Again the cues could be reduced in size as the patients' wandering reduced, with 'booster training sessions' when required. The exact mechanisms by which these cues operate needs further clarification, particularly when they are to be used in rebuilding skills. Intuitively, cues that use more of the dementing person's overlearned knowledge might be expected to be more effective than cues which require the learning of new associations. As yet comparisons have not been made, and there seem to be no reports of their use by other workers.

PSYCHOLOGICAL MANAGEMENT IN PRACTICE

So far we have seen that psychological management of dementia involves attitudes that allow the dementing person human value, dignity and respect, which acknowledge the person's potential to enjoy experiences and to change, and which cater for the dementing person's special needs, by the use of individual care plans, which encourage valued and normal activities as far as is possible, given the person's level of disability. This is a difficult, challenging task; this is not a road that leads to neat simple answers, off-the-shelf packages that can be immediately implemented. Many pitfalls await the unwary. For example, Davies (1982) reported that a year after social interaction at mealtimes had been successfully increased, as described above (Davies & Snaith, 1980), 'only token symbols of the "changes" remained'. The successful toilet-training programme reported by Schnelle et al (1983) continued to be implemented in only one of the two homes after the study finished. Even here the programme's continuation depended on the appointment of a full-time worker to ensure the staff consistency needed. Staff seemed to prefer to change wet clothes than spend the 2.5 minutes per patient per hour needed to reduce the frequency of incontinence. Tarrier & Larner (1983) found that staff did not perceive the objective behavioral changes brought about by a programme which reduced patients calling on nurses for help they did not require. Zarit et al (1982) showed that 'memory training classes' for dementing people at home had little practical value as far as relatives looking after the person at home were concerned.

Many more interventions could be listed of which the implementation has not been continued after the researcher has departed. Often one of the problems is that the sources of reward and satisfaction for the carers are not analysed as fully as they are for the patient. With dementing people the satisfaction of seeing someone improve is rare. Godlove et al (1980) showed that many care staff prefer dependent patients, perhaps because their needs are easier to predict and they are easier to manage. Psychological management involves creating an ethos where staff encourage each other and are encouraged by their managers to develop the attitudes described previously, and to work at the small goals that are attainable, using the individual programme planning approach. Woods & Britton (1985) discuss this important area of institutional change in more detail. If these aspects of the patient's environment are omitted from the behavioural analysis, the intervention is likely to miss its target.

Most dementing people of course live at home, cared for by relatives. Again, in applying the psychological approach with these people, the needs of the carer must not be neglected. Pinkston & Linsk (1984) describe how a behavioural approach can be applied in a family setting with dementing people. It is important that efforts to reduce the carer's stress be part of the plan, and that undue expectations are not placed on them to carry out behavioural procedures. They may already have developed their own coping strategies; care should be taken not to undermine these unless something more useful can be offered. Greene et al (1983) reported that *relatives'* mood improved when their dementing person participated in RO sessions at a day hospital. The onus here should be on partnership between such support services and the family, rather than yet another burden being placed on the caring relative.

This chapter has attempted to show that psychological management does have some current utility and much future promise. We have come some way from thinking that there is no point in such methods because dementing patients cannot learn. Much remains to be done, however, in establishing practical means of applying research findings in both institutional and community settings. The individualized approach described here, backed by appropriate attitudes, represents the most promising way forward for improving the psychological management of dementia sufferers.

REFERENCES

Baltes M M, Burgess R L, Stewart R B 1980 Independence and dependence in self-care behaviours in nursing home residents: an operant-observational study. International Journal of Behavioural Development 3: 489–500

Baltes M M, Honn S, Barton E M, Orzech M, Lago D 1983 On the social ecology of dependence and independence in elderly nursing home residents: a replication and extension. Journal of Gerontology 38: 556–564

Birchmore T, Clague S 1983 A behavioural approach to reduce shouting. Nursing Times 79: 20 April 37–39

Brody E M, Kleban M H, Lawton M P, Silverman H A 1971 Excess disabilities of mentally impaired aged: impact of individualised treatment. Gerontologist 11: 124–133

Brody E M, Kleban M H, Lawton M P, Moss M 1974 A longitudinal look at excess disabilities in the mentally impaired aged. Journal of Gerontology 29: 79–84

Brook P, Degun G, Mather M 1975 Reality Orientation, a therapy for psychogeriatric patients: a controlled study. British Journal of Psychiatry 127: 42–45

Burton M 1980 Evaluation and change in a psychogeriatric ward through direct observation and feedback. British Journal of Psychiatry 137: 566–571

Burton M 1982 Reality Orientation for the elderly: a critique. Journal of Advanced Nursing 7: 427–433

Collins R W, Plaska T 1975 Mowrer's conditioning treatment for enuresis applied to geriatric residents of a nursing home. Behavior Therapy 6: 632–638

Davies A D M 1982 Research with elderly people in long-term care: some social and organisational factors affecting psychological interventions. Ageing and Society 2: 285–298

Davies A D M, Crisp A G 1980 Setting performance goals in geriatric nursing. Journal of Advanced Nursing 5: 381–388

Davies A D M, Snaith P 1980 The social behaviour of geriatric patients at mealtimes: an observational and an intervention study. Age and Ageing 9: 93–99

Gilleard C J 1981 Incontinence in the hospitalised elderly. Health Bulletin (Edinburgh) 39: 58–61

Gilleard C J, Mitchell R G, Riordan J 1981 Ward orientation training with psychogeriatric patients. Journal of Advanced Nursing 6: 95–98

Godlove C, Dunn G, Wright H 1980 Caring for old people in New York and London: the 'nurses' aide' interviews. Journal of the Royal Society of Medicine 73: 713–723

Gray P, Stevenson J S 1980 Changes in verbal interaction among members of resocialisation groups. Journal of Gerontological Nursing 6: 86–90

Greene J G 1984 The evaluation of Reality Orientation. In: Hanley I, Hodge J (eds) Psychological approaches to the care of the elderly. Croom Helm, London

Greene J G, Nicol R, Jamieson H 1979 Reality Orientation with psychogeriatric patients. Behaviour Research and Therapy 17: 615–617

Greene J G, Timbury G C, Smith R, Gardiner M 1983 Reality Orientation with elderly patients in the community: an empirical evaluation. Age and Ageing 12: 38–43

Grosicki J P 1968 Effects of operant conditioning of modification of incontinence in neuropsychiatric geriatric patients. Nursing Research 17: 304–311

Hanley I 1981 The use of signposts and active training to modify ward disorientation in elderly patients. Journal of Behaviour Therapy and Experimental Psychiatry 12: 241–247

Hanley I 1984 Theoretical and practical considerations in Reality Orientation Therapy with the elderly. In: Hanley I, Hodge J (eds) Psychological approaches to the care of the elderly. Croom Helm, London

Hanley I, McGuire R J, Boyd W D 1981 Reality Orientation and dementia: a controlled trial of two approaches. British Journal of Psychiatry 138: 10–14

Help the Aged 1981 Recall — a handbook. Help the Aged Education Department, London

Hodge J 1984 Towards a behavioural analysis of dementia. In: Hanley I, Hodge J (eds) Psychological approaches to the care of the elderly. Croom Helm, London

Holden U P (ed) 1984 Nostalgia. Winslow Press, Winslow, Bucks

Holden U P, Woods R T 1982 Reality Orientation: psychological approaches to the 'confused' elderly. Churchill Livingstone, Edinburgh

Hussian R A 1981 Geriatric psychology: a behavioural perspective. Van Nostrand Reinhold, New York

Hutchinson J M, Jensen M 1980 A pragmatic evaluation of discourse communication in normal and senile elderly in a nursing home. In: Obler L K, Albert M L (eds) Language and communication in the elderly: clinical, therapeutic and experimental issues. Heath, Lexington, Mass.

Jenkins J, Felce D, Lunt B, Powell E 1977 Increasing engagement in activity of residents in old people's homes by providing recreational materials. Behaviour Research and Therapy 15: 429–434

Johnson C H, McLaren S M, McPherson F M 1981 The comparative effectiveness of three versions of 'classroom' reality orientation. Age and Ageing 10: 33–35

Kiernat J M 1979 The use of life review activity with confused nursing home residents. American Journal of Occupational Therapy 33: 306–310

Linsk N, Howe M W, Pinkston E M 1975 Behavioural group work in a home for the aged. Social Work 20: 454–463

Melin L, Gotestam K G 1981 The effects of rearranging ward routines on communication and eating behaviours of psychogeriatric patients. Journal of Applied Behavioural Analysis 14: 47–51

Norris A D, Abu El Eileh M T 1982 Reminiscence groups. Nursing Times 78: 1368–1369

Patterson R L 1982 Overcoming deficits of ageing: a behavioural approach. Plenum Press, New York

Peterson R F, Knapp T J, Rosen J C, Pither B F 1977 The effects of furniture arrangement on the behaviour of geriatric patients. Behavior Therapy 8: 464–467

Pinkston E M, Linsk N L 1984 Care of the elderly — a family approach. Pergamon Press, New York

Pollock D P, Liberman R P 1974 Behaviour therapy of incontinence in demented in-patients. Gerontologist 14: 488–491

Powell-Proctor L, Miller E 1982 Reality Orientation: a critical appraisal. British Journal of Psychiatry 140: 457–463

Reeve W, Ivison S 1985 Use of environmental manipulation and classroom and modified informal reality orientation with institutionalized, confused elderly patients. Age and Ageing 14: 119–121

Rinke C L, Williams J J, Lloyd K E, Smith-Scott W 1978 The effects of prompting and reinforcement on self-bathing by elderly residents of a nursing home. Behavior Therapy 9: 873–881

Rothwell N, Britton P G, Woods R T 1983 The effects of group living in a residential home for the elderly. British Journal of Social Work 13: 639–643

Sanavio E 1981 Toilet retraining psychogeriatric residents. Behaviour Modification 5: 417–427

Schnelle J F, Traughber B, Morgan D B, Embry J E, Binion A F, Coleman A 1983 Management of geriatric incontinence in nursing homes. Journal of Applied Behavior Analysis 16: 235–241

Schwenk M A 1981 Reality Orientation for the institutionalised aged: does it help? Gerontologist 19: 373–377

Seidel H A, Hodgkinson P E 1979 Behaviour modification and long-term learning in Korsakoff's psychosis. Nursing Times 75: 1855–1857

Tarrier N, Larner S 1983 The effects of manipulation of social reinforcement on toilet requests on a geriatric ward. Age and Ageing 12: 234–239

Turner R K 1980 A behavioural approach to the management of incontinence in the elderly. In: Mandelstam D (ed) Incontinence and its management. Croom Helm, London

Woods R T 1979 Reality Orientation and staff attention: a controlled study. British Journal of Psychiatry 134: 502–507

Woods R T 1983 Specificity of learning in Reality Orientation sessions: a single case study. Behaviour Research and Therapy 21: 173–175

Woods R T, Britton P G 1977 Psychological approaches to the treatment of the elderly. Age and Ageing 6: 104–112

Woods R T, Britton P G 1985 Clinical psychology with the elderly. Croom Helm, London

Zarit S H, Zarit J M, Reever K E 1982 Memory training for severe memory loss: effects on senile dementia patients and their families. Gerontologist 22: 373–377

Zepelin H, Wolfe C S, Kleinplatz F 1981 Evaluation of a year long reality orientation program. Journal of Gerontology 36: 70–77

Psychogeriatric and social services for the demented

INTRODUCTION

The object of this chapter is to look at the more specialized provision that may be available for the support of those suffering from dementia. This will entail some discussion of the wide variation in the quality and quantity of such support services and in the extent to which their organization facilitates their availability to the consumer. The main emphasis, however, will be on the ways in which the traditional hospital and social services can adapt themselves to the challenge of the rapid growth in the caseload of demented and other severely disabled elderly people.

It must, of course, be stressed at the outset that the bulk of the caring for patients with dementia is done by a network of family, friends and neighbours. In areas where such traditional links have weakened, the gaps may be partially plugged by voluntary organizations. Likewise the major medical and nursing input is from the primary medical care team. Many aspects of this domiciliary care will be dealt with in the next chapter, but some general points of management need to be reiterated here if we are to work out how best the more specialized (and expensive) back-up services are to be deployed.

Assessment

As will be clear from the earlier sections of this book, the care of the demented person requires a multidisciplinary approach. Central to this has to be the medical diagnosis and assessment based on careful history-taking, physical and mental examination and exclusion of treatable disorders which may mimic dementia. The establishment of a diagnosis of dementia should not, however, close one's eyes to the other physical and psychiatric disorders which so often complicate the clinical picture and course of the illness, and whose treatment and surveillance may do much to alleviate the overall burden of the patient's care. Regular re-assessment, especially in the event of any abrupt change in the patient's condition, is also important. An important task for the specialist psychogeriatric service is the encouragement of such an approach on the part of GPs and the sharing with them of skills in the management of behaviour problems associated with dementia.

These medical aspects only comprise a small part of the assessment necessary to reach a coherent plan for the patient's care. One must also look at the amount of support he or she is getting (and can count on in the future) and the emotional and physical health of any immediate carers. How much reserve is there and how long can the patient's disabilities be compensated for in his/her present environment? Which particular aspects are creating the most stress or risk in the present setting and can they be alleviated? If the carer is handicapped (e.g. by physical ill health, depression, isolation or unsuitable housing), can this be remedied? How soon will things reach a point at which it will cease to be cost-effective (in terms of risk, strain on carers and demand on support services) to maintain the patient where he/she is? Have contingency plans been made and will these minimize the overall number of moves to which the patient will be subjected during an illness which is notoriously exacerbated by them? Finally, how many agencies are going to have to become involved and how easy will it be to get them to cooperate?

A strategy for care

There are two broad groupings in planning care for demented patients based on whether they are living on their own or with other members of their family. For the latter, the main aim will be to support the relatives in their caring role as long as is possible or acceptable. This entails prompt help in crises or exacerbations of the illness and a gradual feeding-in of extra support as the load increases. If this is done well, the point at which long-term institutional care becomes necessary may be postponed till the disease is very far advanced or until death from intercurrent illness. This is a major topic of the next chapter, though I will return to it in discussing the part that the psychogeriatric service plays in that support.

The other group, who create much greater demand on the statutory services, are those living on their own. They can for a while be supported in that setting by help with household tasks and to some extent with self-care; some of the options for such domiciliary support will be discussed later. Eventually, as 24-hour supervision becomes necessary, institutional care will supervene. One of the challenges posed to planners by the rapid increase in the numbers of very elderly people (and thus of those who will be living alone and suffering from dementia) is to get a balance between the types of sheltered living (in the broad sense) that will be both acceptable to the clients and cost-effective. There is certainly an abundance of models and of attractive innovations from which we can learn.

A social or a medical service?

One such model is that of Denmark on which I, and others, have written at length elsewhere (Ammundsen et al, 1982; Godber, 1978a, 1980). The Danes have traditionally valued their elderly much more highly than we in Britain, though it has been uncommon for the elderly to live with their children. These factors have resulted in the building-up of a very high standard of services, particularly in Danish publicly-run nursing homes. It has also been a deliberate policy that responsibility for the support of those with chronic disabilities and handicaps should primarily rest with social services departments. These therefore administer a wide range of domiciliary and day-care services, sheltered housing and all long stay institutional care for the elderly (their nursing homes amalgamate under one roof the range of care of our residential homes and long-stay hospitals). The social work influence is evident in the basic precept that the elderly person has the right to live in his or her own home. If the person insists on doing that literally, he/she can be supported by an extensive package of home help, meals and day nursing care. If the person enters a nursing home, he/she will be entitled to the same privacy, furnishing his/her own room and spending as much time in it as he/she wishes — the patient usually also has his/her own toilet and shower room.

The high standard and quantity of the nursing homes is probably more than the Danes can afford (and certainly much more than we could ever aspire to in Britain). Nevertheless, some other European countries have similar levels of institutional provision, and the 'younger' countries of North America and Australia are already spending much more (per head of the very elderly) on a subsidized private nursing homes sector of which they cannot control the size (Smith, 1982). Because they run the whole range of services, however, the Danish social services are in a position to shift their priorities and alter the criteria for entry to the different sections. They have always, for instance, included a geriatric or psychogeriatric assessment in their selection procedure for sheltered housing and nursing homes, a measure which could very usefully be adopted for any publicly funded residential care in Britain. They are now placing much more emphasis on sheltered housing and have built up a very flexible home-help service capable of round-the-clock supervision if necessary.

SOCIAL SERVICES IN BRITIAN — A PATCHWORK

This contrasts strongly with the system confronting the disabled elderly Briton. The general practitioner is responsible to the Family Practitioner Committee, itself quite separate from the District Health Authority which provides the various other community health services and hospital care. Sheltered housing and some other innovatory schemes in domiciliary support come under the District Council (often not coterminous with the DHA). Home helps, meals on wheels and residential care (for which, unlike health service provision, fees are charged) come under the County Council Social Services Department. There is also a private sector in residential and nursing home care for which many clients' fees are now paid through local social security offices without reference to any medical or social work assessment of need. This arrangement clearly militates against any balanced planning of local resources within a district. There is also a clear contradiction between the stated commitment on the part of the Department of Health and Social Security (DHSS, 1981) towards 'Care in the Community' and its recent runaway subsidy of private residential care. Above all, the system confronts the demented patient and his family with a baffling number of people to deal with and the risk of bouncing unsuccessfully from one to another.

Social services homes (Part III)

Unlike their Danish counterparts, social services homes (Part III homes) in Britain have only catered for the milder end of the institutional sector, leaving the heavier end of the disability range to the long-stay hospitals. This has created a number of problems. Firstly, it can imply more moves as the person's disability increases (e.g. to sheltered housing, to a Part III home and then on to a long-stay psychogeriatric bed). It has also left the Part III homes vulnerable to changes in other parts of the system over which the social services have no control. On the one hand, the exit to hospital care of the most disabled has been restricted by the lack of growth in that sector despite a steady rise in clientele. Indeed, as geriatric and psychogeriatric units have concentrated more on short-term care, their long-stay compartments have shrunk. This has not only meant less movement from the Part III homes, but also more entry to such homes of people whose disability would previously have 'earned' them hospital places. On the other hand, the increasing scope of domiciliary support has filtered out the able-bodied candidates who used to lighten the load for the staff in the homes.

This greater concentration of disability has exposed the inadequacy of staffing levels and expertise in the homes and also the unsuitability of many of the buildings they occupy. There has also been a polarization into those with severe physical handicap and those with dementia, with the latter now accounting for nearly half of the new entrants. These groups often blend poorly and require rather different caring skills and physical environments. With some reluctance many social services departments have set up special homes (or specialized wings within homes) with higher staffing levels to cater for the more difficult cases of dementia.

Homes for the elderly mentally infirm (EMI homes)

Apart from the reluctance to recognize that the Part III sector was being drawn into the care of heavily disabled people, there were other misgivings about this sort of specialization. There were unfortunate early experiences in areas with poor psychogeriatric provision where EMI homes were becoming mini-hospitals without the essential specialized nursing and medical back-up. There was also the fear that they would become stig-matized and that their existence would further discourage the ordinary homes from trying to cope with their demented residents. In areas of low population density, they could also imply long distances for visiting by friends and relatives. On the other hand, there is little doubt that with good liaison with the psychogeriatric service, with the latter helping in the initial assessment and taking over those residents who really needed hospital care, the arrangement was advantageous. Residents could be seen as belonging there rather than face ostracism and heavy tranquillization in the ordinary homes. Since the non-demented residents of the latter are usually physically very frail, the Danish model, split between 'somatic' and 'psychiatric' homes, seems a sensible model to follow.

Care of the severely mentally infirm

Once in a nursing home, the Danish resident need not move again, apart from the need for acute hospitalization. It is rare for a 'somatic' home resident to move to a 'psychiatric' home, since dementia coming on in a known resident is generally well tolerated (as in British Part III homes). As has been mentioned, though, the latter are not geared to nursing the very frail or very demented. When that point is reached, the resident would become a candidate for long-term hospital care. What happens at that point varies widely.

Theoretically he would be transferred to a psychogeriatric bed or, if no longer mobile, to a geriatric bed. If the psychogeriatric service was func-tioning badly, he might end up in a geriatric bed, whether he was mobile or not, and vice versa with an ailing geriatric service. If neither came to the rescue, he would stay put till he died unless things became so difficult that they led to admission to a general medical ward as an emergency (spurious or otherwise) or, following a fall, to an orthopaedic ward. The home would usually then refuse to have him back, and it would be left to the physician or surgeon to lean on the geriatric or psychogeriatric colleague. Because the physician's leaning power would probably be greater than that of the Part III home, one or other would take the demented person over.

If the psychogeriatric (or geriatric) service is also failing to meet its demand from the community, a number of borderline patients will find their way into Part III homes, where they may be too difficult from the start, thus tightening the vicious circle. Another feature of this dismal situ-ation can be the practice of 'swapping', whereby the psychogeriatric unit will only take in a needy case from a Part III home if it accepts a 'reha-bilitated' patient in exchange. This is a bad arrangement all round; it degrades the patient; it leaves the Part III home with little redress if things work out badly; it also leaves the hospital with a long-stay patient in the place of one who would probably have been discharged within the next month or two at any rate.

Fortunately, things need not be as bad as this if the geriatric and psychogeriatric units are functioning well. It is the policy in our unit to keep an eye on what is coming our way from the residential sector and periodically get the homes to indicate which of their clients create the heaviest nursing load. The candidates from the various homes are then considered (in priority of need rather than decibels of demand) as long-stay vacancies come up. Many of the difficult cases turn out to have partially remediable problems (fecal impaction, depression, paranoid symptoms) which can be tackled in the setting of the home or with a short-stay admission. In the latter case it is always understood that the home holds the bed for the patient's return. Likewise, we keep a close eye on borderline patients placed into Part III homes to ensure that they really are manageable in that setting.

There is a little doubt that a system that requires this sort of move at such a stage in the patient's illness is unsatisfactory both when it happens and when it fails to do so. DHSS did flirt with the idea of the Continental-style nursing home but was daunted by the administrative barriers which were exacerbated when it reorganized the National Health Service to the district level (without doing the same to Social Services Departments). The tightening of financial and staffing controls on local government has also deterred Social Services Departments from accepting the realities of their position and staffing the Part III homes to a nursing level.

One other factor in such reluctance is the desire to maintain an atmosphere of homeliness rather than a nursing orientation. Perhaps therefore we should look at the division of the Part III and the hospital clientele on the basis of which patients would benefit most from a domestic/community interaction environment and which would be more in need of skilled nursing/behaviour management. By that sort of framework the homes might cater mainly for the non-demented, however frail physically, with assistance as needed from the district nursing service. The geriatric and psychogeriatric units could then pool their long-stay resources to cater for those whose behaviour and confusion would be incompatible with that setting. This could be much more satisfactory for the customers, would entail much less movement between the two sectors and could help to remove the very arbitrary boundary that separates geriatric and psychogeriatric long-stay patients.

Private residential care

The voluntary and private sectors have had their equivalent to the Part III homes in the form of rest homes. There is also a nursing-home sector, though this has not played a large part in the care of the severely demented. Rest homes have been patchy in their ability to cope with demented patients. Their readiness to do has often increased when the market has been tight, though some proprietors have developed a particular interest and skill in this area and provide a real alternative to the EMI homes. Generally speaking, however, the rest homes have catered for those with mild disabilities, with some being little more than residential hotels.

Paradoxically, at a time when the Part III homes have been grappling with the problem of increasingly frail clientele and DHSS policy has been towards community care, the last few years have seen an explosive increase in the number of rest homes which has been almost entirely funded by DHSS (Godber, 1984). A change in the regulations governing supplementary benefits enabled elderly people with less than £3000 capital to claim the full amount of rest-home fees without the requirement of any medical or social work assessment of need (DHSS, 1983). No such payments could be made, however, to buy extra care to maintain a person at home, and with inadequate growth in sheltered housing and home help services, rest-home admission became the path of least resistance.

The main causes of concern about this development were its rapidity (over a period of three years such payments increased by £200 million nationally and the number of rest homes in many areas more than doubled); the bias towards the mildly disabled for whom less costly options in domiciliary support would have been preferable; the lack of control over standards. More stringent regulations on standards are now being introduced, and DHSS has tried to exert some control over costs and the shape of the clientele by setting price bands for different dependency groups. More needs to be done, however, along the lines of initial assessment of medical and social need (the present system still favours the most mildly disabled).

A welcome concept, though, is that of dual registration of homes (for residential and nursing levels of care). This might be a backdoor way towards the Danish model. It must be recalled, though, that the Danes and others (Smith, 1982) found it very difficult to shape private sector provision in this way and ended up giving the money to the social services department to run the homes themselves.

OPTIONS IN DOMICILIARY CARE

What, then, are the community alternatives and how well can they meet the needs of demented patients living alone? It is of course clear that, barring very acute illness of fatal accidents, these patients will very rarely live out their lives at home. There will, however, be a period of months or even a year or two during which extra support with housework and shopping, the ensuring of an adequate diet, supervision of medication and counteraction of isolation may keep things in equilibrium despite quite marked mental impairment. Such domiciliary support can extend survival at home very much longer still for non-demented but physically very handicapped old people, which can therefore benefit the demented indirectly by reducing the pressure on institutional care.

The traditional domiciliary social services

The traditional services to old people at home are well known. In Britain, primary medical care is well developed, though GP involvement is still too often dependent on self-referral, at which demented patients are bad. Early identification and case-finding is best carried out by nurses, though the use of health visitors for this seems costly and inefficient (in view of their expensive training in child care). The work could be done more appropriately by nurses trained for the needs of the elderly who might also fill some of the vacuum of interest in this group on the part of community social workers.

Home helps have become the mainstay of domiciliary support from social services, carrying out a much wider range of formal and informal tasks than the 'domestic' that the elderly generally expect. As with many other items of social service, the requirement of the client to pay (or subject themselves to a means test) may deter a number in need. Cutbacks in social services budgets have also restricted the service in many areas. In others there have been imaginative extensions of the home help concept to cover periods of absence of caring neighbours and relatives (e.g. weekends) or to provide help at strategic times of the day ('getting up' and 'tucking in' services). Many home helps build up a much more supportive relationship with their clients than their official commitment would suggest and will pop in at other times in the week just to check how the clients are or do some extra shopping.

Home helps are often in a good position to check how much the demented patient is eating, and preparation of a meal may be the most important part of their session's work. The mainstay on this front, however, is through the delivery of cooked meals (meals on wheels) which, if eaten regularly, can just about prevent secondary problems of malnutrition. In some areas, though, the meals are only delivered two or three times a week, and where provision for the weekend is included, it is usually in the form of a cold meal to be heated up later. Many demented patients forget to eat the hot meals, let alone heat up the weekend one, and some extra supervision (e.g. by a neighbour who may also help with certain other meals) may make a vital difference.

Another way of getting a meal into the client may be through attendance at a lunch club or day centre. These also of course combat social isolation and may provide general stimulation, which carries over to the client's overall performance at home. Further mention will be made later of the scope of day care for the demented. Although this stimulating and feeding role has some value, the major contribution of day care in the services of the demented is probably to give spells of respite for caring relatives; that clientele is not always, however, too welcome at day centres.

Sheltered housing

The concept of grouped dwellings, usually flats, with a resident warden to act as a good neighbour and to be available as the first point of call in an emergency (through an intercom) has grown in popularity in the last twenty years. Most have been developed by District Council Housing Departments, but many also by voluntary housing associations (using grants from the government-funded Housing Corporation) and a few by private developers. As with the residential sector, these have encountered the problem of increasing frailty among their clientele, with the load on the warden increasing as the initial cohort ages.

This has led to the concept of 'extra care' sheltered housing ('Part $2\frac{1}{2}$'), with higher staffing levels to enable more to be done for the tenants. This might include help with getting up or preparing meals, supervision of medication and more positive encouragement of communal activity among the tenants. Such schemes would tend to recruit frailer than average clients and support them through to levels of dependency comparable with those in residential care (Godber, 1978b). Demented patients may be maintained to quite high levels of disability, provided they move into the scheme early enough to be able to get their bearings. Many new schemes in the last few years have followed this model, and there has also been the realization that extra staffing and a clearer concept of the role of the warden may considerably increase the scope of existing complexes. At the same time this creates a dilemma for Housing Departments, who find themselves being sucked into providing a social rather than a purely housing service.

Central alarm systems

Despite these reservations, a number of housing departments have embarked on the use of modern telecommunication systems to offer some of the ingredients of grouped sheltered housing to people in their existing accommodation. Such schemes have a central unit which can be alerted by a radio transmitter or adapted telephone installed in the client's home. The alarm can be triggered in the same way as that in a sheltered housing unit, though the system can be modified to check routinely if the person is all right (e.g. by activating a buzzer or light at a regular time of day which the tenant then switches off if all is well).

One such scheme is that in Stockport (Lewis, 1979; Tinker, 1984) which has also been used to provide cover to some blocks of housing for the elderly and also to augment the emergency cover of its existing sheltered housing. When an alarm goes off at the central office, the response is mediated via radio-linked mobile wardens. The latter also do a certain amount or routine visiting of clients of the scheme. After the initial capital outlay it is relatively cheap to install further units (even on a temporary basis for people discharged from hospital). The great attraction of this system for the demented patient is that it saves uprooting her from her familiar home and neighbourhood and of course the support she was already getting there. This has to be offset against possible problems in her operating the alarm. The Stockport scheme met with general satisfaction from its clients and has resulted in a cut in building of new sheltered housing complexes and Part III homes in favour of homes for the very frail to which the alarm-supported clients ultimately graduate.

'Good neighbour' schemes

Another approach has been to formalize or buy in support from neighbours. One of the best-known of these was that operated by Kent Social Services Department, in which social workers were given a budget to buy domiciliary care for old people as a way of avoiding residential home admission. (Two important sources of information on this and other approaches to maintaining the frail elderly at home are by Ferlie (1983) and Tinker (1984).) One approach is to find someone living close to the patient and contract with them to help with housework, provide certain meals and maintain a regular eye on him or her. There may be a basic requirement to call one or twice each day, though the 'neighbour' will often call at other times as well and perform little extra services as part of the relationship and concern that develops. A skilled coordinator is a vital part of such schemes. An alternative approach is to identify people wishing to offer this sort of service (perhaps a home help wanting a more flexible and responsible role) and pay each to act as a 'professional neighbour' to a number of elderly people at risk.

Home Care Attendant schemes

A similar approach but without the immediate neighbourhood context is that of the Home Care Attendant. A variety of such schemes have been developed (Ferlie, 1983; Tinker, 1984), initiated either by Social Services or Community Nursing Departments (the latter merging into the concept of the 'hospital at home'). The aim is usually to provide the sort of care in the client's home that would be available in a residential home. This may be on a one-to-one basis or by a team of Care Attendants who work on a shift system with a number of clients. Many of these schemes were modelled on services of younger chronically disabled people whose requirements would often remain stable over a long period. This is less likely in the elderly, particularly those with dementia, for whom it may therefore be best used for short periods (of illness or to cover absence or sickness of carers) or even temporarily to boost cover in a sheltered housing scheme or Part III home). Care Attendant teams also need a skilled manager whose tasks will include: assessment of the needs of clients; setting the objectives and limits of the care to be provided; recruiting, training and supporting the care staff; coping with the many problems which may arise.

'Boarding out' and 'fostering' the elderly

Following the well-established practice of placing rehabilitated long-stay psychiatric patients 'in the community' in group homes and with individual families, the same approach has also been tried with elderly people (Ferlie, 1983). This can certainly be a cheaper option than full residential care for carefully selected old people. Unfortunately, many of the features of advancing dementia are among those which were found to contra-indicate this sort of placement. There may, however, be some scope for it in short-term relief for relatives as an alternative to hospital admission.

Evaluation

In her book 'Staying at home' Anthea Tinker (1984) describes an extensive evaluation of some of these innovations in domiciliary support. This indicated the capacity of home care, good neighbour and central alarm schemes to support people to a dependency level well into the Part III range. She also made a very thorough analysis of the cost (taking into account that of other health and social service input, pensions, capital outlay etc.) and showed that for these high-dependency clients this was comparable to that of residential care. For those of medium dependency, however, (many of whom are currently drifting into rest homes) the innovatory schemes were much cheaper, particularly the alarms. One point she emphasized strongly was the need for joint planning in such developments because of their impact in terms of extra demand on other parts of the system. It was also clear that these schemes lent themselves better to the physically disabled than the demented.

THE PSYCHOGERIATRIC SERVICE

Is this a specialized field?

As has been mentioned, about a quarter of the long-term institutional care for the eldely in Britain (excluding that of chronically hospitalized schizophrenics) is provided by the geriatric and psychiatric services. It was the steady accumulation of such patients into beds vacated by the more effective treatment of TB and the acute infectious diseases that led to the emergence of geriatric medicine as a specialty. With a painstaking approach to rehabilitation and a move to earlier intervention and greater involvement in the acute care of the elderly, it was shown that the tide could be stemmed.

Somewhat later, a similar impetus developed within psychiatry following reports by a few pioneers of the improvement in service delivery and the satisfaction that could be derived from specializing in the psychiatry of old age (e.g. Arie, 1972; Pitt, 1974). Despite the very limited opportunities for training in this field and the ambivalent attitudes of DHSS and the Royal College of Psychiatrists, there has been a rapid increase in such specialization and a gratifying quality of entrants to the field.

Although services for dementia have been the major priority in the minds of districts setting up these posts, most psychogeriatricians have elected to deal with the full range of old-age psychiatry (though not as a rule the residue of ageing schizophrenics). Offering a service to the over-65s makes referral more straightforward for GPS, and gives the psychogeriatrician a group in which he can expect some 'cures' and (less daunted by physical frailty and the prejudices of ageism) take a more optimistic approach than is used in mainstream psychiatry.

The importance and results of this commitment to the elderly can be illustrated by comparing contact rates and performance in areas with and without a specialized psychogeriatric service. In a community survey of the elderly in Mannheim, Cooper & Schwartz (1982) demonstrated a prevalence of psychiatric disorder of 20%, yet only two of the eighty 'cases' had been in recent contact with the (generalist-based) psychiatric service. Figures from the Southampton Psychiatric Case Register (1982–4), where a 'comprehensive' psychogeriatric service operates, showed that during the year 1983, 3.5% of the over-65 population were in contact with that service. The psychogeriatric service in fact took 35% of all adult psychiatric referrals and 40% of the patients passing through psychiatric beds. Although 50% of the new elderly referrals were suffering from functional illnesses, only 2% were seen by the general psychiatrists. This seems to bear out a more positive approach to functional illness (and dementia) within a psychogeriatric service, also illustrated by the large surge in referral rates which followed the take-over by the psychogeriatric service of an area previously covered only by the general psychiatry service). A recent comparison of the care of demented patients in areas with and without a specialized psychogeriatric service showed clear benefit from the former, and again showed that organic and functional illness referrals were higher with the psychogeriatric service (Ball et al, 1983).

Psychogeriatricians have been claiming these sorts of results for a long time and, like geriatricians, are mildly irritated at the complacency of generalists who feel that they give the elderly a perfectly adequate service — neither specialty would have arisen had that been the case. It is only to be expected that psychiatrists working only with the elderly should become more familiar with the presentations and natural history of dementia. They are therefore more likely to spot the complicating and often remediable factors that can make so much difference to the load on carers. Similarly they learn the variety of ways in which depression may present and the value of a positive and eclectic approach to treatment. Their skills in medical diagnosis and treatment also have to be resurrected, along with familiarization with the actions and side-effects of non-psychiatric drugs. They also amass a great deal of information about local facilities for the elderly and can invest the time in building up the very necessary links with other services. Above all they stake their professional reputation on the care of the elderly (as opposed to seeing it as a sideline or a chore). This is bound to help the morale of the rest of the team and makes it easier to develop and maintain the clear operational policy essential to an effective service.

Operating the service

It is clear from the size of the caseload of old-age psychiatry that the service must be centred in the community. It must be active in assessment and treatment in the home and the support of those looking after the patients there. It must also educate those in other services to manage the many patients who will never come near the psychogeriatric service, and at the same time teach them to pick out those who should be referred. The expensive resource of hospital beds needs to be rationed carefully to facilitate admission for those needing treatment or to defuse crises, and with those that are left to accommodate those most in need of long-term care. In discussing the service as it relates to the needs of the demented patients, I will draw heavily on examples from our own unit, though very similar things are going on in many other psychogeriatric services.

Assessment

Most British psychogeriatricians prefer to assess patients in their own homes if possible. This enables them to be seen more at their ease and with the evidence around them as to how well they are coping or being coped with. We encourage GPs. to phone their referrals so that our secretaries can extract details that will be useful to us (especially ways of contacting friends or relatives who can give further information). As we normally see the patients the same day, they are also able to warn them when we are likely to call. The approach to the assessment is very much along the lines suggested at the beginning of this chapter. In particular, what has been the overall pattern of the illness and has there been any recent exacerbation to suggest a reversible or treatable complication? Are there any symptoms or behaviour suggestive of depression (a common complication of which the treatment may improve behaviour and relieve distress). This initial assessment has to be thorough, as it will be the basis not only for short-term intervention but for the longer-term prognosis and plan for the patient's care and our part in it.

In the case of the demented patient living alone, our main role will be to offer some sort of forecast as to the likely progression of the illness, so that longer-term contingency plans can be made for the time when he/she is no longer able to cope there. At the same time we may also be able to suggest ways of reducing his/her vulnerability in the short term. It may be appropriate to prescribe medication and, if the patient is in an acute flare-up of confusion, he/she may need a short spell in our unit. Apart from that, however, we would expect the GP and Social Services Department to follow the situation and arrange future care.

We would envisage more continuous supportive involvement by the service, however, with those being cared for in a family setting. The initial visit is therefore additionally important in setting the pattern for this future partnership and indicating what sort of help the family can expect from us. Sometimes the situation will have become very fraught, particularly if there has been an acute exacerbation of confusion. Prompt help, backed up if appropriate by short-term admission, will help to restore the family's confidence. Needless to say, we have always encouraged GPs to refer before things reach a critical stage or relatives get to the end of their tether.

Although in many cases it is clear from the GP's story that admission will be necessary, we are still reluctant to by-pass the home assessment. It some-times turns out that the emergency would be better coped with in a medical, geriatric or surgical unit, and every now and then the main problem turns out to be a fracture. In other cases the crisis may simply mark the end stage of a precarious existence living alone for which the most appropriate solution will probably be a direct admission to residential care (which social workers may not think of if the hospital always comes to the rescue). If the GP is right and the patient does need to come into our unit, it is easier to discuss this with the family or friends (not to mention the patient) before the move takes place, so that we can put things into the perspective of a longer-term plan, and so that they can begin to make the arrangements necessary for when the patient is discharged.

The greater the pressure on the unit's beds, the more essential it is to negotiate the discharge in this way before the patient is admitted, while the initiative is still firmly in our hands. Ths helps to counteract the all too common assumption that admission to the psychogeriatric unit is a one-way journey. If things are made clear at the outset without unrealistic promises of improvement and the admission then takes place without delay, it is very rare for the discharge to be vetoed by the carers. When patients are admitted from residential homes, we make no bones about it and expect the bed to be held. Obviously, one cannot always predict what the outcome of the spell in hospital will be, and one's prognosis may sometimes have to span the range from fair recovery to death. Apart from considerations about the discharge, it is a good discipline to try always to admit the patient with a plan for treatment, and I have always discouraged the concept of 'admission for assessment'. This can all too easily become a non-decision (usually based on an inadequate history and examination) and may lead to an unnecessary or prolonged stay in hospital. If that happens frequently, it tends to lead to blocked 'assessment beds'.

Follow-up

This is an essential part of the management of the demented patient in a community orientated service. At a time of acute confusion or just after the discharge, it may be necessary to call two or three times in a week to monitor progress, alter medication and show support for the carers. This is particularly so if beds are tight and one would rather have admitted the patient in the first place; if things get worse, though, it then becomes imperative to arrange admission somehow.

It is the policy in our unit to designate one of the doctors or community psychogeriatric nurses (CPNs.) to visit the patient at home within 48 hours of discharge. This is to ensure that things have gone as planned, that medication is being taken regularly and that any extra services ordered have materialized. It again reassures the carers that our involvement does not end when the patient leaves hospital and can also tide them through the transient increase in confusion that frequently follows the move. Those returning to a precarious existence on their own at home may actually be accompanied by an occupational therapist (who will usually have taken them on a trial visit already) to make sure that they get themselves installed adequately. Patients placed in residential homes also get an early visit, especially if problems are anticipated. My arrival within hours of the patient may give the staff of the home the (perhaps correct) impression that I am expecting trouble, but it is also reassuring. It is also a useful corrective against premature discharge, as one does not encourage the staff to gloss over problems when lining up the placement if one knows one will be reprimanded by the home when things go wrong. Conversely, though, it makes it easier to embark on a borderline discharge in the knowledge that a member of the unit will follow the situation closely and arrange readmission if things go wrong. This 'after-sale service' has certainly helped to build up trust, not only with families but also with the homes, who have overcome much of their earlier reluctance over 'patients from the psycho-geriatric unit'.

These follow-up visits are done by medical staff if the need is mainly one of adjusting medication or otherwise reviewing medical progress. Visits to the residential homes are mainly done by consultant staff to maintain continuity. Our practice is to visit homes with residents 'on our books' every four to six weeks, but more often if there are problems with a particular patient. It has been understood with the GPs that we can get involved with patients previously known to us if requested by the staff, but referral of other cases would have to be initiated by the GP. I might visit ten homes in an average week and see or be asked to see a couple of patients in each (though some of the homes might have a dozen or more of our clients). This can obviously be time-consuming, but with two to three hundred patients annexed in the homes it pays ample dividends in reducing the pressure on our beds. It also gives us forewarning of those heading towards our long-stay beds. The regular contact and advice seems also to help standards and morale in the homes.

The other wing of the community follow-up consists of the CPNs, whose role I will be discussing next. The number of home visits done each year from our unit is about 6000 by medical staff and a similar figure by the CPNs. This can create problems of 'stepping on the GP's toes, and we obviously had to reach a general agreement as to who does what. On visits directly requested by the GP, we will initiate or alter treatment as we see fit and communicate this with him or her in a full letter within a couple of days (or by phone if urgent). If we change medication on subsequent visits, this is also confirmed by letter and we try to avoid tampering with non- psychotropic medication or generally upstaging the GP. Conversely, we make it clear which patients we do not intend to follow. This particularly applies to those seen at home whom we assess as needing residential care but for whom we would leave further action with the GP and area social work team (who automatically get copies of our assessment reports).

Community psychogeriatric nurses

Most psychogeriatric services prefer their CPNs to confine their work to the elderly. Although they have a substantial caseload of patients on depot neuroleptic, we regard ours as specialists, particularly in the support of families caring for demented patients. This involves a continuing counselling role, helping the carers to come to terms with the changes in the patient, the prognosis and the burden of caring for him or her, as well as any feelings of resentment, aggression and guilt towards the patient or the world at large. They offer practical advice on behaviour management, medication and ways of obtaining the extra aids and support to which the clients are entitled. They also act as the informed advocate for the family in chasing up their needs from GPs, social services and other agencies. They can also get the psychogeriatrician to reassess the patient or can line up an urgent or relief admission to the unit if required. Indeed, we rely very much on their assessment of the strain at home in setting the frequency of relief admission or deciding on the eventual need for long-term care. They will frequently spot changes in the health of the carer, such as the onset of a depressive illness, and get this attended to by the GP before things break down. Their involvement will also continue after the death or long-stay admission of the patient, to help the carers with their feelings of loss and guilt.

To fulfil these functions effectively, the CPN should be seen as a member of the primary care as well as the specialist team. For this reason each of ours is aligned to a group of practices and as a rule shares office space with the health visitors for that area. They will frequently be consulted by the latter and the district nurses, as well as GPs and social workers, about patients who may not yet be known to our service. This gives them an important educational role as well as putting them in a position to screen out cases that may need formal referral to our service. They are also in frequent contact with us and come to a weekly meeting (also attended by staff from the short-stay wards) to check over the arrangements for forth-coming discharges and to report on any problems with their patients.

Relative support groups

These comprise another very important part of the support of carers and may originate as part of a self-help organization (e.g. Alzheimer's Disease Society) or at the initiative of the psychogeriatric service. The former model will also serve as a way of spreading information and as a local pressure group, particularly where services are inadequate. We have set up four rela-tives' groups in different parts of our catchment area with varied professional input, but always a CPN. One practical problem is that of making sure the relatives can get there and the patient can be looked after for that period. The benefit obtained from attendance is, however, very clear, despite the range of the problems and severity of illness experienced by the different carers and of their own reactions to it. With careful lead-ership the group can be of great help in sharing the many negative feelings and frustrations as well as practical ways of coping. Another important aspect of the support is that received by those members whose 'patients' have died or come in for long stay.

Day care

As was indicated earlier, I would see the main value of day care for the demented as lying in the respite it offers to caring relatives. Even with the functionally ill elderly, it is difficult to use a day hospital as an area for short-term therapy, and the scope for rehabilitation is much less than at a geriatric day hospital. The major difference, therefore, between day care for the demented as run by voluntary groups, social services and the psychogeriatric unit is that of the severity of behaviour disturbance each can cope with. As day centres are usually more numerous and geographi-cally available to the consumer than day hospitals, this often means that many of the more difficult and thus needy cases cannot be found a niche, while there is often plenty of room for those in less need in the day centres.

This situation may be improved simply by increasing day hospital provision, though this is expensive, usually hampered by transport prob-lems, and fails to attack the problem of the scope of day centre care. A promising approach has been that of the travelling day hospital in which a team of staff set up 'shop' in suitable venues in different parts of the catchment area each day of the week (Hettiaratchy, 1985). This greatly eases the problem of transporting the patient and is particularly useful in rural areas. The value of such an arrangement can be extended if existing day centres are used as the venues and the regular staff (or volunteers) encouraged to help with the 'day hospital' day. This will improve their skills and confidence with the more difficult patients and they may then be readier to accept them on 'day centre' days as well. There is a strong case for widening this approach to incorporate a 'geriatric' day to cater for those chronically physically disabled patients who do not meet the criteria for full day-hospital rehabilitation but are too heavy for the average day centre. In the future we may therefore need to think more in terms of day care centres with specific programmes for different days of the week, with the basic staffing augmented by the appropriate professionals for that day's clientele.

In stressing the respite role of day care I would not wish to deny the obvious value that specific activities, the social environment and the general stimulation bring to the patient. In some cases, however, day care may be counterproductive by muddling or upsetting the patient or by virtue of the hassle for the carer of getting him or her ready for it. In some services the latter problem can be alleviated by sending someone in to help get the patient ready for the transport. Another option is to provide the day care in the patient's home. This has been the principle of the 'sitting service' set up by my colleague Henry Rosenvinge in conjunction with the voluntary organization, MIND. This is operated by a salaried coordinator who deploys a team of volunteers (in fact paid a small hourly rate to underline the contractual obligation to the client) to look after patients in their homes for specified periods to allow the carer to rest or undertake some outside activity. The service is linked to the psychogeriatric unit and therefore complementary to the support available from that quarter. Evaluation of the scheme has shown it to be very well received and to have postponed long-stay admission as shown by survival times in long-stay beds as compared with those not covered by it (Rosevinge et al, 1986).

Relief admission

These form an important element of the respite needed for family carers in their 24-hour, seven-day-a-week commitment. Because relief admissions are disruptive for the demented patient, they should not be started too soon but nor should they be delayed till the relative is exhausted and beginning to harbour feelings of rejection. They may be needed before the patient's disability reaches a level appropriate to a hospital setting, in which case short stays may be arranged in a Part III home, with the psychogeriatric unit taking over later on.

Sometimes the first admission to the psychogeriatric unit will be pre-cipitated by an acute flare-up or an illness on the part of the carer. As mentioned earlier, a quick response is vital and it is likewise essential that dates set for relief admissions should never be cancelled or postponed for lack of a bed. It may, on the other hand, be necessary to extend the period in hospital (from the customary fortnight) if the patient deteriorates or the carer is unwell. In the early stages one sometimes encounters reluctance on the carer's part to have the patient back (often a sign of depression). If the patient does not meet the criteria for a long-stay bed, a sympathetic but firm insistence on the discharge is necessary, though perhaps extending the stay a couple of weeks if the carer needs to go onto antidepressants. (This of course underlines the hardship of the whole matter of dementia care and the fact that a good service may ease the problem somewhat and share it out more fairly, but does not make it disappear.) These teething problems are easier to manage if the CPN has already built up a supportive relationship and if the service has been prompt in its help up to that stage. The interval between the first relief and eventual long stay will be governed by the rate of the patient's deterioration, the resilience and attitude of the carer and the availability of long-stay beds; it may vary from a few months to four to five years. The gaps between admissions would normally start at two to three months and narrow to four weeks or less.

Rationing and use of psychogeriatric beds

It is clear from what has been said that the effectiveness and credibility of the community end of the psychogeriatric service hinges on its ability to help out with admission when things get too difficult for the home setting. The disparity between the numbers of demented patients and beds implies the need for rationing and efficiency. Where services are poorly organized, a backlog develops, intolerable strain is placed on carers, and after admission has eventually taken place it is often difficult to persuade them to take up the task again. In many such cases the patients may be at a fairly early stage in the illness (perhaps a flare-up in a multi-infarct dementia or the complication of a superimposed depression) and may therefore improve somewhat and then survive for several years in hospital, blocking the entry of often much needier cases. Many psychogeriatricians will remember inheriting such situations when first appointed to their posts.

Their reaction had to be put the top priority on short-term care to establish the turnover necessary to cope with the emergencies as they arose. This would involve a temporary embargo on long-stay admissions, a period of very hectic home-based care and strict undertakings from the carers of those actually admitted that the patients would return when things settled. For those clearly needing long-term care the situation could be eased a little with relief admissions as beds permitted. As turnover improved, the criteria for short-stay admission could be eased, planned reliefs could be set up and eventually long-stay admissions could be restarted. Inevitably, a few of the short-stay patients would have proved impossible to discharge (though the better the assessment and the firmer the discharge policy, the smaller that number would be). These have to have the first priority on long-stay vacancies. As the service is seen by GPs to be functioning better, the demand will of course increase and it will be a while before a steady state is reached.

The load will also be influenced by bottlenecks in other services (e.g. delays in transfer to Part III or geriatric unit beds) and a medium-stay area may be needed to avoid these (or some of the more slowly recovering multi-infarct patients) blocking beds in the short-stay wards. Generally speaking, a given population of elderly people will generate a certain demand for acute psychogeriatric care. Only the beds that are left after that demand is satisfied can be afforded for longer-term care. The smaller this residue, the more of these too will be needed for short-term relief to share the support around.

Our experience in Southampton would be fairly typical of the application of these principles. Before the setting-up of the present service (started in 1974 and expanded to cover a wider area in 1979) there were 250 beds, of which only 10–20 were actually functioning in a short-stay role. Admissions totalled 150–200 a year, of which about 70 were for long-term care (with an average survival of $3\frac{1}{2}$ years). With the switch to a comprehensive service the admissions rose, eventually to 950 a year, with a deployment of 55 beds for acute (functional and organic) admissions, 20 for reliefs and 20 for medium stay. Thirty beds had to be taken down for ward changes, and of the 125 that remain for long-term care several are currently empty (though some are on offer to the most disabled of the community patients, but the carers have not yet elected to take them up).

Links with other services

A psychogeriatric service cannot work in isolation, and mention has already been made of the close links that have to be built up with residential homes if they are going to take their increasing share of the dementia caseload — a share which inevitably increases if psychogeriatric units switch beds from long to short-term care.

The other service particularly liable to be affected is the Geriatric Unit, of which the caseload overlaps so much with the psychogeriatrics. DHSS policy (1972) has been that demented patients with major physical illness or disability should be cared for by the Geriatric Unit. It has therefore usually been reckoned that confusion secondary to acute physical illness or the inability to walk would be indications for geriatric rather than psycho-geriatric admission. Many patients of course slip in and out of that category during a demented illness, and the longer the psychogeriatric service maintains people in the community, the more likely is it that mobility problems will supervene — in such instances, though, we would obviously feel obliged to see the case through. In practice the boundary between the two specialties in any one district is mainly influenced by their level of resources and effectiveness. If one is functioning poorly, the GPs merely refer more heavily to the other. This can lead to rather defensive attitudes, especially when both services are hard-pressed or if personalities clash (Ball et al, 1983; Godber, 1978c).

From the consumers' point of view there clearly needs to be very close collaboration between the specialties, not just because of the overlap in clientele but because of their common interest and outlook. If agreement can be reached on operational policies, it is only logical that the long-stay beds should be used as a single resource (with specialization of function between wards) and that there should be substantial joint areas of care in the acute and relief beds as well as the longer-term aspects of day care. A very useful pointer to the direction in which we should be heading is the system operating in the Department of Health Care of the Elderly in Nottingham where the two specialties operate as one service (Arie, 1983). This is perhaps the sort of leap forward that many might expect to accrue from the appointment of a psychogeriatrician to what was envisaged as a Chair of Geriatric Medicine. I hope that it will set the pattern (in services if not Chairs) for the future.

REFERENCES

Ammundsen E et al 1982 The elderly in Denmark: demographic economic, social and health conditions. Danish Medical Bulletin 29: 89–168
Arie T H D 1972 Aspects of the Goodmayers service. In: McLachlan G (ed) Approaches to action. Oxford University Press, London
Arie T H D 1983 Organization of services for the elderly: implications for education and patient care: experience in Nottingham. In: Bergener M (ed) Geropsychiatric diagnostics and treatment. Springer, New York
Ball C, Coleman P, Wright J 1983 The practicalities of achieving collaboration between hospital and community based services for the elderly mentally infirm. Report of a Research Study for DHSS
Cooper B, Schwartz R 1982 Psychiatric case identification in an elderly urban population. Social Psychiatry 17: 43–52
Department of Health and Social Security. 1972 Services for mental illness related to old age. Circular HM 72/71. HMSO, London
Department of Health and Social Security 1981 Care in the Community. DHSS, London
Department of Health and Social Security 1983 Regulation 9, Supplementary Benefit Requirement. Resource and Single Payment Amendment Regulation. Circular 7/143. HMSO, London
Ferlie E 1983 Sourcebook of initiatives in the community care of the elderly. PSSRU, Headley
Godber C 1978a Report on a visit to Danish nursing homes (unpublished — in King's Fund Centre Library)
Godber C 1978b Kinloss Court: an experiment in sheltered housing and collaboration. Social Work Service 15: 42–45
Godber C 1978 Conflict and collaboration between geriatric medicine and psychiatry. In: Isaacs B (ed) Recent Advances in Geriatric Medicine. Churchill Livingstone, Edinburgh
Godber C 1982 A happier old age in Denmark. British Medical Journal 284: 1729–30
Godber C 1984 Private rest homes: answers needed. British Medical Journal 288: 1473–4
Hettiaratchy P D J 1985 The travelling day hospital. Geriatric Medicine
Lewis R J 1979 Flying warden answers 80-year-old's Mayday call. Modern Geriatrics 19(3): 27–33
Pitt B 1974 Psychogeriatrics. Churchill Livinstone, London
Rosenvinge H, Guion J, Dawson J 1986 Sitting service for the elderly confused. Health Trends 18(2):47
Smith T 1982 Old age in the sun. British Medical Journal 288: 1515–17
Southampton Psychiatric Case Register. Annual Bulletins 1982–4, and personal communications
Tinker A 1984 Staying at home: helping elderly people. HMSO, London

Caring for the carers

THE NEEDS OF CARERS

It has been estimated that there are in the UK some 1.25 million people providing care for handicapped adults with whom they share accommodation. Indeed, The Association of Carers estimates that there are now more women caring for frail elderly or disabled persons than there are rearing 'normal' under-16s (Oliver 1984). This figure does, of course, cover the whole range of disability, both mental and physical, but it is an indication of how untrue it is to say that 'the family does not care any longer', and it is certain that, if these care-givers no longer carried the brunt, both health and social services would be quite unable to cope. Many of these carers are very elderly husbands or wives of the sick person, and the bulk of the remainder are daughters or daughters-in-law who are often struggling to provide care for a parent and, at the same time, care for children, run a home, look after other disabled relatives and hold down a job which is essential to the family budget. The task is thus stressful enough even when the person cared for is responsive, grateful and able to cooperate. Those caring for dementia sufferers face the double burden of both emotional and physical stress, and it is exacerbated, especially in the earlier stages of the disease, by almost universal ignorance about the nature and causes of a dementing illness.

In the early stages, loss of short-term memory is usually put down to the normal forgetfulness of old age, and both the sufferer and his/her family may cover up quite severe levels of disorder by reliance on well-established routines and by family members filling in gaps left by loss of capacity for self-care. It is only when a rapid deterioration occurs, or the spouse dies, or some crisis upsets the routine, that it becomes impossible to ignore the disability. Even then it may be denied or misinterpreted; the urge to conceal what is often felt to be a deeply shaming loss of mental capacity can be very strong, especially if it is accompanied by bizarre behaviour and personality change. As the illness develops, the emotional distress of supporters is likely to become increasingly acute. The known and loved individual slowly disappears and a stranger takes his or her place so that

317

he or she becomes only a shell of the former personality: perhaps outwardly conformable but inwardly empty and bewildered; perhaps suspicious, dirty, destructive or aggressive. The supporter may also have to become accustomed to radical role changes, so that an elderly man has to take on the domestic tasks and perhaps the personal care of a woman who has been 'mother' to her family for sixty years, or an old-fashioned elderly woman may have to take on a 'male' role for the first time in her life. All too often the process is accompanied by gradual loss of contact with friends and relatives; increasing financial strains arising from incontinence, destructive habits or irrational use of money; and a deep fear, whether in spouse or child, that this will be their fate, too.

There is certainly ample evidence that supporters tend not to seek help until they are desperate. For example, Gilhooly (1984), in her study of supporters of psychogeriatric day hospital users, found that:

> Because dementia is stigmatised, advice is not sought from other relatives or friends, and often not even from professionals. The first lady I interviewed kept her husband's incontinence and problem behaviour a secret from her daughters for 1½ years; she did not tell her doctor either. It wasn't until a daughter became aware that her mother was on the verge of mental and physical collapse and enquired as to what was bothering her that help was sought. It was not unusual to find that I was the only person that the supporter had ever confided in about the disorder. Although supporters appeared reluctant in many cases to speak to the GP about the dementing old person's behaviour, this does not mean that they did not want information or advice. *Supporters expected the GP to volunteer information which, it seems, at least from my study, they rarely do.* [Present author's italics.]
>
> Furthermore, as Wilkin (1979) noted, the behaviour of the supporters is open to criticism no matter what is done. If the supporter tries to hide the problem and contain it within the home she will be seen as being over-protective. If she tries to continue as normal she will be accused of denying the existence of a problem. If she seeks institutional care she will encounter social disapproval for 'rejecting' the dementing relative or lacking a proper moral obligation.

Even when the problems are well known within the family, there is a strong tendency for one member to be left with virtually the whole responsibility, particularly if there is an unmarried or childless daughter available. The supporter concerned can then develop a defensive mechanism whereby he or she both resents the burden and cannot accept relief from it, perhaps because of guilt about the resentment. In this situation, it can be very valuable for an external professional, whether doctor, social worker or psychologist, to call a family conclave which can talk through the situation and come to terms with the need to share care among the family as a whole.

If the professionals who are in touch with the supporters as the illness develops, and especially the GP, are prepared to face the situation from the supporters' point of view and are willing to talk it through with them, encourage them to approach the right sources of help and be there to turn to in a crisis, a great deal can be done to relieve the pain and stress. It does not make the reality of the illness disappear, but there is much evidence that caring concern, understanding and appropriate help at the right time do a great deal to make the family's task more bearable. With such support they can carry on doing it for as long as is appropriate, and they can also relinquish it without too much guilt when the task has got beyond them.

Apart from grief about a changed and lost personality, there are two main aspects of stress in long-term family care. One of these is the loss of personal privacy and independence. The carer can no longer make any decision, perhaps not even the most personal and trivial ones about when to go shopping or have a bath, without reference to the needs of the person being cared for. Will he be safe? Will he come hammering on the door? Will he keep interrupting the TV programme or the telephone conversation? The parents of a new-born child often say that, to begin with, they never relax even when the baby is asleep — a sixth sense is always on the watch for something going wrong. The same is true, but much more intensely and with none of the compensations, for the supporter of someone whose dementia is becoming severe. For a son or daughter who has taken in an elderly mentally-disabled parent, this constant tension is combined with an acute sense of loss of privacy and personal family life. This loss is well brought out in a report by the Equal Opportunities Commission (1980).

Thus, a woman of 53 caring for a mother of 81 told the researcher, 'I am caring for her full time, I couldn't go into the garden, let alone anywhere else.' And a man of 50 with a dependent mother-in-law said, 'At times it has been disastrous; my wife and I enjoy a close, tranquil relationship, but with the inevitable pressures that arise we have tended to withdraw a lot from each other. Tensions are very high at times. Many of the carers interviewed in this survey talked about loss of social activities, making remarks like, 'It's very hard, you lose friends. They offer to do things, but now they avoid us. Even my best friend, we were inseparable, he just rings up now occasionally'. When the elderly relative is a dementia sufferer, in particular, there are real tensions between his or her needs and those of the rest of the family, and especially those of children who feel that they cannot bring their friends home because they are ashamed of their grandparent's condition and behaviour.

Long-term stresses — and they can last for many years — are serious enough, but it is the acute difficulties which usually break the camel's back. One early and influential study of the aspects of care which give most stress to supporters identified sleep disturbance, fecal incontinence, night wandering, shouting and inappropriate micturition as the most poorly tolerated behaviours (Sanford, 1975), and this has been confirmed by many other writers. More recent studies gave an opportunity to supporters to cite emotional as well as physical causes of stress, and highlighted factors such as personal uncleanliness, bizarre and dangerous behaviour, apathy, bouts of crying and constant demands for attention. In addition, some supporters resent being forced into giving care when there has been a long history of conflict between them and the dependent person, while others feel guilt because the relationship has been close and they feel that they are not doing enough. These problems are probably less severely experienced when the carer does not live with the patient and, if the patient is still living alone, he or she is in any case likely to be only moderately disabled. But even in this situation the life of the carer may be totally dominated by the task, and they may be a constant sense of anxiety and guilt when not actually giving care.

Much detailed evidence about the practical needs of informal carers is provided by a study carried out by the National Institute of Social Work (Levin et al, 1983). The Institute's sample was obtained by selecting two London boroughs and one health district in which a community-based psychogeriatric service was in operation and asking the workers in the health and social services in all three areas to fill in a form for each of the elderly persons on their caseloads or practice lists whom they identified as 'confused'. From this 'census' 50 people, who appeared to be suffering from severe disability, were selected in each area, and interviews were set up with their supporting relatives together with a medical/psychiatric assessment of the confused person. Both interview and assessment were repeated after a year's interval. The researchers found that about three-quarters of the elderly people identified in their census either lived with relatives or had a helping relative living close by, but the social and personal variety within this group of supporters was striking.

> They differed amongst themselves, not only in 'objective' factors such as kinship-tie to the elderly persons, gender, age, marital status, health, the composition of their households and whether or not they had paid jobs, but also in their 'subjective' reasons for undertaking the care of their relatives, for example, whether they did it out of affection, sense of duty or perceived lack of choice. Despite these variations, their wish to care grew out of a pattern of life which was long-established and was reinforced by bonds of affection and obligation. 41% of the supporters were wives or husbands of the elderly persons and 44% were their daughters or sons. Where the elderly persons and the supporters lived together, this arrangement had been established, on average, for 36 years and only 16% of them had lived together for less than ten years.
>
> The supporters were an elderly group — the mean age being 61 years; only one-third of them rated their health as good in the previous year and about one-half had disabilities which limited their activities. Many had other family responsibilities and one in three supporters combined caring with paid employment . . . About one-third of the supporters reported a number of symptoms of acute stress sufficient to suggest a need for psychiatric attention.

The study provides a detailed picture of the supporters' strengths, problems and limitations, and of the way in which services and benefits can promote their capacity to care. It provides factual evidence that the majority of supporters wanted to go on caring, that services were not only needed but appreciated, and that they were effective in preventing the build-up of strain in supporters and so postponing the need for admission to institutional care.

Domiciliary support

The authors suggest that, in developing a comprehensive system of services, attention should be paid to eight key requirements in domiciliary support:

1. *Early identification* — the earlier that support services can be provided, the better. Too often supporters have already reached the point of exhaustion before help is offered.

2. *Comprehensive medical and social assessment* — which covered *all* the main problems which the elderly persons and their supporters face. Whatever the profession or role of the assessor, their contribution was most appreciated if:

* they arranged interviews promptly;
* made it clear who they were, where they came from and why they were visiting;
* showed sensitivity in their dealings with the elderly persons;
* were willing to listen to the supporters and showed concern about their well-being;
* gave clear explanations;
* understood the possible causes of confusion;
* where a diagnosis of dementia was made, through careful questioning, established the precise problems which its management posed;
* agreed a clear and promptly-implemented plan of action.

The authors comment that '*The general practitioners have a key role in ensuring that assessments are initiated, for it is to them that families first turn and, where they played this role, the families appreciated it*' (present writer's italics).

3. *Timely referrals* — when general practitioners, hospital consultants, social workers and so forth could not themselves provide the help required, it was very much valued if they referred on to other agencies which could help, and if they did this *before* the supporters had reached breaking-point.

4. *Continuing back-up and reviews* — the patients concerned inevitably deteriorate, the supporter's health may get worse and family circumstances change. It was very important to supporters that the relevant professionals continued to be involved and were known to be interested both in the patient's condition and in the supporter's well-being, and if they reviewed progress at regular intervals and could be called upon in times of difficulty.

5. *Active medical treatment* — about half the sample of 150 elderly persons with confusional symptoms had physical illnesses which were grave enough to impede the performance of daily living activities, and in many of them the combination of incontinence, falls, unsteadiness and pain would probably have rendered independent existence impossible whatever their mental state. Supporters therefore very much appreciated the regular involvement of doctors and nurses who could and would treate acute illness and other remediable conditions.

6. *Information, advice and counselling* — The report says:

> The supporters made it very clear that they required information, advice and counselling. They liked to know what help was available locally, how to go about getting it, what the particular services could and could not offer, and what benefits they were eligible for. They also liked clear explanations of their elderly relatives' health problems, of the likely course of the illness and what to expect. They wanted straightforward advice on routine care-giving activities and problems: for example, how to lift; how to reduce restlessness, disturbance during the night and repetitious questioning; how to manage incontinence, for example, what pads, sheets or clothing might reduce their workload. They gave high praise to doctors, social workers and nurses who gave them the opportunity to express their feelings about their experience, who recognised what they did for their relatives, and who helped them to come to terms with the changes in their elderly relatives and the associated feelings of sadness and loneliness and, at times, anger, resentment and frustration.

7. *Regular help with household and personal care tasks* — home help, district nursing services and incontinent laundry services were all much appreciated, and the survey found statistical evidence that provision of home help could postpone or prevent admission to institutions.

8. *Regular financial support* — heavy fuel bills, extra washing, need to replace clothing and furnishings and loss of possible earnings all caused financial hardship. It was very important to supporters to be informed about sources of financial help, such as attendance allowance and invalid care allowance. Apart from offsetting expenses, these payments had psychological value in that they were seen as official recognition of the heavy dependency brought about by illness.

It was very evident from the study that supporters although living in relatively well-served areas, were not in fact receiving even a basic level of support. For example:

a. 60% of those with severe dementia had not seen a psychiatrist;
b. 79% of those who also had serious physical illness had not seen a geriatrician;
c. 33% of supporters with high total distress scores had not seen a social worker;

d. 34% of those with severe dementia and 39% of those with a lot of trying behaviours neither attended day care nor had relief care (although in many cases their supporters said they would have accepted this if it had been offered);

e. 47% of those with serious physical illnesses and 45% of those who were heavily incontinent were not visited by the community nursing services;

f. 72% of those with severe dementia did not receive either home help or meals on wheels, and of those not in receive either home help or meals on wheels, and of those not in receipt of the home help service, 65% of supporters said it had not been offered and 26% said that they would accept it if it had been;

g. 95% of the sample did not receive laundry service, though 24% would accept it and 26% of the elderly persons were heavily incontinent;

h. 71% of the sample did not receive attendance allowance, and half of the supporters whose relatives did not receive it had never heard of it. In the research team's judgement one-quarter of those not in receipt of the allowance were definitely eligible for it.

These findings clearly show that they is an immense gap between basic need and efficient service provision which is simply not being filled. GPs in particular have a duty to see that their patients and their patients' supporters have an opportunity to use services which are available and also to take an active part in fighting for provision where these services are non-existent or inadequate. Supporters who are themselves uncared for *cannot* go on caring.

Permanent residential care

The report makes it clear that, however great their goodwill, supporters cannot go on carrying the strain indefinitely without danger of great injury to themselves. It is important that they should not be *forced* to do so by the absence of acceptable institutional provision. If this is not available, they are in effect being blackmailed into caring — a situation which is likely to lead to desperation and perhaps to verbal or physical abuse.

CONSENT, RESTRAINT AND LEGAL COMPETENCE

Both informal carers and supporting professional practitioners face a range of dilemmas in relation to their legal right to give medical treatment to dementia sufferers, ensure their physical safety and safeguard their property. A person suffering from severe dementia is not likely to be capable of giving informed consent to medical treatment, yet under British law it is illegal even to *touch* another person without their consent unless their life is at stake or they are presenting an immediate and serious threat to others.

Doctors have no privileged position in this regard. However, there is virtually no case law which defines the length of time over which an illness may be deemed to be 'life-threatening' or the degree of danger or threat which would justify physical restraint, nor is there any clear definition about the level of mental competence required to make consent valid. Severe dementia sufferers cannot be allowed to suffer unnecessarily from painful or debilitating illness, and so it is common for willingness to cooperate, or at least lack of physical resistance, to be taken as implying consent. It is also common for relatives to be consulted about serious treatment decisions, though they have in fact no legal right to act on behalf of the sick person. Even where there is physical resistance or no relative to consult, a doctor's decision is very unlikely to be challenged in practice because the patient is not in a position to instruct a solicitor in order to take a case to court, and if he or she could do so the court would not award damages unless it was proved that harm had been done or that the treatment had not been carried out in good faith.

In normal circumstances, there is more likelihood of danger arising from neglect of physical illness in a person with dementia than from giving treatment improperly, and it can be argued that it is justifiable to go ahead with treatment if there are good reasons for thinking that the patient would accept the treatment if he or she were able to understand the situation. In some circumstances, however, treatment may be given which a rational patient might well refuse. For example, drugs may be used as a means of restraint or to give the care staff in a home or hospital a quiet life. And life-saving treatment may be used on persons who might well prefer to die if they could understand what was being done to them. As Baker (1976) has said in a famous article, 'Skilled nursing care can maintain life in a frail, elderly patient whose general condition is such that a comparable state in an animal might well lead to prosecution of the owner. Senile dementing processes sometimes lead to a relatively quick and peaceful death. Many, however, particularly under modern conditions of treatment, can be very cruel illnesses indeed.'

There has been some move to encourage the use of a 'living will' which would give a guide to the wishes of people in relation to life-sustaining procedures while they are still mentally competent (Robertson, 1982). The British Medical Association has opposed this idea on the grounds that people might fear being pressurized into signing such a 'will' by their relatives and that anyone is free to express his or her wishes on this matter to the GP without quasi-legal documentation. However, it would take a brave GP to raise this issue with patients who might be at risk and, even if they did express such a wish, it would be extremely difficult for the GP to press its observance once the patient had left his or her care. In any case, the dilemma is not confined to dementia sufferers — we are all at risk of suffering severe brain damage from an accident of one kind or another. There is an immense need for both the caring professions and the general public to become more aware of the issues involved and better able to ensure that these are properly weighed in any particular situation.

The technical risk of a charge of assault is not confined to medical treatment without consent. Such an 'assault' is committed daily by nurses, care staff and relatives, when they tie down restless confused people, confine them in chairs with fixed trays, or keep them in by locking doors. For desperate relatives, such measures may seem to be the only means of ensuring that the patient is out of danger while they do essential shopping or get on with some task. Hard-pressed care staff also often see restraint as the only solution and regard their duty to keep a demented resident safe (and themselves out of trouble) as more important than defending an abstract concept of 'self-determination'. This is another 'grey' legal area in which there is no case law. Undoubtedly, however, exaggerated fears of the risk involved in free movement, unimaginative care regimes and the desire for a quiet life do result in many people being restrained or drugged unnecessarily, and more support to the relatives or better staffing ratios in residential and hospital care would do much to obviate the necessity for physical restraint.

The issue of valid consent is equally important and equally vague in other fields of activity, such as controlling property, signing a will or executing a power of attorney, and there is a comparable dilemma between the need to protect vulnerable people from exploitation and the need to defend the rights of those who are capable of making an informed choice even if that choice happens to be eccentric. There are no clear-cut guidelines or tests in any of these areas. The Court of Protection, which in England and Wales is the agency responsible for protecting the property of people who are not mentally competent, simply requires a referral to include a statement by a medical practitioner to the effect that 'in my opinion the Patient is incapable by reason of Mental Disorder as defined in the Mental Health Act 1983 of managing and administering . . . property and affairs and I base my opinion on the following ground. . .'.

The Mental Health Act 1983, like its 1959 predecessor, defines mental disorder as 'mental illness, arrested or incomplete development, psychopathic disorder or any other disorder or disability of mind'. The issue, therefore, is not the diagnosis but the behaviour or level of comprehension which gives rise to doubts about capability. As with consent to treatment, there is no clear guidance as to what 'incapable' really means, and the responsible medical practitioner may well find him or herself in the middle of a family fight over whether or not the patient should be referred to the Court of Protection. Even when a person has been referred to the Court and a Receiver has been appointed to manage the person's affairs, it cannot be assumed that this will be done in the patient's interest. The Receiver (who is usually a close relative) may, for example, resist the patient's transfer from hospital to residential care because hospital treatment is free in the UK and a transfer, which might be in the patient's interest, would also involve using his or her assets. In this sort of situation, a doctor may well find himself or herself defending the patient's interests against those of the Receiver and even appealing to the Court to have the Receiver changed. It is commonly believed that many of these problems can be avoided by executing a Power of Attorney, but the authority to act under such a Power automatically lapses when a person becomes mentally incompetent, so in law (which again is often ignored in practice), it does not provide an alternative to the Court of Protection. In 1986, however, a new form of authority called an 'Enduring Power of Attorney' came into use. This is a special document which remains valid even if the Principal becomes mentally incompetent. If it comes into common use, it should greatly simplify this aspect of caring for dementia sufferers, though it does not provide any adequate safeguard against misuse of the Power, and in that regard is indeed much less effective a defence than referral to the Court of Protection.

A will remains valid once it is signed, whatever the subsequent mental incompetence of the testator, but again the law is very unclear about the degree of understanding which is required to make a will valid in the first place, and a doctor who is asked to give an opinion on the mental capacity of a testator can find himself or herself in a very difficult position. Much more common in daily life, however, are dilemmas arising from action taken by relatives or care staff to prevent a demented person from losing or giving away valuable jewellery, putting his or her pension money down the lavatory and so forth. There is no clear dividing line between assuming charge of someone else's possessions in his or her own best interests and the exercise either of a ruthless paternalism which assumes incapacity in all areas of choice or, still worse, the appropriation of goods to someone else's benefit. Doctors who are genuinely concerned for their patients' interests, especially those who look after people in long-stay institutional care, can be an invaluable defence (and are often the sole resource) in protecting their patients against abuses of this kind. Often simple alertness to the fact that a patient is no longer wearing her rings, for example, or the asking of questions about opportunities for shopping and obtaining new clothes or luxury foods will alert care staff and relatives to the fact that an eye is being kept on their activities and help to prevent abuse. If there is any serious cause for concern, there is a moral responsibility for the doctor concerned to report the matter to the Court of Protection or to the Health or Social Services Authority which is responsible for providing care or registering the facility concerned. In private residential homes, procedure for making complaints against any abuse of the recognised Code of Practice in residential care is now built into the British system (Avebury et al, 1984).

ADMISSION TO INSTITUTIONAL CARE

It is well known that change of environment and loss of well-established routines can be very distressing and damaging to dementia sufferers, and there is a great deal to be said for keeping people going in a familiar environment for as long as possible, especially if that is, so far as can be ascertained, their own wish. On the other hand, much anxiety is generated amongst neighbours and relatives of people who are living alone and who are felt to be at risk from wandering, lack of adequate self-care and inappropriate behaviour, especially if they are a nuisance to their neighbours or are thought to create a fire hazard. One or more members of the medical profession (the GP, the geriatric or psychogeriatric hospital consultant, and, in some circumstances, the Community Physician) are likely to have a decisive part to play in the decision-making process about whether long-stay care is really essential, and they have a commensurate responsibility to ensure that all aspects of the situation are properly taken into account. Indeed, when the proposed admission is into private care, there is no automatic social work involvement, so a doctor may be the only person who is in a position to try and make sure that the patient's interests are fully defended. This may involve being prepared to take responsibility if the person is allowed to go on living at home and an accident occurs. In any situation of this kind, it is important to weigh the potential dangers and corresponding gains of removal against the dangers and gains of maintaining the status quo (taking the needs of the supporters as well as the patient into account). All too often, however, a hospital doctor who is anxious to clear his bed or a general practitioner who is anxious to get a tiresome patient off the list is tempted to go along with admission procedures without asking any questions, even if they do not actively promote and encourage admission to care when it is not in the patient's best interests.

If a patient with dementia is actively refusing consent to admission to residential or nursing home care and there are sufficient grounds for acting, legal action to compel admission can be taken through the use of Section 47 of the National Assistance Act 1948 and its 1951 Amendment (a very unsatisfactory piece of legislation which is falling into disuse) or under the guardianship powers available to the Local Authority under Section 7 of the Mental Health Act 1983; (neither of these powers gives a right to enforce treatment). All too often, however, neither of these legal processes is used and the patient is quite literally 'taken for a ride', with no effective means of protest. Here again, the responsible doctor, who will probably have been asked to provide a medical report to the admitting institution, has a real duty to see that the situation is explored as fully as possible with both the patient and the supporters, and that the patient is not illegally shanghaied.

CONCLUSION

Throughout this chapter the primary emphasis has been on the defencelessness of both dementia sufferers and their supporters. The greater their need and the more severe the illness, the less they are in a position to fight for effective help or to defend their civil rights. Carers are themselves commonly either elderly and themselves unfit, or are carrying other responsibilities, and the love which makes them wish to go on caring and to do it as effectively as possible often makes their task harder through the guilt, anxiety, sense of bereavement and stress from which they suffer. They are in no position to verbalize their anxieties, to fight for support services, and to pursue the tortuous paths which lead to welfare benefits. And of all groups of patients, dementia sufferers are perhaps most defenceless and at greatest risk. Year by year they slide, slowly and inexorably deeper into their disability, deeper into incapacity and deeper into the awareness that their mind is giving up on them and their world is becoming an unfamiliar, unpredictable place which no longer makes sense. In the process of incurring this loss, they may experience much fear and depression as well as antagonism from family and friends who do not realize what is happening. As the disease worsens, they are virtually at the mercy of whatever care or lack of care society chooses to accord to them. They can make no demands and defend no rights. They are, as Professor Arie (1979) has well said, their own worst enemy. 'A paralysed polio victim who can only twitch one eyelid but is of sound mind, can call for help when he needs it; he is his own monitor. A demented person, on the other hand, far from being her own monitor, is the agent of her own undoing. It is she who leaves the gas on, she who neglects to feed herself or keep herself warm, she who persistently disturbs the family or the neighbours to the point that their spirit breaks and they reject her.'

If their doctors, whether family practitioners or specialists, do not help dementia sufferers, both by insisting on the provision of effective support services (Norman, 1982) and by giving competent, concerned, on-going care, both they and their carers are, indeed, defenceless.*

---

* As well as providing or involving professional help, it is often useful to refer caring relatives to a voluntary agency concerned with supporting supporters. In the UK, a local branch of MIND or Age Concern can often provide advice and assistance and, nationally, help can be obtained from The Association of Carers, Medway Homes, Balfour Road, Rochester, Kent ME4 6QU and the Alzheimer's Disease Society, Bank Buildings, Fulham Broadway, London SW6 1EP. Similar organizations elsewhere are: The Societé Alzheimer's Society (Canada); the Alzheimer's Disease and Related Disorders Society (USA); and the Japanese Association of Families Caring for the Demented Elderly (Japan). Information on the relevant Australian society is obtainable from the Australian Council on the Ageing.

REFERENCES

Arie T 1979 Psychogeriatrics: how and why? Fotheringham Lectures in the University of Toronto, unpublished
Avebury K et al 1984 Home life: a code of practice for residential care. Centre for Policy on Ageing, London

Baker A A 1976 Slow euthanasia or 'She will be better off in hospital'. British Medical
    Journal 2: 571–2
Equal Opportunities Commission 1980 The experience of caring for elderly and
    handicapped dependents: survey report. OEC, Manchester
Gilhooly M L 1984 The social dimensions of senile dementia. In: Hanley I, Hodge J (ed)
    Psychological approaches to the care of the elderly. Croom Helm, London
Levin E, Sinclair A I C, Gorbach P 1983 The supporters of the confused elderly at home.
    Extract from the Main Report: Families, services and confusion in old age. Allen &
    Unwin, London
Norman A 1982 Mental illness in old age: meeting the challenge. Centre for Policy on
    Ageing, London
Oliver J 1984 The informal carers. Action Baseline, Spring 1984, p 9 (using data compiled
    by the Association of Carers and the Equal Opportunities Commission)
Robertson G S 1982 Dealing with the brain-damaged old — dignity before senility. Journal
    of Medical Ethics 8: 173–179
Sanford J R A 1975 Tolerance of debility in elderly dependents by supporters at home: its
    significance for hospital practice. British Medical Journal 3: 471–3
Wilkin D 1979 Caring for the mentally handicapped child. Croom Helm, London

Epilogue: research prospects

The Editor kindly invited me, as an old hand, to read the typescript of this book and to add a chapter on research prospects. This I have attempted, though I can only do so from the point of view of a clinical psychiatrist whose attempts at research have been almost entirely confined to the so-called functional disorders of late life: there is thus no need to declare an interest.

SECONDARY AND SUBCORTICAL DEMENTIAS

Not all of the chapters of this encyclopaedic book raise research problems, beyond presenting the reader concerned with the care of the aged with a full and up-to-date picture of dementing illnesses. Many of these are secondary to deficiencies and diseases affecting organ systems other than the brain. The mechanisms by which they produce dementia are fairly well understood, and research will have to be directed towards the causes and the treatments of these primary conditions, and specifically, in one of the commonest dementias of later life, towards the prevention of cerebral infarction. In the much rarer dementias associated with the names of Pick, Creutzfeldt-Jakob, Binswanger and others the pathological changes are primarily confined to the central nervous system. In their case considerable understanding of pathology and aetiology has been achieved by highly expert workers, and to suggest lines of future research is quite outside my capacity.

Far commoner are dementias related to disease of the basal ganglia and other subcortical structures such as Huntington's chorea and the various kinds of Parkinson's disease. In Chapter 13 relevant further research needs are clearly formulated. In summary, it is suggested that the neuropsychological defects of subcortical dementia still have to be more convincingly defined (Chapter 13) in both these and other conditions, and that if subcortical dementia does in fact exist it should be compared with that of Alzheimer's disease. These defects should also be correlated with neuropathological findings. In addition to underscoring the need for cooperative research, it should also be noted that the beneficial effects of levodopa therapy on the motor and cognitive symptoms of Parkinsonism have turned out to be only temporary (Chapter 13), and that for this reason research aimed at discovering different therapies, and if possible causal rather than replacement, ought to be envisaged.

SENILE DEMENTIAS OF ALZHEIMER TYPE

Several authors contributing to this volume have once again stressed that senile dementia has assumed epidemic proportions, and that this threatens to undo the benefits gained by geriatric medicine to a considerable extent. In the oldest age groups, therefore, Alzheimer's dementia presents an even greater research challenge than cardiovascular degeneration and cancer.

Replacement therapies

By an odd coincidence, on the very same day on which this book in typescript landed on my desk, I had come across a note by the health correspondent of a leading daily newspaper. In this he reported a well-known and much respected researcher in neuroscience as having said that major advances in understanding the chemistry of the brain offered the possibility of treating both Parkinson's disease and senile dementia. He is further quoted as saying that scientists had identified a chemical compound usually found in the cerebral cortex which was missing from brain tissues taken posthumously from senile dementia victims. Work was now going ahead with the possibility of replacing this chemical in the brains of incipient sufferers. He expected clinical trials to start within six years, followed by at least four years of assessment, before the treatment might become generally available.

I have been given to understand by people in touch with this worker that he was not referring to an as yet unpublished discovery, but almost certainly to the well-documented deficits in the cholinergic system of the brain. Readers of this book will have been made aware of the great difficulties ahead. Like in other degenerative diseases of the central nervous system, there is selective damage, and in Alzheimer's disease this affects most obviously the cholinergic system (Chapter 8). This is almost certainly due to the reduced activity of the enzyme choline acetyltransferase in certain cortical neurones. However, other transmitters, such as noradrenaline and serotonin, are probably also reduced. One must, therefore, carefully note the last sentence of Chapter 8 which stresses that the results of further studies to define the clinical correlates of the cholinergic and also of other transmitter deficits in Alzheimer's disease are awaited.

In the meantime, work aimed at replacing the cholinergic deficit must continue, and the possibility that loading with choline substances like lecithin may benefit a certain subtype of Alzheimer dement (p 272) should be confirmed or negated by further studies. The conservation of acetylcholine by medication with anticholinesterases seems a more promising procedure, and one can only echo the statement (p 267, 268) that developing a long-acting preparation of an agent with good brain penetration and possibly some selectivity towards the cortical cholinergic system must be seen as a major challenge for researchers. The pursuit of further studies in the use of cholinemimetic agents by continuous injection into the CSF via an implanted pump system (Chapter 16) would seem a promising endeavour. This mode of delivery may also be worth looking at in the case of other therapeutic agents.

There is tacit recognition that replacement therapy will not cure well-advanced dementia, and that its application is only likely to be effective in early cases. The discovery of patients during the incipient stages of the disease is fraught with great difficulties. To apply prospectively controlled trials to apparently normal samples of the elderly population seems quite impracticable. Case-finding will have to be limited to old people not only with memory deficiencies but also with other psychiatric problems of recent origin. Clinical assessment will obviously have to be supplemented by psychological testing, and there is thus an urgent need for the further development of screening tests for the detection of early dementia (Chapter 4). The claim that the items making up the Kendrick Cognitive Tests for the Elderly (Chapter 4) do differentiate between dementing, pseudo-dementing, depressed and normal modes of responding needs to be confirmed by other workers, and it is reassuring to note that this further assessment is under way. For gauging the results of therapy there is additionally the need for specific tests measuring changes in the various target abilities, both in cognitive and behavioural areas. Needless to say, these measures will have to be suitable for serial use and allow for practice effects. Initial and follow through assessments would be very much facilitated if computerized tests could be used, but much work will be needed before this form of presentation can be employed in the case of dementing elderly persons (Chapter 4).

Before commencing trials which are directed towards the replacement, conservation, or enhancement of cholinergic transmitters, the desirability of including in any therapy strengthening of other transmitter systems (e.g. noradrenalin or serotonin) should be more fully assessed. It seems, therefore, imperative to discover whether neurones of transmitter systems other than the cholinergic are affected in early dementia, or whether their deterioration occurs only later during the progress of Alzheimer's disease, in a secondary fashion.

In this context, further examination of the cognitive defects encountered to a varying extent in late life depressions seems strongly indicated, with the aim of confirming more definitely that the psychometric pattern of cognitive impairment is of an entirely different nature from that of Alzheimer's dementia (Chapter 15). The need comes to mind for a further development of the Kendrick test procedures (Chapter 4) and of their serial application to elderly depressives after their index attack has passed, as well as that for further work along the lines reported in Chapter 15 (pp. 256–260), especially perhaps on evoked cortical potentials, computerized tomography, and e.e.g. sleep patterns. If it should emerge that the cognitive defects and other abnormal findings in some elderly depressives did, after all, come to approximate to those found in Alzheimer's dementia, and thus the term of depressive pseudodementia was a misleading one (Chapter 15, p 256) then, and only then, a closer study of transmitter defects in these depressives might be indicated in order to discover substances which should be added to the cholinergic replacement therapy of early dementia.

To halt, or even only to retard the progression of incipient and of moderately advanced senile dementia, would be an achievement well worth considerable research efforts. It might even be possible to keep within the timetable forecast in the above-quoted newspaper item. At the same time workers in the field should be aware of the diminishing effects of replacement therapy in Parkinson's disease (Chapter 13), and of the likelihood that this disappointment may be repeated in the case of Alzheimer's dementia, possibly because the deteriorating neurones become no longer capable of producing acetylcholine or other transmitter substances, even when supplied with the missing enzymes and building materials. Research into the primary causes of neuronal degeneration should, therefore, be envisaged, even though the difficulties are truly formidable.

More causally directed therapies

Comparatively speaking, it should not be too difficult to determine whether or not external factors were principal and potentially remediable causes of the Alzheimer type of neuronal degeneration. The plea made for increased cooperation between epidemiologists and other researchers (Chapter 13) should be taken very seriously. There would be a strong indication for an important role of environmental aetiology if it could be confirmed that Alzheimer's disease is less common in Japan (Chapter 13) and very rare in largely non-urbanized developing countries, but that at the same time it is equally common in North American blacks as in whites, and that senile dementia tends to cluster in certain areas of cities.

Another relatively-speaking manageable task concerns the alleged heterogeneity of Alzheimer's dementia. If it could be definitively confirmed that early onset was more associated with temporal-parietal defects, a more rapid downhill course and a higher family prevalence of the disorder, while later onset was characterized by mainly memory loss, a more benign course and less by family history (Chapter 6, p 111, Chapter 11, p 203), then this would be useful not only for selecting the appropriate replacement therapy, but also as a lead towards more basic research. In complementary fashion, the discovery of differing patterns of transmitter defects would considerably strengthen the case for the existence of different forms of Alzheimer's dementia.

As far as environmental causal agents are concerned, there is probably little point in pursuing further the role of aluminium or of immune mechanisms (Chapter 6). The claim of having produced Alzheimer changes by the transmission of a conventional type of virus seems to have been exploded (Chapter 6, pp. 113–114).

Interest has now been directed towards a possible association of slow viruses and prions (Chapter 6), and as these may affect the gene apparatus, we are thus led to the centre of things, the neurone cell's nucleus. There is need to clarify our understanding of the relationship between the Alzheimer's and the Down's syndromes and of the status of chromosome abnormalities in the senile condition (Chapter 6). Even more fundamental and difficult would be research into the regulation of expression of nerve growth factor genes conceived of as stimulating enzymes, which among other actions regulate the synthesis of proteins in neurones at the transcriptional level (Chapter 6). These are indeed deep waters, even right down to genetic engineering, which may have to be explored if environmental causes of Alzheimer's dementia cannot be found.

MANAGEMENT OF AGED DEMENTING PERSONS

At a time of rapid progress in so many areas of microbiology and molecular biology, it was tempting to speculate rather wildly, especially because at any moment unforeseen and Utopian approaches may become possible. This seems unlikely in the subjects treated in the book's last chapters on psychological management, services and the roles and problems of families and friends. While the results of research into causes and somatic treatments of senile and other dementias of old age are awaited the psychosocial management of the sufferers will continue for some time to come to remain a challenging and most difficult task. In spite of many efforts, progress has been slow. Two problems have retained their central position, and very much as they had first presented themselves to me when I was associated with one of the first experimental studies of rehabilitation of dements some thirty years ago: the improvements achieved in some skills and behavioural defects can be quite useful and even significant. However, not only is there little carry-over to other impairments, but also the results achieved prove evanescent, and the successful measures have to continue to be applied indefinitely. Whether in dementia there is loss of a central motivational function is a question which needs to be answered. Beyond this I cannot think of any fresh suggestions for future research which, as I see it, will have to proceed by trial and error of methods directed at individual disabilities.

A few more general observations may not be out of place. Rigorous evaluation of results should become an absolute rule — not just by rating the impressions of care staff and families, but by serial examinations of the patients with appropriate and quantified instruments. This is not advocated mainly from the point of view of science: the point is made several times (e.g. Chapter 17) that carers find the application of measures designed by researchers tedious and very time- consuming, so that it often seems that they prefer to continue old chores, such as frequent changing and washing in the case of toilet training. Or, where initial enthusiasm had been kindled, it often tends to be evanescent. There will be better perseverance in carrying out new routines, and promotion of the carers' cooperation in research, if ultimate time-saving can be demonstrated by continuing only with measures of proved efficacy in specific patients. The aim should be to promote the carers' work from drudgery to a professional activity, even for those who by some, and often also by themselves, are at present regarded only as pairs of hands.

As a final point, there is still much resistance on the part of some members of the community to carry out research on old people. This problem is especially often encountered when attempts are made to recruit the essential normal control subjects, even for the most innocuous procedure. Of this form of oddly anachronistic paternalism a telling account was recently given by Prof. Raymond Levy in his inaugural lecture (to be published). Propaganda and education in the narrow sense are unlikely to combat this attitude successfully, but it is hoped that clearly demonstrated and documented effects of the various somatic, psychological and social therapies as outlined in this book and achieved in the future will increase public support as well as funding.

Index

Abbreviated Mental Test (AMT), 81
Abulia, 32
Acalculia, 97, 210
Acetyl choline, 8, 13, 19, 142, 143–144,
   147, 247, 248, 266, 271, 333
Acetyl cholinesterase, 13, (29), 126, 143,
   148, (219), 272, 332
ACh, see Acetyl choline
ACTH, 277
Activating the demented, 286
Activities of daily living (ADL), 82
Acute organic states, see Delirium
AD see Alzheimer's disease
Adenosine triphosphate, see ATP, 275
ADL, see Activities of daily living, 82
Adrenergic receptors, alpha (α) and beta
   (β), 144
Advocacy for the demented, 283
Affective disorder, 38, 65, 185, 186, 192,
   203, 253, 255, 257, 260
   in Huntington's chorea, 235
   in Parkinson's disease, 232
   in subcortical dementia, 236
   see also Depression
Age and delirium, 246
AGECAT, 65
Ageing, 53, 70, 71, 73, 85, 91, 92, 97, 119
Ageism, 307
Agnosia, 27, 28, 32, 37, 39, 58, 180–182,
   210, 236
Agraphia, 30, 210
Akinesia, 144
Alarm systems, 304–306
Alcohol, 62, 246
Alcoholic dementia, 4, 56, 59
Alexia, 30, 210
Allowances
   attendance, 192
   for carers, 322, 323
Alpha rhythm, 96
Aluminium, 13, 34, 112–113, 118, 123,
   124, 126, 129, 135, 334
Alzheimer, 5, 6, 174, 193
Alzheimer's disease (AD), 6, 7, 10, 11, 12,

13, 14, 15, 20, 22, 40, 41, 57, 61, 64,
   74, 85, 91, 92, 96, 97, 98, 102, 104,
   105, 109–208, 212, 213, 215, 216, 217,
   218, 219, 220, 229, 230, 234, 235, 236,
   237, 238, 243, 248, 249, 260, 261, 262,
   265, 266, 268, 270, 271, 272, 273, 274,
   276, 278, 330, 331, 332, 333, 334
AD 1 & 2, 31, 167 203
   duration, 188
   familial, 133
   immunological factors in, 111–112
   incidence, 160–162, 168
   senile dementia, Alzheimer's type
      (SDAT), 7, 12, 28, 31, 74, 85, 133,
      154, 155, 156, 157, 158, 160, 161, 162,
      163, 167, 175, 197, 198, 199, 200, 201,
      203, 206, 213, 214, 216, 277, 278
Alzheimer's Disease Society, 312
Amantadine, 37
Amentia, 3
American Psychiatric Association, 7
Amino acids, 145–6
Amnesia, 39, 40, 176, 178–180, 189, 191,
   192, 193, 210, 211, 241
Amphetamines, 39
Amygdala, 133, 144
Amyloid, 112, 114, 120, 121, 128, 131,
   135, 140, 141, 212
Amyotrophy, 83
Amyotrophic lateral sclerosis, 127
Angiography, 220
Angiotensin, 29
Angular gyrus, 97
   syndrome, 6, 29, 210
Anomia, 175, 182, 191
Antiobiotics and survival, 203–204
Antibodies, monoclonal, 119
Anticholinergic drugs, 85, 167, 233, 234,
   247, 272
Anticholinesterase, 266, 270, 271, 272
Anticoagulants, 223, 225
Antidepressants, 232, 247, 266
Antigens, 112
Antihistamines, 266

Aphasia, 3, 11, 22, 27, 28, 29, 31, 32, 34, 35, 37, 38, 39, 55, 158, 175, 176, 182, 186, 189, 190, 191, 209, 210, 217, 236
  jargon, 185
  paraphasia, 182
Apraxia, 27, 28, 30, 31, 32, 34, 37, 39, 55, 58, 59, 175, 180–182, 189, 190, 209, 210, 218, 236
  dressing, 181, 192
Arecoline 270, 271, 272
Aretaeus of Cappadocia, 1
Argyrophilic inclusions (Pick's disease), 31, 32
Arousal, in depression, 42, 257
Arterial disease, 56
Arteriosclerosis, 12, 20, 56, 59, 120, 123
  see also Atherosclerosis
Aspartate, 145
Aspirin, 223
Astrocytoma, 25, 101
Asymbolia (visual), 31
Ataxia, 215
Atherosclerosis, 37, 38, 63, 133, 134, 209, 211, 213, 220
  see also Arteriosclerosis
ATP, 275
Atrial fibrillation and multi-infarct dementia, 217
Attention, 69, 72, 78, 255
  seeking, 319
Attitudes, 70, 280, 284
Auditory evoked potentials, see Evoked potentials
Automated testing, 169
Autopsy, 158, 160, 162, 189, 190, 204, 215
Avicenna, 2
Axon, 123, 126, 128

Babinski sign, 183
Baglivi, 5
Baillie, 5
Basal arteries, 39
Basal ganglia, 42, 97, 104, 212, 229, 231, 232, 235, 236, 238, 330
Bayle, 3, 4
Bayle, François, 5
Beck depression inventory, 252
Behaviour (in dementia), 69, 82, 284, 291–292
  modification, 291–292
Benign senescent forgetfulness, 9, 10, 22, 156, 159
Benzodiazepines, 34
Benztropine mesylate, 233
Berkson's bias, 155
Beta rhythm, 90
Betahistine, 274
Bethanechol, 270, 273
Bieschansky stain, 6
Binswanger, Otto, 6, 330

Binswanger's disease, 6, 39, 91, 96, 98, 101, 104, 221, 219
Blessed score, 134, 217, 218
Blocq, 5
Blood brain barrier, 99, 164, 247, 267, 276
Boarding out, 306
Boissier du Sauvages, François, 2
Brain, 160
  failure, 241
  syndrome, 241
  volume, 119
  weight, 119, 121, 122, 135
British Medical Association, 324
Broca, 3, 22
  diagonal band of, 143
Bruits, 59, 217
BSF see Benign senescent forgetfulness

Calcium, 26
Camdex, 168
CAPE see Clifton Assessment Procedures for the Elderly
Capsule, internal, 211
C (carbon) 150_2, 95
Carbon monoxide poisoning, 40
Cardiovascular disease, 217, 223
  signs in multi-infarct dementia, 217
CARE, see Comprehensive Assessment and Referral Evaluation
Care attendants, 305–306
Carer(s), 184, 192, 193, 285, 292–293, 307, 308, 310, 311, 314, 315, 317–328, 335
  Association of, 317
  concealment of dementia by, 317–318
  stresses on, 318
Case control studies, 155, 160, 169
  recognition 157, 159
CAT, see Computerised axial tomography
Cataract, 164
  extraction, 246
Cathepin A, 129
'Catastrophic reaction', 184, 186
Catatonia, 185
Caudate nucleus, 37, 92, 104
Cavum septum pellucidum, 33
Cerebellum, 144
  atrophy of, 93
Cerebral amyloid angiopathy, see Congophilic angiopathy,
Cerebral atrophy, 2, 5, 6, 22, 31, 33, 91, 93, 94, 104, 122, 147, 219, 245
Cerebral blood flow (r CBF) 37, 95, 96, 99, 220–221, 222, 223, 224
Cerebral metabolic rate of oxygen (CMRO$_2$), 95, 96, 99, 221, 222
Cerebroactive substances, 270, 274–277
Cerebrospinal fluid, 26, 27, 93, 148, 332
  shunting, 27, 63
Choline, 143, 270, 271
  acetyl transferase, 13, 127, 132, 134,

142, 143, 146, 147, 148, 331
Cholecystokinin, 146, 147, 148
Cholinergic deficit, 31, 118, 132, 135, 143, 149, 203
  neurones, 143, 146, 147
  system, 132, 135, 142, 143, 144, 145, 148, 149, 247, 270, 331, 332
  transmission, 28, 29, 144, 149, 332
Cholinomimetics, 266, 270, 272, 273
Chromosomes, 21, 164, 334
  abnormalities in Alzheimer's disease, 111
Cingulate gyrus, 120
Cirrhosis, 247
Claustrum, 141
Cleveland, Ohio, 204
Clifton Assessment Procedures for the Elderly (CAPE), 65, 80, 81, 85
Clinical dementia scale, 10
Clinical trials, 268–269
'Closing in' phenomenon, 181
Cobalamin, see Vitamin B$_{12}$
Co-dergocrine mesylate (Hydergine), 224, 274, 275, 276
Cognitive assessment, 76–82
  impairment, 9, 10, 11, 14, 72, 73, 82, 185, 191, 209
  in depression, 252
  in Parkinson's disease, 231, 235, 237
Colchicine, 126
Community physician, 327
Comprehensive Assessment and Referral Evaluation (CARE), 168
Computerised axial tomography (CAT), 11, 14, 26, 28, 60, 90, 93–95, 100, 160, 210, 212, 215, 216, 219, 245, 257, 258, 333
  diagnosis, 65, 72, 83–85
  testing, (72), 332
Confabulation, 243
Confusion, acute, see Delirium
Confusional states, see Delirium
Congophilic angiopathy, 122, 123, 131, 134, 213
Consciousness, clouding of, 60, 62, 167, 168, 243, 244
  impairment of, 241
Consent to treatment, 323–326
Constipation, 187
Contingent negative variation, see Evoked potentials
Contractures, 189
Corpus callosum, 25
Cortical atrophy, see Cerebral atrophy
Cosin, Richard, 2
Court of Protection, 325, 326
Craniopharyngioma, 25
Creutzfeld Jakob Disease, 13, 35, 36–37, 60, 64, 91, 104, 113, 114, 131, 135, 330
Crichton Royal Hospital, 200, 206

CSF, see Cerebrospinal fluid
Cullen, William, 3
Cyclandelate (Cyclospasmol), 224, 274

Day care, 298, 303, 304, 312–312, 323
Day hospital, travelling, 312
Daytime lucidity in multi-infarct dementia, 214
Deafness, 55
Deanol, 270, 271
De-differentiation, 71
Deep vein thrombosis, 189
Delirium, 2, 3, 20, 21, 23, 27, 38, 62, 66, 178, 187, 205, 241–249, 310
  tremens, 243, 244
Delta rhythm, 91
Delusions, 59, 61, 66, 94, 176
Dementia, 1, 2, 3, 4, 6, 7, 19, 69, 71, 82, 155, 186, 209, 241, 242, 243, 248, 249, 253, 258, 259, 260, 261, 265, 281, 282, 283, 286, 299, 306, 307, 308, 309, 312, 313, 317, 323, 326, 327
  dialytic, 33
  early, 64, 65
  hereditary dysphasic, 32
  hippocampal, 7
  limited, 66–67
  mild, 156, 157, 158, 167, 169
  multi-infarct, 7, 37–39, 55, 57, 59, 61, 62, 63, 85, 91, 94, 96, 98, 99, 103, 104, 105, 157, 158, 161, 185, 198, 199, 200, 201, 203, 205, 209–227, 242, 243, 255, 261, 262, 314, 315
  neurosyphilitic, see Neurosyphilitic dementia
  pervasive, 66–67
  praecox, see Schizophrenia
  pre-senile, 6, 7, 8, 12, 21, 53, 66, 95, 110, 111, 133, 156, 160, 162, 175, 177, 188, 189, 235, 255, 260
  primary degenerative, 7
  pugilistica, 33, 56
  reversible, 23
  senile, 3, 4, 5, 6, 7, 8, 10, 11, 12, 15, 19, 63, 66, 91, 95, 110, 111, 161, 185, 189, 197, 198, 204, 205, 260, 261, 333, 334
  senile, Alzheimer's type, see Alzheimer's disease
  sub-cortical, 7, 39–46, 64, 210, 211, 230, 235–237, 238, 330
  traumatic, 127
  vascular, see Multi-infarct
  'vesanic', 20, 21
Demoralisation, 184
Demyelinisation, 23, 39, 100, 101, 123, 211
Dendrites, 118, 120, 123, 126
Denmark, 297, 298, 299, 300, 302
Department of Health and Social Security, see DHSS
Dependency, 186

Depression, 6, 9, 27, 54, 55, 56, 57, 58, 59, 60, 61, 62, 63, 66, 70, 71, 79, 85, 148, 164, 165, 166, 167, 168, 178, 185, 205, 213, 214, 232, 233, 266, 278, 301, 307, 308, 314, 332, 333
   cerebrovascular disease and, 257
   dementia and, 251–262
Developmental psychology, 70, 71, 77, 84
Dexamethasone Suppression Test, 28, 258, 259
DHSS, 2, 7, 299, 301
Diabetes, 56, 219, 224
Diagnostic criteria, standardised, 157, 165, 166–167
Diagnostic Interview Schedule (DIS), 167
Diagnostice and Statistical Manual, see DSM III
Diazepam, 34
Diethylaminoethanol, 275
Digit span, 80, 252
Dignity, 282, 283
2-Dimethyl aminoglycol, see Deanol
Disorientation, 60, 61, 64, 182, 189, 191, 192–193, 210, 241, 242, 243, 244, 256, 288–290
   see also Orientation
District Health Authority, 298
Domiciliary assessment, 54, 56, 58, 308
Domiciliary care, 156, 297, 302–303, 314, 321–322
'Don't know answers', 256
DOPA, 13, 29, 142, 144, 148, 236, 273, 275
Dopamine-beta-hydroxylase, 13, 132, 144, 147
Dopaminergic, 41, 141
Dose, response curve, 267, 272
Down's syndrome, 13, 30, 110, 127, 162, 163, 165, 334
Driving, incapacity for, 191
Drug intoxication, 62
   toxicity, 31
DSM III, 6, 7, 65, 66, 166, 169, 241, 243, 258, 262
DST, see Dexamethasone Suppression Test
Duration of Alzheimer's disease, 188
DVT, see Deep vein thrombosis
Dysarthria, 33, 175, 176, 183, 211, 214
Dyscalculia, see Agraphia
Dyslexia, see Alexia
Dysphagia, 214
Dysphasia, see Aphasia
Dyspraxia, see Apraxia

Ebers papyrus, 1
Echocardiography, 219
ECG, see Electrocardiogram, 219
Echolalia, 22, 32
ECT, see Electroconvulsive therapy
Edinburgh, 197
Educational achievement (influencing dementia), 56

EEG, see Electroencephalogram
Elderly, 70
Elderly mentally infirm, homes for, 300, 302
Electoral rolls, 165
Electrocardiogram, 219
Electroconvulsive therapy, 28, 253
Electroencephalogram, 34, 60, 64, 90–92, 215, 216, 255
   in delirium, 245, 247, 249
Emboli, 38, 217, 223
EMI homes, see Elderly mentally infirm, homes for
   in delirium, 243
Emotional disturbance, in dementia, 57, 61, 176–177, 185–186, 209
   incontinence in multi-infarct dementia, 214
Encephalins, 277
Encephalopathy, dialytic, see Dialytic dementia
   mink, 36, 110
   spongy, 35–37, 119
   subcortical arterio-sclerotic, see Binswanger's disease
   Wernicke's, 59, 245
Encoding, 9, 72, 73, 235, 252
Endorphins, 277
Environment, 284, 290
Environmental agent, 135
Epidemiology, 19, 333
Epilepsy, 25, 56, 99, 183, 187, 193
   temporal lobe, 62
Epileptic dementia, 4
Ergot derivates, 224
   see also Co-dergocrine mesylate (Hydergine)
ERP, see Event related potentials
Erythrocytic sedimentation rate (ESR), 218
Esmarch, 4
Esquirol, 3, 4
ESR, see Erythrocytic sedimentation rate
Etàt lacunaire, see Binswanger's disease
Ethics, 269
Ethnicity and dementia, 159
European Transplant and Dialysis Association, 34
Evodeviation, 159
Evoked potentials, cortical, 90, 92–93
   auditory, 92, 94, 259
   contingent negative variation, 92–95
   event related, 259
   long latency, 92
   motor, 92
   P300 latency, 92, 93, 259
   sensory, 92, 259
Extrapyramidal features in dementia, pugilistica, 33
   phase in Alzheimer's disease, 31

Face–hand test, 183
Factor analysis, 76, 82
Faecal impaction, 301
Falls, 187, 193, 322
Family history, 162, 333
  in multi-infarct dementia, 216
Family Practioner Committee, 298
Family, see Relatives
Fernel, 2
Fertility, 154
Fever in delirium, 245, 249
Fingerprints, 162
Finland, 230
18-Fluorodeoxyglycose (FDG), 96, 99
Focal signs in MID, 215, 216
Folate deficiency, 24, 60
Fornix, 33
Forgetfulness, see Memory impairment
Fractures, 187
Free oxygen radicals, 164
Freud, Sigmund, 6
Frontal lobe (cortex), 25, 41, 62, 94, 95,
  97, 99, 119, 133, 181, 184
  atrophy, 31

GABA, 8, 29, 145, 146, 147, 148, 275, 276
Gag reflex, 218
Gait disturbance, 27, 30, 33, 63, 181, 183,
  211, 218
Ganser state, 254
Gegenhalten, 183
Genetics, 13, 334
  in Alzheimer's disease, 110–111, 162,
  163, 164
  engineering, 334
Geniculate body, lateral, 120
Geriatrics/geriatric medicine, 70, 197, 306,
  307, 313, 314, 316, 323
  mental state, see GMS
  psychiatry, see Psychogeriatrics
Gerontology, 69, 70, 74, 84
Gerontologists, 71
Glia/glial cells, 120, 128, 129, 140
Global deterioration scale, 10
Glucose, 13, 96, 97, 274, 275, 276
Glutamate, 145
Glutamic acid decarboylase (GAD), 145
GMS, 65, 80, 165, 167
Goals in psychological management, 285
Goldstein, 185
'Good neighbours', 305, 306
GP, 296, 298, 307, 308, 310, 311, 314, 315,
  318, 321, 324, 327
  lists, 165, 166
GPI, see Neurosyphilitic dementia
Granulovacuolar changes, 6, 29, 120, 130–131
Grasp reflex, 183
Graylingwell Hospital, 200, 201
Griesinger, 2, 3, 4,
Group sessions for dementia, 289, 290

Guam, 127, 129
Gyri, 122

Hachinski ischaemic score, 63, 158, 262
Haematocrit, 224
Haemorrhages, intracerebral, 123, 212
Haematological malignancies, 30, 110, 162,
  163
Hallucinations, 28, 59, 61, 242, 243
Halstead Reaction Battery (HRB), 77, 78,
  253
Hamilton (Max) scale, 260
Homonymous hemianopia, 215, 218
Haslam, 4
Health visitors, 303, 311
  associations, 304
  Departments, 304
Herxheimer reaction, 35
Herpes simplex, 26, 30
Hippocampus, 6, 9, 118, 124, 127, 131,
  132, 141, 148
Hippocrates, 1
Hirano bodies, 120, 129, 130
History, 54
3H Ketanserin, 145
Hobart, Tasmania, 166, 169
Home help, 298, 303, 322, 323
Homes, see Residential care
Homocysteine, 23
Hospital(s), mental, 197
  beds, 311, 314, 316
  long stay, 298, 299, 300
Hounsfield units, 95, 25, 28
Housing, sheltered, 298, 304, 305
3HQNB, 143
Huntington's chorea, 40, 41, 56, 59, 63, 91,
  97, 104, 229, 234–235, 237, 238, 330
Hydergine, see Co-dergocrine mesylate
Hydrocephalus, 39, 104
  communicating, low/normal pressure, 6,
  22–27, 40, 59, 62, 93, 104
5-Hydroxyindoleacetic acid, 144, 145
Hypercalcaemia, 34
Hypertension, 27, 38, 39, 56, 63, 123, 211,
  212, 214, 216, 223
Hypnotics, 278
Hypothyroidism, 23, 24, 59, 63, 226, 278
Hysteria, 27, 253

ICD-9, 7, 66
ICD-10, 166
Idiotism, 3
Illinois, 242, 243
Illusions, 242, 243
Immune system, 135
  in survival, 204
Immunological factors in Alzheimer's
  disease, 111–112
Incidence of Alzheimer's disease, 160–162,
  168

Incontinence, 27, 63, 187, 189, 278, 287–288, 322, 323
faecal, 319
laundry services, 322, 323
Individual care plan, 284–286
Infarction
cerebral, 93, 134, 209, 219, 244
lacunar, 94, 96, 211, 223
myocardial, 56, 134
watershed, 220
Infarcts, 100, 101
Informant, 54, 56, 74, 175–176, 187, 241
Information processing, 72, 73, 80
Inoculation studies, 36
Insight, preservation in multi-infarct dementia, 184, 214
Institutional care, 297, 298
Intelligence, 69, 81–82, 96, 167
International Classification of Diseases, see ICD 9 and 10
Inversion recovery (IV) image, 100, 101
Investigations in dementia, 60, 177–178
IQ, see Intelligence
Ischaemic heart disease, 219
'Ischaemic score', 38, 212, 213–16, 209, 220, 225
see also Hachinski ischaemic score
N. Isopropyl[123] iodoamphetamine (IMP), 99
Isoxsuprine, 274

Japan, prevalence of SDAT and multi-infarct dementia in, 158, 333
Jaw jerk, 218
Jessen, 4
Judgement, 66
Juvenal, 2

Kahlbaum, 3
KCTE see Kendrick
KDCT see Kendrick
Kendrick, Battery (KBDE), 77, 332
Cognitive Tests for the Elderly (KCTE), 77, 78, 79, 81, 85
Digit Copying Test (KDCT), 77, 78, 79, 80
Object Learning Test (KOLT), 76, 77, 78, 79, 80, 81
Kent Social Services Department, 305
Kingston, Ontario, 201
Korsakoff, 179, 185, 245
Kluver-Bucy syndrome, 189
KOLT, see Kendrick
Kraft Ebbing, 4
Kraepelin, 4, 5, 6, 7
Kuru, 13, 36, 113

Lability, affective in multi-infarct dementia, 217, 262
Language disorder, 21, 97
Learning, 8, 69, 76, 283, 289–290

verbal, 78, 25, 252
Lecithin, 270, 271, 272, 331
Levy, Raymond, 335
Lexicon, 22
L-dopa, 39, 41, 230, 233, 278, 330
'Life threatening' illness, 323–324
Ligands, 143, 145
Limbic encephalitis, 26
dementias, 41
system, 30, 186
Lipid solubility (of drugs for dementia), 267
Lipofucsin, 113, 120, 123
Lipohyalinosis, 211
'Living well', 324
Locus coeruleus, 31, 132, 133, 134, 141, 144, 147, 148, 248
Logoclonia, 183
London, 255
Lundby, 161, 201
Lunch clubs, 303
Luria Nebraska Neuropsychological Battery, 78
Lymphomas, see Haematological malignancies

Macular degeneration, 164
Magnetic gait, 27
Malpighi, 5
Manganese, 234
Mania, 1, 3, 27, 244, 254
Mannheim, 307
Marinesco, 5
Maudsley, Henry, 5
Meals on wheels, 298, 303, 323
Melancholia, 1, 3, 21
Membrane modification, 274
Memory/memory impairment, 3, 8, 9, 55, 58, 61, 66, 69, 71, 72, 133, 159, 166, 167, 175, 178–186, 190, 191, 209, 210, 211, 236, 243, 244, 251, 252, 253, 256, 281, 317, 332
logical, 252
long term, 72, 251
primary, see short term
processing, 72, 73, 79, 159
recall, 252, 256
registration, 179
retrieval, 71, 72, 73, 79, 159
rote, 252
sensory store, 72, 79
short term, 72, 179
traces, 72
training classes, 293
transmission, 85
Meningioma, 25, 101, 219
Meningitis, 27, 63
Mental handicap, 20, 56
Mental Health Act 1983, 325, 327
Mental State Examination, 56–59, 176–177
Mental State Questionnaire (MSQ), 81

Mental state assessment, 80–81
Mesocortical systems, 144
Methionine, 23
11-Methionine, 97, 99
Microtubules, 126, 127
Mill Hill Scale, see Vocabulary tests
MIND, 313
Mini mental state, 11, 58, 64, 81, 157, 167, 168, 169, 218, 252
Mirror sign, 181
Misdiagnosis, 74
Mitral valve, 219, 223
Moria, 184
Moore, 5
Mortality, 9, 154, 161, 189, 199–203
Motivation, 71, 133, 334
   in depression, 253
Motor stereotypes, 189
Multidisciplinary assessment, 296
Multiple scelerosis (MIS), 101
Muscarinic receptors, 28, 32, 143, 273
   M1, 143
   M2, 143, 144
   agonists, 272
Mutism, 31, 33
Myocardial infarction, see Infarction, myocardial
Myoclonic phase
   in Alzheimer's disease, 31
   in dialytic dementia, 34
   in Creutzfeld Jakob disease, 36
Myxoedema see Hypothyroidism

NA, see Noradrenaline
Naftidrofuryl (Nafronyl), 224, 274, 275, 276
Naloxone, 270, 277
Naltroxone, 278
National Adult Reading Test, see Vocabulary tests
National Institute on Ageing, 15
Necropsy, see Autopsy
Needs of the demented, 281, 282, 283, 284, 285, 292
Neumann, 3
'Neural noise', 247
Neurites, 128, 129, 140, 147, 148
Neuroblastoma, 126
Neurofibrillary tangles, 6, 10, 12, 27, 29, 32, 33, 112, 118, 120, 123, 124, 125, 127, 131, 132, 135, 140, 141, 147, 148, 160, 237, 249
Neurofilaments, 125, 126, 127, 141
Neuronal loss, 118, 119, 123, 127, 132, 133, 141, 147
   vulnerability, 140, 141–142
Neuropeptides, 142, 146, 270, 277
Neuropeptide Y, 146, 148
Neuropsychology, 177, 218
Neurosyphilitic dementia, 3, 4, 5, 20, 34–35

meningovascular, 35
   parenchymatous, 35
Newcastle, 197, 260, 205, 260
New York, 201, 204, 255
New Zealand, 230
13 NHS, 99
Niacin, 274
Nigeria, dementia in, 159
Nissl, 5
NMR, 14, 90
Nocturnal confusion in multi-infarct dementia, 214, 215
Noguchi, 5
Noradrenaline, 29, 132, 142, 144, 178, 247, 248, 273, 275, 292, 331, 332
Noradrenergic neurones, 248
   system, 144
Normalisation, 282–283
Nottingham, 316
Nuclear magnetic resonance, see NMR
Nucleus, basalis of Meynert, 29, 32, 41, 131, 132, 134, 141, 143, 147, 148, 237, medial septal, 143
Nuchocephalic reflex, 30
Nursing, community, 305, 310, 311–312, 314, 322, 333
Nylidrin, 274

Occipital cortex, 96, 119
Occupational therapist, 310
Oculomotor nuclei, 127
OER, 95, 96, 221
Olivary nuclei, inferior, 120
Onset of mental illness, 55
   age at, 203
   delirium, 242, 244
   multi-infarct dementia, 214, 216
   pseudodementia, 256
'Organic orderliness', 184
Oribasius, 2
Orientation/disorientation, 30, 58, 80, 288–290
   scale for geriatric patients, 81
   test, 81
Orofacial dyskinesia, 184
Oxypentifilline, 275

P300 latency, see Evoked potentials
Paired Associated Learning Test (PALT), 76
Paired helical filaments, 112, 113, 127, 140, 141
Pallilalia, 183
Palmomental reflex, 183
Panencephalitis, subacute sclerosing, 127
Papaverine, 274
Papulosis atrophicans maligna (of Kohmaier Degos), 35
Paralysis, 55
Paranoia, 4, 186–187, 191, 193, 255, 301

Paraphrenia, 205, 206, 254
Parasagittal cortex, 119
Parietal lobe, 62, 96, 97, 99, 119, 203
Parkinson's disease, 13, 40, 41, 60, 63, 91,
    104, 118, 132, 134, 135, 141, 142, 181,
    182, 183, 189, 229–232, 235, 238, 278,
    330, 333
  dementia complex of Guam, 127, 129,
    234
Parkinsonism, 182, 183, 230, 234, 331
  'arteriosclerotic', 229, 234
  post-encephalitic, 229, 230
Part III accomodation, 299, 300, 301,
    306–316
Pascal's law, 26
Perception, 69
Performance, 69, 71
Perplexity, 184
Perseveration, 22, 29, 57, 60, 61, 183, 185,
    189
Personality
  change in dementia, 184, 209
  disorder, 254
  previous, 185
PET, 11, 14, 90, 95–97, 210, 215,
    221–223, 224, 225
PHF, see Paired helical filaments
Philothermal responses, 30
Phobias, 39
Phosphatidyl choline, see Lecithin
Physical examination, 59–60
Physostigmine, 247, 270, 271, 272
Pick's disease, 12, 20, 31–32, 91, 229, 230,
    234, 235
Pinel, Philippe, 2, 3
Piperazine, 275
Piracetam, 275
Pirenzipine, 273
Pixels, 94
Placebo effect, 266–267
Plantar response, extensor, 215
Plaques, senile, 5, 6, 10, 12, 29, 32, 110,
    114, 118, 120, 121, 124, 126, 128–129,
    133, 134, 140–141, 147, 148, 160, 213,
    237, 249
Platter, 2
Pneumonia, 189
Polyarteritis nodosa, 219
Polycythaemia rubra vera, 218, 224
Pons, 211
Positron emission tomography, see PET
Post mortem examination, see Autopsy
Power of attorney, 325, 326
Praxilene, see Naftidrofuryl
Prealbumin, 128
Prednisone, 35
Presbyophrenia, 20, 21
Present state examination, 65, 167
Presentation of Alzheimer's disease,
    190–191

Pressure sores, 187
Prevalence of multi-infarct dementia,
    212–213
  SDAT, 156–160, 168
Prichard, James Cowles, 3, 154
Prions, see Virus-like agents
Private sector, 298, 301, 302
Problem solving, 69
Procaine penicillin, 35
Progressive supranuclear palsy, 6, 40, 127,
    236
Prognosis in delirium, 245
Propanolol, 248
Prosody, 22, 33
Prosopagnosia, 177, 180, 192
Protein synthesis, 97, 118, 119, 124, 126
Protons, 95, 99, 100
  density (PD), 100, 101, 104
Pseudobulbar palsy, 39, 59, 61, 215, 217,
    218
Pseudodelirium, 244
Pseudodementia, 6, 27–28, 34, 40, 74, 79,
    85, 91, 178, 232, 332, 333
PSE, see Present state examination
Psychiatric status schedule (PSS), 65
Psychogeriatrics, 71, 197
  services, 296, 297, 300, 306–316
Psychological tests, 65, 69–90, 332
Psychoses, psychotic symptoms, 4, 21, 23
Ptal Hotep, Prince, 1
Pulmonary embolus, 189
'Punch drunk' syndrome, see Dementia
    pugilistica
Purkinje neurones, 120
Putamen, 97, 141
Pyramidal cells, 120, 127, 131

Quality of life, 282

Radiation therapy, 25
Radio frequency pulse (RF), 99, 100
Raphe, 132, 134, 141, 145, 147, 148
Rating scales, 82
Raven's progressive matrices, 177
Reality orientation less therapy, see RO
Reasoning, 69
Redlich, 5
Regional extraction ratio of oxygen, see
    OER
Registration, see Memory
Relatives, 293, 309, 313, 324, 334
  support, 297, 312
Reliability, 75, 79, 84, 160
Relief, see Respite
REM, see Sleep
Reminiscence therapy, 290–291
Renal failure, 34
Research, 330–335
  Diagnostic criteria (RDC), 66
  spending on dementia, 109

Residential care, 197, 198, 309, 310, 311, 315, 322–323
Respite, 312, 313–314, 323
Rest homes, 301, 302
Restraint, 325
Reticular formation, 122
Reversibility in delirium, 245–246
Ribot, 20
Ribot's law, 243
Richet, 20
Risk factors for Alzheimer's disease, 162–164
RNA, 124
    messenger, 124, 142
    ribosomal, 124, 126
RO, 71, 82, 83, 288, 289, 291, 293
    group, 289
    24 hour, 288–289
Robin, 33
Roth and Hopkins Test, 81
Royal College of Psychiatrists, 307
RS86, 270, 273

Saccadic latencies, 30
Salmon, William, 2
Sampling, 165–166
Saxondale Hospital, 200
Schizophrenia, 4, 21, 38, 42, 54, 57, 61, 235, 254, 255, 307
    paranoid, 187
Schneiderian first rank symptoms, 61
Scrapie, 30, 36, 113, 114, 129, 131, 135
Screening, 168–169, 332
Section 47 (of the National Assistance Act), 327
Self-care skills, 286–287
Senility, 12, 13
Sensation, 69
Serial 7s, 80
Serotonin (5HT), 13, 29, 132, 144–145, 147, 248, 273, 275, 278, 331, 332
    serotonergic neurones, 145, 248
    projection, 145
    receptor binding sites, 145
Sheltered housing, see Housing, sheltered
'Shifting aptitude', 231
Short Portable Mental Status Questionnaire (SPMSQ), 81
Shunt, ventriculoatrial, 63
Side-effects of drugs for dementia, 267, 268
Silicon, 113, 135
Simchowicz, 6
Signposts, 289
Single photon emission tomography (SPET), 90, 97–99
Sitters, 313
SLE, see Systemic lupus erythematosus
Sleep, 91, 260
    disturbance (insomnia), 266, 278, 319

REM, 21, 28, 91, 248, 260
    wake cycle, 242, 243, 248
Snout reflex, 183
Social class, 164, 166
Social Security, 299
Social Services, 298, 299, 301, 305, 308, 317, 323
Social work, 298, 303, 308, 311, 321
SOL, see Space occupying lesion
Somatic complaints in multi-infarct dementia, 214
Southampton, 315
    case register, 307, 315
Space occupying lesion, 23, 24, 59
Spasticity, 183, 188, 189
Spin echo technique, 100
    lattice relaxation time (T1), 100, 101, 104
    transverse relaxation time (T2), 100
    warp, 100
Staff resistance, 292–293
Stages of Alzheimer's disease, 189
Steele Richardson Olszweski syndrome, 127
    see also Progressive supranuclear palsy
Stepwise deterioration in multi-infarct dementia, 214
Stereotypes, 21
Stockholm Psychiatric Hospital, 199
Stockport, 304, 305
Stockton Geriatric Scale, 65
Strengths, residual, 285
Striatum, 144, 211
Stroke, 39, 57, 212, 213, 216
Subarachnoid haemorrhage, 27, 63
Subcortical nuclei, 118, 132, 147
    white matter, 141
Subdural haematoma, 23, 26, 63, 93, 101, 134, 187, 219
Substance P, 29
Substantia nigra, 33, 127, 141, 236
    nigro-striatal pathway, 236
Suicide, 57, 190
Sulci, 122
'Sundown' phenomenon, 242, 256
Superoxide dismutase, 164
Survival, 199–203, 204, 205
'Swapping', 300, 301
Sydenham, 2
Synapses, 126
Syphilis, 4, 5, 6, 60
Systemic lupus erythematosus, 219

T1/T2, see Spin lattice and transverse relaxation time
Tachycardia in delirium, 245, 249
T-cell, 131, 135
Telephone, 304
Temporal arteritis, 218
    lobe, 62, 94, 95, 96, 119, 141, 143, 146
    atrophy, 31
    epilepsy, see Epilepsy, temporal lobe, 62

Tempero-parietal defects, 333
Test batteries, 76, 77–80
  see also Psychological testing
Testamentary capacity, 191
Tests of Mental Impairment (TMI), 81
Thalamus, 39, 40, 41, 211, 212
Theta rhythm, 91
Thiamine deficiency, 247
Thyroid disease, 30, 56, 162, 163, 164, 165, 187
  tests, 218
Thyroxine, 266
TIA, see Transient ischaemic attacks
Toiletting, 287–288
Toronto, 201, 255
'Toxic confusional state', 246
  see also Delirium
Transient ischaemic attacks, 214
Transmissible agents, see Virus-like agents
Transport, 312, 313
Trauma, head, and Alzheimer's disease, 30
  and Pick's disease, 32
Tryptophan, 128
Tuberous sclerosis, 127
Tumours, cerebral, 25, 59, 62, 99, 100
Twins, 161, 204
  studies, 110
Tyrosine, 128
  hydroxylase, 147, 148

USA, ageing population in, 14
US–UK Diagnostic Project, 53, 67, 167–168

Validity, 75, 76, 79, 84, 160
  construct, 75, 76, 79
Variability in delirium, 242
Vascular surgery, 220, 225
Vasodilators, 38, 224, 270, 273–274, 275
Vasointestinal peptide, see VIP
Vasopressin, 277
VDAL, 218, 219
Ventricular dilation, 5, 26, 31, 33, 93, 94, 212, 257

peri-ventricular white matter, 101, 104
Vertebrobasilar syndromes, 38, 39
Vinblastin, 126
Vinburine, 273
Vincamine, 274, 275
Vinci, Leonardo da, 5
Vincristine, 126
VIP, 127, 128, 146, 147, 148
Virchow, 5, 33
Virus-like agents, 13, 29, 37, 113–114, 123, 128, 131, 135, 164, 334
Visual field defects, 215
Visuospatial difficulties, 97, 175, 189, 190, 209
Vitamin B$_{12}$, 23, 24, 60
Vitamin deficiency, 59, 63
Vocabulary tests, 81–82
  Mill Hill Scale, 81
  National Adult Reading Test, 81–82
Volunteers, 812–813

Wakefulness, disordered, 242, 248
Wandering, 184
Wardens, 304
Waugh, Evelyn, 242
Wechsler, 70, 78
  WAIS, 79, 177, 178, 233
Wernicke's aphasia, 22, 25, 38, 178, 182
  encephalopathy, see Encephalopathy
Western Aphasia Battery, 22
WHO, 159, 166
Will, 5
Willis, Thomas, 2
Wilks, 5
Wilson's disease, 40
World Health Organization, see WHO

Xanthene, 275
133-Xenon, 37, 97

Zichens, Theodor, 4
Zinc, 113
Zung questionnaire, 261